Outside the Walls of the Asylum

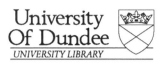

University
Of Dundee
UNIVERSITY LIBRARY

School of Nursing and Midwifery
Fife Campus

Date of Return

2 2 FEB 2002

1 2 MAR 2002

0 1 JUN 2002

1 3 NOV 2002

2 4 FEB 2003

2 0 JUL 2004

3 0 APR 2007

Outside the Walls of the Asylum

The History of Care in the Community 1750–2000

Edited by

PETER BARTLETT & DAVID WRIGHT

THE ATHLONE PRESS
London & New Brunswick, NJ

First published 1999 by
THE ATHLONE PRESS
1 Park Drive, London NW11 7SG
and New Brunswick, New Jersey

© The Athlone Press 1999

British Library Cataloguing in Publication Data
*A catalogue record for this book is available
from the British Library*

ISBN 0 485 11541 7 hb
0 485 12147 6 pb

Library of Congress Cataloging-in-Publication Data

Outside the walls of the asylum : on "care and community" in modern
Britain and Ireland / edited by Peter Barlett and David Wright.
    p. cm.
    Includes bibliographical references.
    ISBN 0–485–11541–7. – – ISBN 0–485–12147–6 (pbk.)
    1. Psychiatric hospital care – – Great Britain – – History.
2. Psychiatric hospitals care – – Great Britain – – History   3. Mental health
policy – – Great Britain – – History.   4. Psychiatric hospital care –
– Ireland – – History. 5. Psychiatric hospitals – – Ireland – – History.
6. Mental health policy – – Ireland – – History. I. Bartlett, Peter.
II. Wright, David, 1965–
RC450.G7098   1999
362.2′1′0941 – – dc21   98–54264
                                                    CIP

Distributed in the United States, Canada and South America by
Transaction Publishers
390 Campus Drive
Somerset, New Jersey 08873

Typeset by Ensystems, Saffron Walden

Printed and bound in Great Britain by
Cambridge University Press

Contents

Preface

Care in the Community constitutes one of the most contested programmes in contemporary social policy. While most commentators denigrate the era of institutional confinement, a confinement typified by the old Victorian mental hospitals, few seem at all comfortable with the notion of the mentally ill 'at large' in society. Recent scandals of discharged patients committing suicide, perpetrating acts of violence, or generally falling through the net of community services, have fostered a perceived crisis of care. Research in the history of 'madness', however, has focused almost exclusively on the emergence of a state-supported system of mental hospitals and its foundation for an institutionally-based psychiatric profession. We still know relatively little about responses to madness in the community over the course of modern period, whether in the domicile or in the changing and complicated network of poor law, charitable, private and community provision.

Based on workshops sponsored by the Wellcome Trust held at Oxford University and the University of Nottingham, *Outside the Walls of the Asylum* explores for the first time in one book this complex historical phenomenon. Experts in medical and legal history, and social policy, investigate the history of community care both as a social phenomenon and as a distinct government programme. The remit of this book is Britain and Ireland from 1750 to the present, including original research on the care of those classified as idiots, lunatics, mentally defective, developmental handicapped or mentally ill.

Much of current social policy rests on the belief that the history of society's response to insanity in the modern era can be narrowly understood within the context of the rise and fall of the asylum. As this book demonstrates, the historical relationship between institutions, the community and the mentally ill and mentally handicapped is far more complex. From the mid-nineteenth to the mid-twentieth century, institutions did play an ever-increasingly important role in the complex possibilities of caring and controlling the 'insane', but mental hospitals never *replaced* community care. Rather psychiatric institutions were only part of an increasingly complex array of provision. In fact, this volume suggests that care outside the walls of the asylum remained the primary response of industrial societies to the problem of the mentally disordered from 1750 to the present day. As a result, this book adds a critical new voice to the reappraisal of Care in the Community and to the changing historical understanding of the role of institutional medicine in the treatment of mental health problems.

The editors would like to thank several individuals and institutions for their assistance in the genesis and gestation of this edited volume. David Allen, former Director of the History of Medicine Programme of the Wellcome Trust, first suggested a specialist colloquium on the history of madness in 1994. Under his support, and that of the Wellcome Trust more generally, two small conferences were held – one in Linacre College, Oxford, in 1995, and another at the University of Nottingham in 1996. These specialist conferences have now become a semi-annual event and are marked by a high degree of camaraderie and good-will. The chapters contained in this volume come largely from these two colloquia. Many academics leant their support to these proceedings and deserve special thanks: Anne Digby, Len Smith, Elizabeth Malcolm and Peter Nolan. We would also like to thank the staff of Linacre College and the University of Nottingham for their assistance and hospitality. Jonathan Andrews and Pauline Prior kindly read drafts of the Introduction to ensure proper weight was given to Scotland and Ireland. Isabel Allen diligently proof-read the entire manuscript before submission. Lastly, we would like to thank Brian Southam and The Athlone Press for their support and Sheila Jones for better secretarial assistance than we deserve.

DW & PB
Nottingham

Notes on Contributors

Richard Adair is Research Fellow in the Department of Economic and Social History at the University of Exeter where he works on the Exminster Project with Bill Forsythe and Joseph Melling. His doctoral and post-doctoral research was mainly concerned with illegitimacy and courtship in the early modern period and his study *Courtship, Illegitimacy and Marriage in Early Modern England* was published in 1996.

Dorothy Atkinson is Lecturer in the School of Health and Social Welfare at the Open University. She is joint organiser of the Social History of Learning Disability Research Group, and has published widely on contemporary and historical issues concerning people with learning disabilities. She has co-edited (with Jan Walmsley and Mark Jackson) *Forgotten Lives: Exploring the History of Learning Disability* (Kidderminster, 1997).

Peter Bartlett is Lecturer in Mental Health Law in the University of Nottingham. He received his Ph.D. from University College, London, exploring the interface between the poor law and the administration of the lunacy acts. His thesis will shortly be published by Cassells under the title – *The Poor Law of Lunacy* (1999).

Jim Campbell received his PhD from The Queen's University of Belfast. His doctoral thesis focused on the concept of violence in the history of social and political thought. He has published in the fields of mental health social work, social policy and mental health law in Northern Ireland, and social work and sectarianism. He is a lecturer in the Department of Social Work at The Queen's University of Belfast.

Bill Forsythe is Reader in Historical Criminology at the University of Exeter and Dean of the Faculty of Academic Partnerships. He is a joint director (with Joseph Melling) of the Wellcome-funded project on the history of Devon County Lunatic Asylum, 1845–1914. He has published a number of books and articles on prisons and the social history of crime.

David Hirst is Lecturer in Social Policy in the School of Sociology and Social Policy, University of Wales, Bangor. His main research interest is in nineteenth-century and twentieth-century social policy. In addition to his current work on mental illness and mental deficiency, he has published articles on the School Medical Service and juvenile employment policy.

Rab Houston is Professor of Early Modern History in the University of St Andrews. He has published extensively in the fields of European education and literacy, historical demography, and Scottish social history. The archival research for this chapter was carried out during a Leverhulme fellowship in 1996–7. A monograph study of perceptions of mental incapacity (rather than their care) will appear in due course: R. A. Houston, *Madness and its Social Milieu in Eighteenth-century Scotland* forthcoming (Oxford University Press, 2000).

Hilary Marland is Wellcome Lecturer at the Centre for Social History, University of Warwick, Research Associate at the Wellcome Unit for the History of Medicine in Oxford, and is an editor of *Social History of Medicine*. She has published on the history of midwifery, women doctors, infant welfare and nineteenth-century medical practice, and edited volumes on early modern medical practice, midwives, maternal and infant welfare and alternative healing, most recently *Midwives, Society and Childbirth: Debates and Controversies in the Modern Period* and *Illness and Healing Alternatives in Western Europe*. She is currently engaged in two projects: the study of puerperal insanity in nineteenth-century Britain and Dutch midwives 1897–1941.

Joseph Melling is Senior Lecturer in Economic & Social History and Director of the Centre for Medical History at the University of Exeter. Joint director of the Wellcome project on Devon Asylum, he is also directing the Medical Record Survey of hospital and community health records within Devon and the South West. He has researched different aspects of state welfare and business welfare history including housing provision.

Pamela Michael is Welsh-medium Lecturer in Sociology and Social Policy in the School of Community, Regional and Communication Studies, University of Wales, Bangor. She has research interests in the social history of medicine and women's history. She was previously Research Fellow on a Wellcome funded project on Madness and Society in North Wales, from which she is currently preparing other work for publication.

William Parry-Jones was Professor of Child and Adolescent Psychiatry at the University of Glasgow until his untimely death in July 1997. His principal clinical and research interests included psychological traumatisation in children, the effects of war trauma and displacement and chronic illness in adolescence. Author of *The Trade in Lunacy* (1972), and numerous articles and chapters on the history of psychiatry, he had a long-standing research interest in the historical aspects of institutional provisions, childhood insanity and eating disorders.

Sarah Payne is Lecturer in Social Policy in the School for Policy Studies at the University of Bristol. She has published on aspects of gender, health, and poverty, mental illness and gender issues, in relation to both in-patient psychiatric treatment and care in the community for people diagnosed as mentally ill. She is currently engaged in two projects – researching aspects of poverty and deprivation in rural areas, and researching gendered aspects of suicidal behaviour.

Sheena Rolph is doing doctoral research in the School of Health and Social Welfare at the Open University. Her research interest includes the social history of learning difficulties, and she is currently completing her Ph.D. on the history of community care for people with learning difficulties in Norfolk, 1930–1980. She has published in the area of ethical dilemmas and historical research with people with learning difficulties.

Harriet Sturdy was awarded her PhD in 1996 from the University of Glasgow, having undertaken a study of boarding-out insane persons in nineteenth-century Scotland under the sponsorship of the Wellcome Trust. She has recently collaborated with William Parry-Jones on a study of private madhouses in Scotland, also funded by the Wellcome Trust. Her particular research interest is the provision of non-institutional care for the mentally ill over the last two centuries in Britain and across the world.

Akihito Suzuki completed his PhD on medical concepts of madness in the eighteenth century at the Wellcome Institute for the History of Medicine in 1992 after having studied history of science at University of Tokyo. He received a post-doctoral research fellowship at the Thomas Reid Institute for Interdisciplinary Research, University of Aberdeen. In 1997 he became Associate Professor in History at Keio University in Tokyo. He has published numerous articles on the history of psychiatry.

Jan Walmsley is Senior Lecturer in the School of Health and Social Welfare at the Open University. She is joint organiser of the Social History of Learning Disability Research Group, and has published widely on the history of community care and learning disabilities. She has co-edited (with Dorothy Atkinson and Mark Jackson) *Forgotten Lives: Exploring the History of Learning Disability* (Kidderminster, 1997).

Oonagh Walsh is lecturer in history and director of women's studies at the University of Aberdeen. Educated at Trinity College, Dublin and Nottingham University, she has just received her Ph.D from Trinity College. She has published articles on Irish women and colonial consolidation, female philanthropy, and female political activity. Her current research is centred in the field of nineteenth-century Irish psychiatry. Her publications include "A Lightness of Mind': Gender and the Psychiatric Service in Ireland' in *Separate Spheres* (Irish Academic Press).

John Welshman studied social history as an undergraduate at the University of York, and his Oxford D. Phil thesis examined the School Medical Service in England and Wales, 1907–39. He has published articles on aspects of the social history of medicine in twentieth-century Britain in journals including *Medical History*, *Social History of Medicine*, *Twentieth Century British History*, and

Urban History. He is currently a Research Fellow in the Department of Health Sciences at the University of York.

David Wright received his D.Phil. in Economic and Social History from the University of Oxford in 1993. After a post-doctoral research fellowship at the Wellcome Unit, Oxford, he was appointed Wellcome Lecturer in the History of Medicine at the University of Nottingham in 1996. He has publications in the history of psychiatry and the history of the family, and recently co-edited (with Anne Digby) *From Idiocy to Mental Deficiency: Historical Perspectives on People with Learning Disabilities* (Routledge, 1996).

Tables and Figures

CHAPTER ONE

Community care and its antecedents

Peter Bartlett and David Wright

The typical response to the deranged underwent dramatic changes in English society between the mid-eighteenth and mid-nineteenth centuries. At the outset of this period ... the societal response to the problems posed by the presence of mentally disturbed individuals did not involve segregating them ... The overwhelming majority of the insane were still to be found at large in the community. By the mid-nineteenth century, however, virtually no aspect of this traditional response remained intact. The insane ... found themselves incarcerated in a specialized, bureaucratically organised state-supported asylum system which isolated them both physically and symbolically from the larger society.[1]

This dramatic opening paragraph launches Andrew Scull's *Museums of Madness*, arguably the most influential monograph on the history of psychiatry in Britain. In stark juxtaposition Scull contrasts the open and tolerant care of the insane in pre-industrial communities with the restrictive incarceration of the Victorian period. Building on the thesis of the 'rupture' between pre-modern and modern approaches to insanity enunciated in Michel Foucault's *Madness and Civilisation*[2] and David Rothman's *The Discovery of the Asylum*,[3] Scull argued that the rise of the asylum in England represented a fundamental transformation in the position of the mentally disordered in modern society. The mental hospital replaced the family and community as the epicentre of care and control as a new regime of discipline and surveillance replaced social tolerance and individual liberty.[4]

The centrality of the asylum to the social history of madness, however, was not a theme invented by 'revisionist' historians of the 1970s. Kathleen Jones, writing in the 1950s and 1960s, also saw the emergence of a public asylum system in Britain as the centrepiece of society's response to the problem of the mad.[5] More recently, Mark Finnane, in his study of the insane in post-famine Ireland, focused on the county asylums in his exploration of why institution-alisation should be so advanced in what was a relatively unindustri-alised country.[6] Of course, Jones, Scull and Finnane differ on the social uses of the asylums. For Jones, asylums were a reflection of a new humanitarianism and the manifestation of the state's 'recog-nition' of its responsibility for the mentally ill; according to Scull, the asylum system was encouraged by a group of medical 'entre-preneurs' who claimed expert knowledge over the cure of the mad and championed institutional treatment as a means of professional consolidation and advancement; by contrast, Finnane stressed the importance of asylums to the administration in Dublin as a con-venient way of imposing social order in the absence of a developed poor law.[7] Nevertheless, ever since their monographs, the construc-tion of asylums, and the incarceration of the insane, remain para-mount to our understanding of public responses to mental disorder in the modern period.

Several factors have contributed to an institutional focus within the historiography of madness. Some of the histories of psychiatry were written by practising physicians, so it was unsurprising that medical men would focus upon the mental hospital in searching for their professional roots.[8] When the anti-psychiatry movement coalesced into a recognised entity, many of the early treatises were anti-institutional rather than strictly anti-psychiatry. Russell Barton argued that the mental hospital exacerbated, or indeed created, mental disorder, whilst Erving Goffman popularised the conception of the mental hospital as a 'total institution'.[9] Pinel's Bicêtre and Tuke's York Retreat were the institutional sites where Michel Foucault located the new regime of surveillance. Thomas Szasz identified involuntary hospitalization as the prime evil afflicting contemporary society's response to madness.[10] These works con-centrated the minds of researchers on the efficacy of contemporary mental hospitals and, by extension, the historical origins of these institutions.

There are also archival factors which have shaped and informed this institutionally-oriented tradition. Hospital records are often held in collections, conveniently organised for doctoral students[11] and other researchers to explore a discrete subject for theses or major monographs. The anniversaries of mental hospitals, and the importance of publicity to newly-formed National Health Service Trusts in Britain, proved to an impetus to the writing of institutional histories.[12] Social policy historians have most often looked to Parliamentary Papers for sources, evidence which dealt overwhelmingly with the regulation, licensing and inspection of institutions.[13] As we shall see below, laws established in the nineteenth century were created to regulate existing institutions and lay the groundwork for new public asylums, giving a distinctly institutional bias to the history of mental health policy and the history of psychiatric law.[14] As a result of these various interests and constraints, institutional case studies figure prominently in the proliferation of literature on the history of madness.[15]

The preoccupation with the lunatic asylum has led undoubtedly to excellent monographs on individual institutions in Britain and Ireland: Hunter and MacAlpine on Colney Hatch, London, Anne Digby on the Quaker Retreat near York, Charlotte MacKenzie on Ticehurst Asylum in Sussex, Elizabeth Malcolm on St. Patrick's, Dublin, to name just four notable works.[16] Ironically, it has been these institutionally-oriented studies, many of which have been devoted to detailed examinations of patient populations, which have alerted modern historians of psychiatry to the persistence of extramural care, control, treatment and supervision during the so-called 'asylum era'. Studies of individual institutions, such as John Walton on Lancaster, Allan Beveridge on the Edinburgh Asylum, and Laurence Ray on Brookwood in Surrey, revealed a high turnover rate of patients.[17] Approximately 40–50 per cent of patients admitted to public (lunatic) asylums in the nineteenth century stayed twelve months or fewer. Only about one in five patients were ever readmitted, and admission orders reveal that the 'attack' of insanity had often been underway for months, if not years, before confinement took place.[18] These arresting findings imply that situations of 'care' in the community existed long before a crisis precipitated institutional confinement, and continued after discharge. Care outside the walls of the asylum was therefore a reality, not only for those suffering from madness who were never admitted at all, but also for those patients who were confined in mental hospitals only for short periods of their illness. This research signalled a vast history of 'community', or non-institutional, care of the insane which had yet to be written.

Interest in the history of care in the community has not merely been triggered by the excellent work on the social history of institutional patients. Historiographical innovation has also coincided with a move in medical history more broadly away from institutional foci for welfare provision. This seam in the history of psychiatry has been mined by two groups of researchers. First, there has been the influence of early modern historians, such as Michael MacDonald and Roy Porter, who have revealed a complex history of madness which predated, and persisted parallel to, the coming of the asylum.[19] Further work by Peter Rushton, Akihito Suzuki and Jonathan Andrews traced the use of boarding out by Overseers of the Poor in seventeenth- and eighteenth-century England.[20] Secondly, there has been the impact of historical demographers who have investigated the prevalence of disability in communities over the course of the last two hundred years. The recent book *Locus of Care*, for instance, constitutes a re-interpretation of accepted norms within the history of 'welfare' by challenging accepted assumptions about the decline of family support and the recent rise of state-supported institutions. Three chapters in particular confront the question of extramural care and control of the insane during the period of the emergence of the asylum and challenge the primacy of the institutional model.[21] Articles on the relationship between household care and institutional confinement have also recently appeared in journals devoted to the history of the family.[22]

This volume builds on the new interest in the history of care outside the walls of the asylum. The eleven chapters which follow focus on Britain and Ireland from the eighteenth through the twentieth centuries, and investigate both the social history of extramural care of mentally disordered persons, and the historical evolution of Community Care as a government policy. These chapters demonstrate that the history of modern responses to the insane is far more complex than previously assumed. They provide further evidence that the asylum, though increasingly important in the range of options open to communities, did not *replace* the family as the central locus of care of the insane. Rather, the household remained an important locus of care for the insane, and families maintained a central role in the decisions over treatment and supervision. Furthermore, there existed no simple inverse relationship between asylum and community provision since the definition and conceptualisation of 'asylum', 'community', 'care', and, for that matter, 'insanity', varied both over time and between regions. Chapters in this volume discuss these definitions within the context of particular case studies. This introduction highlights some of the major themes which run across the book as a whole: the persistence of community care in the era of the asylum; the social dimensions of care within and without the household; the breaching of the walls of the asylum; and social control and surveillance in the community. We hope that it provides a starting point, a springboard, to future research and contributes to a reconsideration of the place of the asylum within the historiography of madness.

COMMUNITY CARE IN THE 'ERA OF THE ASYLUM'

Britain and Ireland, at the turn of the nineteenth century, incorporated three legal jurisdictions for the care, supervision, treatment and control of disordered persons: England and Wales, Ireland, and Scotland. Before the First World War, most of the statutes within these jurisdictions which affected insane persons were dedicated to regulating existing institutions or laying the groundwork for new ones. England and Wales fell under a permissive act of 1808 allowing magistrates to establish rate-aided (publicly-funded) pauper asylums. Two Acts of 1845 made such accommodation mandatory at the county level. Nine county asylums were constructed before 1828; another seventy followed before the end of Victoria's reign.[23] Shortly after the Union with Britain, Ireland constructed its first purpose-built public institution, the Richmond Asylum, in 1814. Three years later, the Irish administration in Dublin was empowered to impose asylums at will, and twenty-one county institutions were erected before 1871.[24] Communities in Scotland began to establish charitable and rate-aided asylums for their poor insane in the second half of the eighteenth century and early nineteenth century, starting with the construction of the Montrose Asylum in 1781.[25] Other regions followed suit, before an 'English-style' compulsory act was imposed on the country in 1857. Following the Lunacy (Scotland) Act of that year, Scottish District Lunacy Boards oversaw a dramatic increase in the number and size of district and parochial asylums.[26] By the end of the nineteenth century, Scotland, Ireland, and England and Wales, each had a comprehensive system of public, rate-aided asylums, supplemented by a patchwork of charitable subscription institutions and an uneven distribution of private licensed homes. The institutional backbone of the mental health system had been established.

The nineteenth century, then, witnessed the rapid construction of purpose-built asylums and a dramatic rise in the number of the insane resident in licensed institutions. Returns to the Lunacy Commissions in England and Wales, the Lunacy Board in Scotland, and the Irish Lunacy Inspectors testified to this social phenomenon. Ireland had a resident insane population of 0.5 per cent of total population by World War I; England and Wales had 0.37 per cent by 1909, and Scotland had similar rates of residence.[27] This much is well-known. What is less often highlighted is that annual reports sent by government agencies, acknowledged that mental disorder continued to be cared for outside of the new asylums on a significant scale. The 1871 Census of England and Wales, for example, was the first census to ask householders, or superintendents of institutions, to list all people who were 'lunatics', or 'idiots or imbeciles'. The total number of said persons was 69,019, of which only 39,734 were residing in institutions licensed by statute.[28] Moreover, the Census Commissioners believed that there was widespread underenumeration of idiots, imbeciles and lunatics not resident in institutions, by as many as a half.[29] Thus, twenty-five years after the imposition of the asylum system, and after more than two decades of apparently rapid incarceration, there was no convincing evidence to suggest that the majority of people in England and Wales recognised as insane by their communities were in what Andrew Scull coined the new 'Museums of Madness'.

Some of the 30,000 insane persons in England and Wales not in asylums were resident in workhouse accommodation under the new (post-1834) poor law. Only dangerous insane persons had to be removed from workhouses to county asylums within 14 days. 'Harmless' cases were permitted to remain in workhouses indefinitely.[30] In Ireland, the lunatic asylum system operated independently of the poor law, being regulated in the first half of the century by the Inspectorate General of Prisons, and in the second half by the Inspectorate of Lunacy under the auspices of the Lord Lieutenant. Prior to 1867, dangerous lunatics (who formed the bulk of admissions to public asylums throughout most of the century) had to be admitted to gaol in the first instance and then transferred to the asylum. Many insane people spent long periods of time in gaol waiting for a place in the asylum system, which was severely overcrowded by the mid-century. This overcrowding could not be relieved by transferring people to workhouses or to private mad-houses as was the case in England. Transfer to workhouses was legally permitted only at the end of the century.[31] Thus Ireland had a 'colonial' system of confinement similar to Canada and Australia.[32]

Scotland adopted a unique approach, widely acknowledged throughout the English-speaking world, to the regulation of extra-mural care. As Sturdy and Parry-Jones highlight, boarding-out was official policy following the 1857 Lunacy (Scotland) Act. Up to one-quarter of registered pauper and private patients were relo-cated to households where (usually non-related) families were paid to care for a mentally disordered person. Houston, in the next chapter, reveals that such boarding out developed over the course of the proceeding century. Irish authorities, by contrast, apparently resisted attempts to impose a state-sanctioned system of boarding out before World War I.[33] Within England and Wales, different practices seem to have been adopted within the structures of the 'new' poor law. Poor law unions in England permitted 'out-relief' (poor law payments of money or payments in kind) to families with illness and disability, and some poor law unions arranged for the care of the insane in other households – a form of poor law boarding out. The number of people accommodated in this manner amounted to only half as many as those relieved under Scotland during the same period (Sturdy and Parry-Jones). Moreover, the frequency of this measure must have varied enormously between different poor law unions. Hirst and Michael reveal that the 'farming out' (boarding out on farms) of idiots and lunatics in Welsh poor law unions continued to be widely used, despite the erection of purpose-built institutions, confirming the English Lunacy Commissioners' views that this practice was more prevalent in the principality.[34]

In Ireland, England and Wales, and Scotland, inspectors had responsibility not only for the public asylums, but also for houses where lunatics were being kept for profit.[35] We also know that all the lunacy inspectorates throughout Britain and Ireland at this time were understaffed and felt incapable of properly fulfilling their

statutory function.[36] In practice, then, large purpose-built institutions and madhouses were given priority, and small, informal
arrangements for caring outside of the insane person's household,
though sometimes officially disapproved of, were only investigated
if there was reason to assume neglect or mistreatment. The degree
to which paid out-nursing, for a fee, existed is thus very difficult to
determine, as it was not systematically recorded, and there was a
disincentive for families to admit that this practice was going on.
Research on the care of 'idiot' children, however, shows that
domestic servants were being paid to care for them within households.[37] Similarly, the extent of neighbourhood sharing,[38] an informal market of reciprocal services in working class neighbourhoods,
impinged upon the care of the insane remains to more fully
researched. Bearing these limitations in mind, chapters in this
volume support the contention that the household had an important role in regulating the treatment and care of the insane during
the eighteenth and nineteenth centuries.

COMMUNITY CARE WITHIN AND WITHOUT THE HOUSEHOLD

In a reconsideration of his seminal monograph on post-famine
Ireland, Mark Finnane acknowledged that he had placed too much
emphasis on the state, and too little on the family and household
as active participants in the social organisation of the insane during
the industrial revolution.[39] Since then, historians have been taken
up his thesis that the family was active in the pattern of confinement throughout the British Isles and elsewhere.[40] Chapters in this
volume have explored several aspects of this family participation:
the legal prerogative of families, the household as a locus of care,
the family as purchasers of care, and the sexual division of caring
in the community. Rather than passive recipients of state support,
the family is seen as a unit which negotiated with authorities over
the conditions and locus of care, often from a position of power.

The deference in law to this family power was considerable. A
husband, for instance, could not be convicted under the cruelty
sections of the Lunacy Acts for assaulting his wife. In *R v. Rundle*
it was held that those statutes did not intend to interfere with care
and charge arising out of relations of a purely domestic nature, and
to superadd to the ordinary obligations under which any master of
a family lies.[41] The perception of families as having the right to

conduct their affairs outside the scope of the asylum acts is noted by Melling *et al.* Family power is also emphasized by Walsh, in her discussion of admissions to the Ballinasloe Asylum in Galway, where admission might be based on a desire to protect familial property rights as much as on the condition of the insane person. Families negotiated with local authorities in eighteenth-century Scotland (Houston) and Victorian Wales (Hirst and Michael) over the conditions of the care of relatives. In the event of institutional confinement, the family further had the right to insist on the release of lunatics confined in asylums so long as they would not be a charge on the poor rates, and so long as the asylum superintendent did not certify the lunatic to be dangerous.[42] The family thus had power over the locus and duration of care, and even, as Marland suggests, the type of treatment.

The apparent 'sanctity' of the household, and prerogative of the family, did not, however, go unchallenged. In some cases the social history of community care during the era of the asylum might involve an outside agency transgressing the 'private sphere' of the household, through visitation and inspection of the insane person. As Suzuki suggests, control within the household might be informed by concerns over etiquette and propriety, and how the transgression of these appeared to the outside world. The household sometimes became a place to enclose, rather than disclose. Hirst and Michael find a similar tendency to hide the insane person from the public gaze in their study of boarding out of paupers in Wales, although here it is ambiguous whether it is the family or the local officials who wish to conceal the presence of the lunatic. Melling *et al.* remind readers that care within the household was not necessarily more humane than the asylum. Their chapter identifies asylum provision as in part a policy response to family care which might be substandard, painful, or even cruel. The meeting of public and private, as well as lay and professional, resonates well with Marland's investigation of puerperal mania. The household in this context can be understood as a contested space between the family and medical professionals.

In the nineteenth century, as in the twentieth, caring for the insane had profound economic consequences for families. Not only did poor households lose the economic contribution of vital members, but caring and supervision of a disabled household member reduced the contribution of the carer(s). Families often had to make calculative choices as to the viability of paid care both within and without the home, or the desirability of institutional confinement. Although historians of medicine now appreciate the remarkably diverse occupational backgrounds of patients sent to public asylums, there has been comparatively little work on the economic factors which impinged upon the decision to confine, for how long, and when. How did local economic changes affect the ability or desirability of families to care for the insane within the household or in the local community? To what extent did grants of outdoor relief to a lunatic's family affect the calculus of care? Did government subsidies, such as grants-in-aid to English parishes for the resident insane, promote institutional confinement by altering the desirability of non-institutional care?

Researchers have tended to locate the purchase of care within the network of for-profit madhouses which constituted the 'Trade in Lunacy'. Such private provision was indeed very important in certain regions of Britain and Ireland, and did not cease with the rise of the public asylum. In England, it was not until 1890 that a policy decision was made to restrict the number of new licences granted for private madhouses.[43] Were these private licensed homes 'institutional' or representative of local, community care? While subject to regulation, they otherwise operated outside the public sector. While the larger ones might be 'institutional' in character, smaller houses might bear considerable similarity to boarding out of the poor insane to 'strangers', as described in papers by Sturdy and Parry-Jones and Hirst and Michael, except that the bills would be paid by the family rather than the poor law authorities. Although the public, county asylum system had been designed for, and largely restricted to, the insane poor[44] recent research has shown, however, that in counties where there was limited scope for private care, public institutions often responded by offering private accommodation. Clearly more research is needed on the relationship between the demand for local caring resources for the insane (nursing), changes in work patterns, the availability of private care and the use of public accommodation.

BREACHING THE WALLS OF THE ASYLUM

The traditional image of the asylum, reflected in the title of this volume, is of a walled fortress, an impregnable barrier separating the insane and society. This image distorts as much as it reveals. Chapters in this volume suggest that the conceptualisation of, and boundaries between, 'asylum' and 'community' have always been contested. Out-patient clinics in England and Wales were formed pursuant to the Mental Treatment Act 1930, and distinctions between in-patients and out-patients have been less and less clearly defined since that time. This legislation also allowed informal admissions[45] in England and Wales for the first time. After the creation of the Republic of Ireland, Northern Ireland followed the 1930 Act with similar legislation. The Irish Republic, and Scotland, were later in implementing voluntary admission continuing until the 1960s with in effect, legislation dating from the mid-Victorian period.[46] These acts removed a significant symbolic barrier between asylum and other forms of care.

The shifting boundaries of 'asylum', however, predates the twentieth century. Throughout the nineteenth century, routine visits to asylum wards were made not merely by asylum governors, but also by representatives of the poor law unions which paid for the care of patients and, by mid-century, official commissioners and inspectors. For the remainder of the public, there was a tension created between the privacy of the individuals contained in the asylum, and concerns that the management of the asylum be known to be appropriate. Some institutions, such as the York Retreat, appear to have welcomed visitors; in other cases, such as the York Asylum in 1813, respectable members of society were required to subscribe to the asylum in order to force disclosure of the asylum's operations, but subscribe they did. Annual reports of asylums were often published, and at least occasionally reported in the press. Reports of annual inspections by the official lunacy commissioners were a matter of public record, and lunacy and asylums policy was a matter of fairly steady public debate. While the nineteenth-century asylum was certainly not a public space, it was also not outside the public gaze.

If society could at least occasionally look in, so a number of the inmates could look out. Trial discharges in England were expressly provided for in legislation commencing in 1845.[47] These allowed patients, with the approval of the Visiting Committee running the asylum, to be absent from the asylum for up to a month. In 1866 at the Leicestershire and Rutland County Asylum, 17 per cent of the asylum population was permitted to leave the asylum unattended on probationary discharge or day passes.[48] In addition, work on the asylum farm and occasional special outings would take at least some of the inmates out of the asylum and into the public view. Legislation in 1862 (affecting England and Wales) allowed inmates to reside in approved workhouse wards without formally being discharged from the asylum.[49] While this may appear a mere movement from one institution to another, it does re-enforce that asylum boundaries were not cut and dried.

The mechanisms by which the walls were breached will strike resonance with twentieth-century readers. Pressure on hospital beds has now made leaves of absence, the very technique used by the Victorians, now last for days, weeks or months at a time, blurring the line between asylum treatment and care in the community even more than in the Victorian period. Indeed, until 1986, it would seem that some hospitals were using the leave provisions to allow the patient to live in the community, but to remain legally confined, so that control over the individual, including forcible medication, would remain available.[50] Some aspects of this have now been struck down by the courts, but it would still appear that hospitals rely on the leave provisions in order to function 'efficiently'. Payne describes how some London psychiatric wards have recently been operating at 117 per cent capacity, a figure suggesting reliance by hospitals on the ability to place considerable numbers of patients on leave as a matter of necessity. This form of community care has thus become a manifestation of the evolving hospital system itself. Similarly, the extension of the 1983 English Mental Health Act[51] to mental nursing homes registered under section 23 of the Registered Homes Act, 1984, bears more than passing similarity to the extension of the nineteenth-century asylum protocols to workhouse wards. Once again, the boundaries between the asylum and community are vague and uncertain.

The reasons for the granting of leave in the nineteenth century are under-reseaerched, but one case study of Victorian Buckinghamshire suggests that visiting magistrates used probationary discharge as a means of monitoring, through poor law medical inspectors, ex-patients. Patients who were not able to cope in the community were returned to the asylum; patients whose households could show that that the ex-inmate was properly cared for and not a danger to themselves or others were fully discharged.[52] The precise reasons why some patients were selected for probationary discharge, and others not, remain elusive. It may be that probationary discharge was granted to assist in acclimatisation of patients prior to permanent discharge; or it may be that it was to place inmates with specific behavioural problems on 'long leashes', to ensure proper behaviour. Although after-care planning for persons confined in psychiatric facilities became mandatory in England in 1983, the practice of monitoring ex-patients in the community is as old as the asylum itself.[53]

SOCIAL CONTROL, SURVEILLANCE AND CARE IN THE COMMUNITY

If some dimensions of the modern asylum system can be portrayed in the context of 'community', so services outside the asylum can be understood in institutional terms. In his 1985 book, *Visions of Social Control*,[54] Stan Cohen argued that the late twentieth century has moved social control out of the realm of the asylum, into the community at large, led by a vanguard of professionals and experts. Decarceration has not meant, according to his thesis, a reduction in social control, but an increase, for it no longer stops at the asylum door. The rise of increasingly controlling programmes and legislation for those released into the community, discussed in the twentieth-century papers in this volume, is consistent with this view; yet as will now be clear, there is a long history of surveillance outside the so-called 'total' institution before the 'decarceration movement' which serves as Cohen's point of transition. The papers in this collection can be seen as charting different forms of social control, and providing the conceptual roots of some of the forms of control continuing at the end of the twentieth century.

Some of this control can be seen as the extensions of professional hegemony. As Hirst and Michael point out, local poor law officials in Wales (and England) were required to compile registers of insane persons in their jurisdictions as early as 1828. In 1853, a fee became payable to the poor law medical officer for each insane person contained on the list. While Hirst and Michael suggest that even this fee was insufficient to induce diligence of medical officers in completion of the register, the lists which were created would suggest that the state had already moved to a posture of surveillance. Welshman indicates that few mid-twentieth-century local authorities employed psychiatric social workers or other specialist staff, suggesting something of a reduction in the scope of that particular form of surveillance in that period, but it can be seen on the rise again at the end of the century, in the insistence that aftercare be provided, generally by community psychiatric nurses.

It is not merely the insane person who has been subject to surveillance. Marland's paper suggests that puerperal mania provided a mechanism by which obstetricians could enter the broader domestic sphere, being potentially critical of the family environment of the patient. In Scotland, Sturdy and Parry-Jones detail an ornate system of official inspections of nineteenth-century boarding out. At issue in this inspection is as much the suitability of the carers as the state of the insane person, a suitability enforced by the reliance of carers on payments from the authorities. As the paper by Melling *et al.* suggests, the reports of the Lunacy Commission in England and Wales reflect that the difficulties of supervision of care of lunatics outside larger institutional settings was one of their reasons for encouraging the asylum option. Further study of the relations between local authorities and carers is necessary, to determine the degree to which the insane person can be seen as an entry point, by which the state controlled the entire household of the lunatic.

The behaviour of the carers was pivotal in instituting the day-to-day mechanisms of social control which kept in check any deviant behaviour of the insane person. While the authorities might have administrative mechanisms to ensure the standards of the carer, both through surveillance and through economic controls, this does not answer the question of how the insane person was actually controlled by the carers. Suzuki identifies cases where the individual might literally be locked in a darkened room, but he stresses that this was not the typical approach: privacy did not mean cruelty. Sturdy and Parry-Jones suggest that the objective of the Scottish system of boarding out was to make the insane person as much as possible part of the family of the carer, creating resonance with the twentieth-century ideology of Normalization. In both papers, it does seem that what could be provided in small-scale settings was an intensive level of surveillance by the carers. With insane people lodged in families, the control mechanisms of the family itself could be used to ensure appropriate conformity. These might in their way be as restrictive as any asylum.

COMMUNITY CARE AND THE HEALTH CARE PROFESSIONS

Control, care, surveillance and treatment of the insane in Modern Britain and Ireland were increasingly entangled in the multiplicity of professions claiming expert knowledge over the insane. Asylums have been seen, quite rightly, as midwives to the psychiatric profession. But the psychiatric profession has not been always been unanimous in its attitude to the locus of care. There were debates within the ranks of medical superintendents of asylums over which groups should be confined, and battles between alienists and other medical professionals over clientele. As early as the 1850s, during the peak in asylum construction, medical men were questioning the efficacy of large 'warehouses' for the insane. John Bucknill and Alexander Morison, for example, believed that a prudent policy of care of the mentally ill should include both institutional and community options, and allow for flexibility at the local level.[55] More needs to be known about the debates within the ranks of asylum superintendents over the appropriate locus of care for different sub-groups of the insane.

Changing theoretical approaches to the treatment of insanity could also alter the balance of care. Janet Oppenheim has shown the rise of 'nervous clinics' for the middle classes who wanted to avoid the stigma of certification and the social trauma occasioned by confinement.[56] Psychotherapeutic models of medical interaction led to a preference on behalf of family members and practitioners to locate treatment outside the asylum during the first decades of this century. The adoption of Freudian psychoanalysis, though less influential in Britain and Ireland than in the United States, further challenged the institution as the most appropriate and efficacious locus of medical treatment. The capture of drug and alcohol addiction in the community, eating disorders in households and shell shock at the front, have greatly expanded the profession's territory, and accelerated the transition of treatment into clinics, households and general hospitals.[57]

Where families were once the central actors in the provision of care, and are still sometimes pivotal to the provision of care in the community, professional interests and roles have developed an expertise to eclipse, at least in public policy and perception, family providers. This is not just a result of the changing cultural values concerning who should care. The NHS, as with the welfare state more generally, created the expectation that the state will provide care. It is also, in part, the result of a move to new (drug) therapies which are easy to administer in the community. And in part it is the result of changes in professional status: doctors, and psychiatrists in particular, are far more respected than they were a century ago; nurses and social workers compete for similar prestige. Thus while the family of the patient continues to enjoy a legal place in English confinement legislation, they are now more likely to find their views overridden or contested.[58] The driving force in psychiatric confinement now flows from professionals. The result is that care in the community is more likely now to be viewed in medical (or at least, professional) terms, rather than in an essentially residential context a century ago.

The twentieth century has witnessed a greater separation of the ideas of care and accommodation. In many post-war facilities, daytime occupation or medical treatment may be provided, with the expectation that the individual will reside elsewhere. Welshman's paper provides a study of such facilities. Under the vision of community care of the 1950s and 1960s, facilities would be provided for daytime activity only. No long-term residence was provided in Leicester, his local study. In the absence of other provision, families were expected to provide residential support, as they always had. As the chapters by Campbell and Payne highlight, a variety of social factors have transformed the stereotype of the insane person. At the close of the twentieth century, insanity is associated in the public consciousness with homelessness, a homelessness seen as the visible of failure of Community Care. This contrasts with the stereotype of the rootless lunatic in pre-industrial society, so often idealised in revisionist critiques of modern asylums.

CONCLUSIONS

In the closing years of the twentieth century 'Care in the Community' holds the dubious distinction of being universally supported in principle, and universally condemned in practice. And there is much to condemn. Chronic underfunding from governments, poor co-ordination of service providers at the local level, rivalry amongst professional bodies, lack of continuity of care, and a general misunderstanding and resistance by the public are just some of the most recognisable problems inherent in this contested programme of social engineering. What's more, since Community Care has never been properly defined, there is no standard measurement to evaluate its success and to remedy its shortcomings. This book hopes to contribute to a more complex understanding of Community Care by examining the historical roots of this phenomenon both as a government policy, and as a crucially important dimension of the social history of madness.

This introductory chapter has suggested that the history of modern responses to the insane has too often been portrayed in the light of institutional care and treatment. The dominance of the institutional paradigm can be seen in the major works on the history of social policy. Kathleen Jones's *Asylums and After*,[59] Peter Barham's *Closing Down the Asylum*,[60] as well as books in comparative and British mental health policy,[61] accept without question the premise that the history of social responses to the mad can be seen primarily in a history of the 'rise and the fall of the asylum'. Images of chained and furious madmen, the public outcry over wrongful detention, and the emergence of a new psychiatric nosology which pathologised women's reproductive stages, have fuelled the fascination with this historical institution. The virulence of the debate over the role of psychiatry in the modern period, and the obvious relationship between the formation of psychiatry and the establishment of lunatic asylums, has forced scholars into placing themselves in one of the many rival camps in the debate, thereby inhibiting, in Mark Micale's estimation, a more extensive philosophical reconsideration of the methodology of psychiatric history.[62] Part of such a reconsideration must include a re-evaluation of the centrality of the asylum to the complex of care for the insane which has existed in the modern period. As the following chapters will show, care outside the walls of the asylum has a long and varied history which must be studied in parallel to that of institutional treatment.

Community Care as a social policy also has a long history; it has repeatedly been 'rediscovered' as a solution to the proliferation of asylums. In the 1880s and 1890s, in response to the dangers of urban degeneration, farm colonies for epileptics, the feebleminded and the consumptive were in vogue. These colonies bridged the gap between asylums and communities by creating rural, enclosed self-sufficient communities of themselves. Although the notorious Mental Deficiency Act of 1913 would become associated with institutional solutions, in reality local authorities used enhanced powers under the act to engage in their own form of care in the community for mental defectives.[63] And experience of military men with shellshock showed that non-institutional therapy could prove beneficial. Tempting as it may be to represent Community Care as a post-war development, the intellectual roots of an alternative to the asylum deep lie in the Victorian period.

Researchers need to be more aware of this historical legacy, rather than assume that care in the community has recently appeared on the landscape of social policy. Chapters in this book recognize that a range of 'caring' possibilities for the mentally disordered has always been provided. But the boundaries between private and public, institutional and community, voluntary and statutory, were never fixed: their relationship remains complex. Furthermore old clichés must be abandoned. Neither institutions nor the community had a monopoly over kindness or cruelty, beneficence or malevolence; each had a set of rules and regulations governing the care of those disordered in mind. We therefore must move to an historical evaluation of mental hospitals which compares their care and treatment with that offered outside the walls of the asylum. For, inevitably, 'to understand what was happening within the asylums, we should know what treatment insane people received outside them.'[64]

CHAPTER TWO

'Not simple boarding': care of the mentally incapacitated in Scotland during the long eighteenth century[1]

R. A. Houston

INTRODUCTION

Until the nineteenth century, Scottish idiots, imbeciles, and mad people can be found in a wide variety of circumstances. They might be cared for in their families of origin; boarded out on an individual basis with other families; maintained in workhouses, 'hospitals' or jails; housed temporarily in the infirmaries of the larger cities; placed in the few private madhouses which existed around Edinburgh; or, from 1743, incarcerated in one of the still rarer public asylums. Other lunatics and idiots were left to their own devices: 'at large' in the words of late-Georgian reformers like Dr Andrew Duncan. This chapter explores the familial and other contingencies which determined where a person who was mentally incapable might be accommodated. It examines the place of private and public madhouses among other options for care in an age before widespread institutional provision. Welfare was available from (local) government, commercial sources, community, and household.[2] Finally, the kinds of men and women who looked after lunatics and idiots are considered.

In view of the scarcity of secondary literature on any except medical and institutional aspects of care in historic Scotland,[3] this study relies to a considerable extent on primary documentation. The sources used are civil court cognitions of mental incapacity, criminal court records involving an insanity defence, and early official investigations of the 1810s into the nature of care. These are supplemented by family papers, further civil court documents about marital breakup and disputed inheritance, newspapers, and the records of the Kirk Session – the parish body comprising clergyman, and lay elders and deacons who policed poor relief, and moral and religious life. These documents allow different forms of support to be analysed, and sometimes offer an insight into the changing types of care which individuals experienced. Most sources will be familiar to historians of madness, except perhaps for the civil court processes, which resemble proceedings before Chancery in eighteenth-century England. If a person was allegedly unable to manage their own affairs, their relatives could ask for a formal legal procedure to test whether they were 'furious' or 'idiotic'.[4] Relatives purchased a brieve or writ from Chancery ordering a judge to hold inquest by jury into the questions raised in it, and to return or 'retour' the answers. A retour named the court, judge, jury, and subject; it offered a legal term for the nature of his or her ailment plus the duration of time it had been suffered; it concluded with the name of the next of kin charged with their care. The person petitioning for the inquest generally also entered a claim to be the guardian ('tutor' or 'curator') of the person if he or she was found to be *incompos mentis*. Proof depended on witness statements, which were usually delivered in person but might be submitted in writing, and (normally) a personal interrogation of the brieve's subject by a jury of 15 laymen. Recorded witness statements list instances of why the deponent thought the subject deranged or stupid. In doing so they also outlined the care and treatment of the sufferer. The process was known as 'cognition' or 'cognoscing' someone as an idiot or lunatic. Between 1701 and 1818 a total of 164 individuals became the subject of tutories and curatories on the grounds of idiocy or furiosity, producing 500 often lengthy depositions.

Certain conventions are followed in this exposition. 'Care' is defined as attention, custody, protection, supervision, or support rather than medical treatment. The concern is less with the sources of finance for welfare than with the spectrum of choices or strategies available, and their meanings for communities, families, and individuals. For the sake of brevity, when not employing contemporary labels such as troubled (in mind), idiotic, or furious the phrases 'mentally incapacitated' or 'mentally impaired' are used to describe the spectrum of afflictions from violent lunacy to mild imbecility.

These phrases summarise most accurately the reasons why people became visible in historical documents. While some statistical information is presented, much of the analysis is necessarily qualitative.

LOCATIONS FOR CARE

'In the eighteenth century, madmen were locked up in madhouses: in the nineteenth century, lunatics were sent to asylums: and in the twentieth century, the mentally ill receive treatment in hospitals.'[5] So writes Kathleen Jones in her seminal study of English social policy. However, Jones does accept that individual care with an attendant or in the family was also an alternative for rich and poor respectively.[6] Indeed, available sources indicate that the latter options were far more common than institutionalisation during the eighteenth century. However, the distinctions between the categories are blurred. A public asylum can be identified by the sources of its funding and its admission policy, but the licensing of private madhouses in Scotland was not put in place until the early nineteenth century.[7] Even then, some owners applied to the Sheriff for licenses even though they had only one inmate, whereas other singleton establishments known to us from other sources did not.

Nor does the community/institution dichotomy always survive close investigation. Placing a person in an 'institution' did not necessarily mean cutting them off from 'care in the community'. George Weir, sawer, petitioned the managers of Paisley Town's Hospital in the summer of 1793 'for having his wife Mary Brown who has for some time past been deprived of her reason admitted into the cells upon his paying for her maintenance . . . considering the very clamant and distressing situation of the woman and that the man is by constant attendance upon her prevented from earning subsistence they agree to admit her for some time into the cells of the house'.[8] George was to pay for her 'and also to give all due attendance himself in furnishing her with victuals at meal time and in being aiding and assisting at all other times in taking care of her so as to give the house as little trouble and inconvenience with her as possible'. This example, one of a number from this establishment in the late eighteenth and early nineteenth centuries,[9] reminds us that those in institutions were not necessarily 'institutionalised'. Some workhouse environments might be an extension of the family, an idea and a practice reinforced by the tendency of administrators to use the vocabulary (and the authoritative rhetoric) of family life.[10] When the prestige public establishments of the early nineteenth century sought a keeper and a matron, husband and wife or brother and sister teams were preferred, recreating the sort of family-run madhouses which had characterised private care in eighteenth-century Scotland.[11]

We should bear in mind the permeability of categories of care when we analyse early-nineteenth-century surveys. In his *General view* of 1828 Andrew Halliday calculated 'that, in 1826, there were six hundred and forty-eight individuals in the public and private asylums in Scotland, and ten in public gaols; but this bears no proportion to the actual number of insane persons in that kingdom'.[12] Using returns provided by clergy from 800 of 900 parishes Halliday claimed there were some 3,700 insane persons and idiots in Scotland. Of these, 146 were in private asylums or madhouses, 50 in the public asylum, and 60 in Bedlam[13] – all in or close to the city of Edinburgh. Other public asylums and workhouses accommodated 387 people.

> One thousand one hundred and ninety-two are confined with private individuals, principally with small farmers and cottagers, and twenty-one are in gaols – making the number of persons actually in a state of confinement, one thousand eight hundred and sixty-one; while upwards of sixteen hundred are allowed to be at large, most of them wandering over the country, and subsisting by begging.[14]

A similar survey for 1818 (based on approximately 850 parishes) showed 2,304 males and 2,324 females of whom 416 were in asylums or madhouses, 1,357 with 'friends' (relations), and 2,855 were at large (of whom 2,419 were maintained wholly or partly by the parish).[15] Halliday, like others who were promoting public asylums, suggested various multipliers to correct omissions and provide 'real' figures of mental incapacity. What matters for our purposes is that those outside institutions would more likely escape notice, reinforcing the point that non-institutional care massively predominated even at this date.

National investigations give the opportunity to discover whether the insane were more likely to be in the community or confined, and who among them were cared for wholly or partly by parish funds or by relations. What is lacking in most sources is any detailed idea of how a cross-section of local society was maintained. For that we have to look to evidence contained in the report to the Parliamentary Committee on madhouses of 1816.[16] Here we find 33 individuals, mostly named, who were cared for in five Renfrewshire parishes (tabled below). Unless stated, all were receiving some money from poor funds and the sterling sums specified were to help with, or wholly to provide, maintenance. The recently-opened Glasgow asylum had been built on subscription, and some neighbouring parishes contributed, allowing them to place paupers there more cheaply than the normal rate for non-Glaswegians. The table (Table 2.1) shows that there was a patchwork of public and private provision rather than a 'system' of care, and that the location of care shifted with changing 'medical' condition, funds, and familial circumstances.

Appearing in one support category or another in such cross-sectional evidence is directly related to the amount of time spent receiving that kind of care. Thus, the early-nineteenth-century surveys accurately represent the experience of care for sufferers *at that point in time*. Sometimes, as above or in asylum admission petitions, the documents give a history of provision or attempted cure. Yet, these sources do not always reflect the changing types of care used for fatuous and furious people. Nor do they tell us much about the circumstances which led to that form of maintenance being selected. The further away we move from institutions and official surveys, the harder it becomes to quantify information. Generalisations become less robust and we are forced to rely on qualitative evidence about the choice of care, and how it was perceived by those who had mentally impaired relatives. What we find is that pragmatism and fluidity are the key to understanding the options for care.

The case of Jean Marshall illustrates the difficult choices and limited facilities available to carers in mid-eighteenth-century Scotland. Jean's relations squabbled over her inheritance before the supreme civil court in Scotland, the Court of Session, from 1756 until just after her merciful death in the spring of 1758. Those who cared for her until her demise were her maternal niece, Mary Gillespie, and Mary's husband, Gilbert Lawrie of Crossrig, surgeon in Edinburgh. Their interest was in retaining control of an annuity, left to Jean by her mother, against the efforts of her cousin, who was her legal curator or guardian. Never very bright ('originally but of mediocre understanding'), Jean Marshall's physical and mental health had been declining for years before her plight was

Table 2.1 *Name, age, mental condition, occupation, place and means or amount of support[17] (where available) of insane or idiotic people in part of Renfrewshire, 1816.*

Greenock West or Old parish

Name	Age	Condition	Support
James Watson	48	Insane	Resides with his mother here. £7–10–0 a year from parish funds.
James Stewart		Partially insane	Wife. £3–12–0
John McMillan	33	Insane	About to be sent to Glasgow Asylum
Eliz. McArthur	26	Insane	Resident with John Chalmers in Greenock. £6.
Agnes McKenzie	14	Idiot	Mother in Greenock. £4–16–0.
John Wilson	18	Idiot	Father in Greenock. £7–4-0.
Robert Lyon	49	Idiot	Sister in Greenock. £3.

Middle or New parish

Name	Condition	Support
Isobel Downie		Formerly in Greenock Bridewell now Glasgow Asylum. £21–2-0.
Graham Campbell		Glasgow Asylum since January. £21–2-0.
Daniel Cameron		Glasgow Asylum since May. £21–2-0.
Mrs McBryde		Greenock Bridewell 'where she has become in some sort an inmate of the Jailor's family, and useful in working.' £20.
Eliz. McAllester	Insane	John McArthur, farmer in Luss parish. £15–10–0.
James McCulloch		Sister here. 4/- monthly.
Joseph McAllester's son	Idiot	Mother, a widow here. 32/-.
Donald MacDonald	Lately become insane	Father. 5/- monthly.
widow Campbell's son		Mother. 3/- monthly.

East parish

Name	Condition	Support
Janet Telfer	Insane	John McArthur, farmer in Dumbartonshire. £36–6-0.
Ann Murray	Idiot	James Roger, smith in Greenock. £2–8-0.
Clementina Parker	Idiot	James Parker, shoemaker in Crawfords-Dyke. £2–8-0.
Robert Rankin	Idiot, orphan	Mrs MacDonald in Crawfords-Dyke. £9.
Carolina Allan	Idiot, orphan	Mrs Sage in Crawfords-Dyke. £6.

Port Glasgow

- McKellar   former soldier Glasgow Asylum. 9/- a week.
- Donald   'a barber, resident in Port Glasgow, is subject to occasional fits of insanity when overtaken in liquor.'

'Joseph Thomson, formerly a smith in Port Glasgow, is deranged, lives in his own house, and is taken care of by his wife, and is supposed at present to be dying. He is supported partly from parish, and partly from the funds of charitable societies. He was for some time in Greenock Infirmary, but was discharged as incurable and insane.'

'George Lane, a negro, is deranged and at large, without any fixed abode, sleeping in stairs and closes through the town from choice; is sometimes a bishop, and at other times a duke, as the mania operates; quite harmless.'

James Park, tide-waiter, sent to Glasgow Asylum. Returned cured.

Angus McFie, mason, sent to Glasgow Asylum. Returned cured.

'David Hutcheson, a cooper, had been sent from thence to the Asylum, where he remained some time, but got out, and has not been heard of; and that Mrs Walker, a person subject to intermittent fits of insanity, is at present lucid, and resides with her son in a house of Bailie Gillespie, from which the some became obliged to remove, if his mother should relapse.'

Innerkip

A reply from the minister mentioned 'a married woman boarded at Glasgow Asylum at her husband's expense' and Janet Boag 'kept in the parish by her own relations, who had for a long time, unaided, provided for her'. £4–4-0.

recorded in the court papers. In particular, the convulsive fits Jean began to experience left her very poorly in the mid 1740s. Her predicament worsened when her mother died in 1746. Gilbert and Mary, faced with the problem of who was to look after Jean,

> with much importunity, prevailed upon a good friend of her mother's, one Mrs White, to take her into her house and board her at a rate of £5 sterling per quarter; but at the end of one quarter she grew so wearied of her that no arguments could prevail upon her to keep her any longer, though the petitioners were willing to give any addition to her board that she could demand.[18]

However financial the reason for their petition, and however overstated their submission, Mary and her husband seem genuinely to have cared about Jean. Indeed, nobody else would take her. The Royal Infirmary wanted £20 sterling a year plus another £12 a year for constant attendance by a servant, 'which with the expense of keeping her decent in clothes' would cost more than her annuity would bear.[19] For this reason, the petitioners rented a house for her at £6 a year with 'a servant who had been 14 years with her mother and her', and another woman. This too did not prove a permanent solution. At the end of two years the woman 'wearied of her charge' and refused to continue on any terms, with the result that Jean was taken into the petitioners' house in the country.

By the early 1750s Jean was in a dreadful state, racked by convulsive fits which left her in 'a state of absolute idiotry' and 'devoid of all sense and understanding'. She was also covered in 'loathsome ulcers'. The main reason for the ulcers was bed-sores since Jean was too weak to turn herself where she lay. When helped from bed, she also tended to sit too close to the fire if left unattended and her clothes caught alight. Once, she had fallen into the fire and the resulting burns had turned septic, adding to her bodily discomfort. Her sores had to be dressed regularly and, to cap it all, she was incontinent: 'her bodily infirmity was at all times so great that she constantly spoiled her bedclothes, which, besides a perpetual attendance and trouble that no servant cared to submit to, occasioned a great waste and consumption of bedding'.[20] While Lawrie was a surgeon and could provide medicines and advice, it was his wife who did most of the day-to-day caring and 'it has been great part of the work of the whole family to look after and wait on her'. However exaggerated their claims, it would be hard to deny their argument that such a person made 'a disagreeable boarder', and that care of her 'is not simple boarding'.[21]

An institution, Edinburgh Royal Infirmary, was considered as an option by Jean Marshall's relatives. It was rejected as too expensive. Bedlam is not mentioned, probably because it housed lunatics rather than the incurable and fatuous. It too was thought an expensive destination.[22] Yet, all public institutions of our period which took in the mentally troubled – asylums, infirmaries, towns' hospitals, or workhouses – consistently had more applications than they had places. From the early nineteenth century, campaigners like Halliday and Duncan argued that only public asylums could provide proper care for lunatics. By definition, therefore, those who appeared in the columns of reports and pamphlets headed 'at large' were sadly neglected. Those cared for in families were said to be only slightly better off. Modern observers have condemned late-nineteenth- and twentieth-century institutions as dumping grounds for society's victims: 'warehouses of the unwanted'.[23] However, during the transitional period dealt with here, a range of attitudes towards care co-existed. The decision to send a person to a madhouse or asylum was not taken lightly, and those who took this course cannot simply be written off as uncaring or failing. In the absence of proof that one regime or location of care was superior to another, it seems better to try to understand the reasons why an option was chosen rather than to judge it.

At a moral or emotional level, there was a clear preference for family care. Mr Wood, a friend of James Boswell, opposed placing John Boswell with Mr Campbell at Inveresk because he was said to be harsh and, in any case, 'the plan [was] by no means consistent with a proper concern for a relation'.[24] In the end, John was sent to Newcastle. Other examples point to the same values. Widow Pollock spent three months in Glasgow Town's Hospital some years before becoming wholly deranged. However, 'in consequence of some of her friends making reflections on her daughters for putting her there and their own desire to attend to her and keep her with themselves she was taken out, after which she appeared calmer for a short time ... but she did not continue long so'.[25] Motives were complex. Stuart Moodie, the Paterson family's 'advocate' or lawyer, recalled the progress of the banker David Paterson's derangement. 'At one time, it was talked of to send David Paterson to an asylum, but Mrs Paterson was extremely averse to let him go out of the house. The deponent at one time proposed that David Paterson should be cognosced, but Mrs Paterson was so much shocked with the proposal that the deponent did not urge it.'[26] The Patersons were extremely rich, but financial considerations were necessarily present for some relatives, as they had been for Jean Marshall's. David Blair proposed to his father that his sister Ann be sent to a madhouse 'where she could be boarded for a much less sum than the provisions he had bequeathed her. This most revolting proposition was received in the manner it deserved.'[27] Rendering the final deposition about the evident incapacity of Archibald Coats, Robert Buchanan, civil engineer in Glasgow, said that he was never 'ill used in the family and the deponent's opinion was and is that they had done themselves injustice and Archibald more than justice in keeping him so long in it as he had been'. A man in his fifties, Archibald had been mad for at least 20 years.[28] The stated preference was to care for mentally incapable kin in the family.

Brieves of idiocy and furiosity were, of course, designed to prevent a deranged or incapable person from dissipating their assets. The interest was economic. This source bias pervades most types of document which contain references to the mentally impaired. Very obvious for well-off landowners, this emphasis is also true of the poor and middling ranks of society. Idiots and others who appear as objects of charity do so because they were an economic burden. Parish poor records contain only rare mentions of lunatics and idiots, suggesting at first glance that this category of the poor was not well provided for by agencies other than the family.[29] In the early nineteenth century, at least, idiots could not obtain a settlement in their own right, even if separately resident from their parents, because they were unable to act for themselves. To this end, even someone aged 14 years or above was treated as a pupil 'if it necessarily remains a member of the parents' family, unemancipated, from imbecility or bodily weakness'.[30] The Scottish poor law prior to 1845 was highly discretionary and claimants had no unambiguous right to relief.[31]

Mentions of pauper lunatics or idiots are sparse even in sources exclusively concerned with the poor. Among the blind, lame, shipwrecked, orphaned, abandoned, and merely poor we rarely find instances where the recipient of relief was troubled in mind. The detailed Kirk Treasurer's Accounts for Edinburgh from

1663–1743 run to over a thousand pages. A single relevant entry for 1664 reads 'clothes to John Kennedy madman' as one of 236 'disbursements to ordinary poor ones'. This figure is of 'present supports to poor ones' and does not include quarterly pensioners of the city.[32] In 1667 we find recorded 'a chist [coffin] and sheet to John Kennedy mad-man'. Then in 1669 there is 'a distracted woman' and in 1672 'Agnes Plenderleith distracted, her entertainment [maintenance]' £42 – a figure which stands out in columns where £1 or £2 was the most common disbursement. Mentally impaired paupers were generally more expensive to lodge than others partly because they required more attention, but more because they were usually unable to contribute to their own upkeep – as was expected with almost all other poor.[33] The city spent £1–4-0 in 1682 'for burying a mad-man'. The only other entry where the mental condition of a recipient is given in this source before it ceases in 1743 is in 1694: 'by act of council for a distracted student' £26.[34] This was Archibald Campbell 'a poor student at the college who had fallen in a distraction and since into perfect stupidity'.[35] A different type of source provides evidence that mental disability was rarely encountered. Of 177 individuals who entered into obligations to desist from begging within the city of Edinburgh between 1743 and 1758, only one was described as an idiot.[36]

Close analysis of charitable sources for another Scottish town reveals a similar picture. Two surviving volumes of Dumfries burgh chamberlain's accounts 1773–78 and 1779–85 contain only two mentions of insanity, each involving the transportation of a mad person back to their home parish.[37] In 1773 town officers were paid to take a 'mad woman' outside the boundaries of the burgh of Dumfries.[38] Wanderers who showed signs of derangement might be treated in the same way as other poor people who looked as though they might become an enduring burden on a community's exiguous poor relief funds. The insane and stupid were treated in the same way as other paupers, even if (depending on the extent of disability) their care was generally more expensive.[39] This shows not a lack of discrimination, but a willingness to care for the mentally incapacitated within the limits of available charity. Thirty more volumes covering the years 1669–1729 at Dumfries are similarly sparse in mentions of madness or idiocy.[40]

These summary accounting documents often lack detail, and we cannot be sure that the lunatic and idiot were as rare as they suggest, or that they were not well provided for by agencies other than the family.[41] The position may be more complex than the apparent neglect which seems evident from poor relief records. For one thing, deserving poor were generally those who had limited means of their own and insufficient family support. In eighteenth-century Scotland, relief was often denied to the able-bodied unemployed, meaning that someone with mental problems who could work to maintain themselves might never appear in receipt of funds.[42] For another, the parish accounts may not reveal all administrators' attempts to help the mentally impaired or troubled. Given that Scottish poor relief was based principally on voluntary donations and informal charity throughout our period, those whose mental problems rendered or kept them indigent may never have entered the ambit of record-keeping bodies like the Kirk Sessions.

Some of those we are describing as mentally 'incapable' and indigent were able to look after themselves, up to a point. James Fullarton, one-time radical and a former merchant in Greenock, came to the shop of a former political associate to collect one shilling a day contributed by other like-minded men who had known him 'in his better days'.[43] James received his doles on a daily basis directly from his acquaintances, and had done so for some years. He had his own accommodation, as did Charles Simpson, a blind man subject to delusions and furious fits who nevertheless had modest private means and his own lodging close to his siblings in Midlothian.[44] Such non-residential forms of support from kin and strangers are particularly difficult to uncover in most sources. Neighbourhood support for non-financial reasons is difficult to document but seems in most cases to have extended only to the toleration of certain types of behaviour which would not have been acceptable from a stranger.

We should not underestimate the significance of passive acceptance of the mentally troubled or impaired as sources of support. Those born into a lower station of life might be able to subsist on their own because they were good workers and had practical skills. During the very hard winter of 1798–99 *The Edinburgh Weekly Journal* carried a report: 'a poor man, weak in his intellects, who usually brought milk to Edinburgh, was on Saturday [9 February 1799] found dead among the snow, a little way north of the New Town'.[45] Among John Kay's 'characters' of eighteenth-century Edinburgh were simple men who seem to have made a living by 'amusing' passers by.[46] Outside the city, a pauper lunatic called 'Daft Jamie' or 'Anderson Reid' 'infested the parish of Dalkeith' for two years prior to being arrested and moved to Edinburgh in 1818. Reid slept in barns and outhouses, and lived on casual charity from strangers.[47]

The examples we have just given are of people 'at large'. During the 1800s Fullarton had spent time in a madhouse on an island in Loch Lomond before he lived on his own in Glasgow. Reid took the opposite path from being very much in the community to a 'tolbooth' or jail, and thence to Bedlam. Early nineteenth-century surveys show a handful of lunatics confined in jails, a situation which reformers invited the reading public to deplore, for if the law gave the nearest male agnate (i.e. related on the father's side) care of those found mentally incapable before a civil court, other laws were designed to protect the community against violent or disruptive behaviour. Reid was arrested and imprisoned not for being mad but for using threatening behaviour. Those labelled insane by a criminal court might be incarcerated to protect society from them until someone else came along to fulfil that function. Those who locked up a furious criminal were, according to the jurist Sir James Balfour, acting in place of kinsmen.[48] If nobody came to claim the criminal insane, they might languish for years in jail.

Sending the criminal insane to an institution to be cared for '*in loco amicorum*' (so to speak) only later became the norm. In the 1800s and beyond, the criminal insane might be sent straight to Edinburgh Bedlam or to one of the asylums which took paupers (as convicted felons often were), rather than languishing in a jail.[49] The Sheriff-Depute's report on Aberdeen Hospital of 1816 noted how: 'The court of justiciary have been of late years in the practice of ordering lunatic convicts to be confined for life'.[50] The Justiciary Court (approximately equivalent to an English Assize) had no legal right to order the committal of convict lunatics to public madhouses. An attempt by the Justiciary Circuit Court at Aberdeen to do this was successfully resisted by the managers of the asylum there.[51] They were initially reluctant to take a convict so condemned into the hospital, but reassurances about funding ultimately persuaded them to accept elements of the criminal insane, turning that into one *de facto* destination for such people. The 'state' was beginning to accept direct responsibility for certain types of insane poor, rather than simply passing prescriptive or proscriptive legislation.[52]

Whatever the significance of this development for the future, most provision was private. It may be that areas well provided with medical and other service facilities encouraged more local people and strangers to bring their mad relatives for care. Parts of England with other provisions for lunatics tended to have more licensed private madhouses too.[53] East and Mid Lothian had the largest number of licensed private mad-houses in Scotland. Edinburgh was by far the richest city (and region) in Scotland prior to the Industrial Revolution, but during the seventeenth and eighteenth century it was also the area where rural wet-nursing was most prominent. One reason for this phenomenon, apart from the existence of a large pool of urban families who might want to put their infants out to a wet-nurse, is the absence of alternative employments for women in the receiving parishes.[54] The Edinburgh area had a tradition of wet-nursing stretching back into the seventeenth century and probably one of care for the insane too. Robert Porteous was kept at a private madhouse at Drumsheugh in the early 1720s. He was then moved to his sister's house, and thence to Inveresk where 'he was put in the custody of a person that had the reputation of a person useful to such furious persons and likeways under the close attendance of a keeper'.[55] From Inveresk he was moved to Slipperfield, Peeblesshire, 'at the desire of his friends and in company with his two brothers'. Robert Porteous beat his landlady's mother while there and was returned to Inveresk soon after.

Economic reasons may have been behind the prevalence of boarding the mentally abnormal in particular regions. Halliday noticed that Argyll and Bute had a large number of mad people, while the Hebrides and Western Isles had 'scarcely any'.[56] The reason for the surplus in Argyllshire and Bute lies in the housing of the mentally incapable. Abuses of the system of farming out pauper lunatics were uncovered in the 1844 'Report by Dr Hutcheson of the Royal Lunatic Asylum at Glasgow, on the state of the insane poor in the Island of Arran.'[57] Hutcheson found that the big towns of the west were housing mad people cheaply on farms in Arran. Paisley was paying 9d a week for some unfortunates: too little even for subsistence.[58] Farmers on the island had long found this an easier way of making a living than adjusting to improved farming. Another set of statistics, once again incomplete, shows the approximate geographical distribution of types of care (Table 2.2).[59]

Table 2.2 *Andrew Halliday's estimate of mentally incapable persons in regions of Scotland, 1817.*

			Region				
Type	1	2	3	4	5	6	7*
A.	78	312	226	118	169	198	61
B.	12	106	6	-	65	52	223
C.	-	2	3	6	2	2	6
D.	159	554	409	262	239	250	93
%@	7	27	18	11	13	14	11

A. Confined with relations or private persons.
B. Confined in public institutions such as asylums and infirmaries.
C. Confined in public jails.
D. Idiots or fatuous persons not confined.

1. Dumfries, Wigtown, Kirkcudbright
2. Glasgow, Ayrshire, Lanark, Renfrew, Dumbarton, Argyll, Bute, Stirling, Clackmannan
3. Perthshire, Inverness, Nairn
4. Thurso, Ross, Cromarty, Sutherland, Caithness, Orkney
5. Aberdeen, Banff, Elgin
6. Montrose, Dundee, Forfar, Kincardine, Fife, Kinross
7. Edinburgh, Berwick, Roxburgh, Selkirk, Peebles, Lothians (* A. includes Berwicks, Roxburgh, Selkirk only. B. includes 132 in private asylums in Midlothian, 19 in Edinburgh public asylum and 72 in the cells of Edinburgh poor house. C. is the county Bridewell at Jedburgh. D. includes only Berwicks, Roxburgh, Selkirk.)

@ total percentage of 101 is due to rounding error.

LAY AND 'PROFESSIONAL' CARERS

Options for care were numerous in later Georgian Scotland and the number of institutional places was growing, albeit from a low base. Dumfries Infirmary was completed in 1778 with a room set aside for four cells for lunatics. In 1791 a separate building was added with six cells.[60] Until the very end of our period, workhouses or 'towns' hospitals' like Paisley or Glasgow which had cells were very reluctant to admit anyone without external funding, or indeed to let in anyone who was a potential danger to other inmates.[61] On 5 July 1803 Canongate Charity Workhouse, Edinburgh, similarly ordered that nobody of unsound mind was to be admitted,[62] though

St Cuthbert's (on the other side of the city) had made such admissions since it opened in the 1760s.

At one level, paucity of places may not have been a problem given the apparent preference for care by relatives, and the legal responsibilities placed on male agnates. Family care was the norm. Those responsible made decisions about care based on their financial resources and those of the deranged person (assuming they had independent means); their own age, marital status, and domestic arrangements; their responses to social values; and the extent of the insane relative's disability. In a sense, their choices were restricted. In contrast, strangers who took in lunatics, idiots, and imbeciles did so voluntarily in exchange for payment. A wide variety of people of no known relationship took in the mentally troubled or impaired. The first few lines of a deposition generally give the name, occupation, place of residence, marital status, and approximate age of the witness. A number of witnesses were involved in the care of the subject. Beyond this, there are incidental references to their maintenance in the present and past from other witnesses, who numbered in all 500 men and women. They seem to have been drawn from a range of occupations from 'gardeners' and farmers to craftsmen and tradesmen. In this section we explore the issue of who other than relatives actually attended to the needs of the troubled and impaired.

Writers on seventeenth- and eighteenth-century England have stressed the significance of doctors and clergy in the provision of care for the better off. 'The private madhouse trade in fact started with the practice of doctors taking private patients into their homes.'[63] According to Parry-Jones, English 'lunatics from the more affluent classes were cared for individually, often in the custody of medical men or clergymen'.[64] The importance of the latter social group should not be overstated for Scotland. Only four clergymen entered a claim to be tutor or curator to a subject or were asked by Scottish Sheriff Courts to care for a relative. Of these, one refused: Mr Robert Stark, minister at Torryburn, who was named as next of kin to George Stark of Gartsherrie.[65] Another clergyman did end up caring for George but he was also an uncle.[66] Indeed, in all cases where we can identify actual care (as opposed to the legal claimant or person designated as guardian by an inquest), the ministers were kin to the deranged person. Mr Dugald Campbell, minister at Southend of Kintyre, was the claimant in the case of his brother Duncan Campbell of Kildallaig.[67] One claimant described as 'reverend' was the subject's father Dr James Couper, professor of astronomy in the University of Glasgow.[68] Such appointments necessarily followed lines of kinship and do not always show how the brieve's subject was actually cared for. The fact that a person was named as tutor or curator does not mean they had the day to day charge of a subject. However, depositions and additional papers allow us to examine how the person had been cared for up to the point of cognition and sometimes beyond. Clergy are no more evident behind the legal forms.

Nor are doctors, and indeed the other profession mentioned by Parry-Jones has similarly limited relevance to Scotland. Five surgeons or physicians claimed or were nominated as tutor or curator to a mentally incapable person. Dr Robert Grahame of Boquhaple, physician in Stirling, was appointed tutor to his cousin William Govan of Drumwhastle in 1767, but the arrangement was temporary until William's younger brother came of age, which duly happened in January 1775.[69] Graham himself clarified the arrangements and their justification in 1775. Setting the scene, he told how he had visited the family 'as a friend [cousin] in his earlier life and frequently both as a friend and physician for a good many years past'. William 'was taken ill of the disorder under which he now labours' around 1761 when 'the deponent was called to him as a physician and his disease quickly increased so as to deprive him of his judgement and render him at times furious, and at all times fatuous'. Then, 'soon after his father's death in January 1767, it was concerted among his friends for the preservation of his estate and means that the deponent as then his nearest agnate should be served tutor to him as being an idiot' which was done on 4 March 1767.[70]

Yet, as stated for the clergy, even when the care of a subject is described in witness statements or other papers relating to the recent past, it is rare to find medical practitioners lodging people, and equally unusual to find them in the houses of men of God. An example of the former is John Stewart of Lassintullich who was placed with William Menzies, surgeon at Broomhall in Perthshire, between 1802 and 1804.[71] Two examples of the latter are Robert Brisbane of Milton, who was cognosced in March 1800 and died at the manse of Strathblane in September 1807,[72] and James Arbuthnot of Nether Kinmundy who was residing at the manse of Liff in

1818.[73] The minister of that parish since 1817 had been George Addison, formerly a tutor to David, Earl of Airlie, for 12 years. David Ogilvy of Airlie had been insane for a number of years before he was cognosced in 1804 and he died in 1812.[74] Addison may have been especially well qualified for his charge. Furthermore, Liff was the place where Dundee Lunatic Asylum was opened in 1820. Four licenses to keep private madhouses within the sheriffdom of Forfar were taken out in May 1816 and again the following year.[75] Each was a singleton establishment and three were run by clergy: Rev. William Ramsay at Cortachy; Rev. George Addison, now at Liff (formerly at Auchterhouse); Rev. Peter Jolly, episcopal clergyman at Glenesk in the parish of Lochlee.[76] The fourth was Thomas Spence, farmer at Garth in the parish of Forfar, whose lodger was described as 'silly and simple'. With larger parishes and stricter controls on non-residence and neglect of duty, Scots clergy had to work much harder at their pastoral duties than their English counterparts. The relative absence of a tradition of clerical care for the insane may explain why one titled Scot in our sample was sent to England to be cared for by a man of God: Reverend John Townsend, curate of Braunton in Devonshire.[77] Interestingly, all the examples cited above are from the early nineteenth century, possibly suggesting that the practise was an importation from south of the Border.

Furthermore, few of those whose cases mention sojourns away from their family of origin ever lodged with a doctor until the early nineteenth century. One reason for chosing a doctor is that professional care was being substituted for that of close family. However, that assumes that there was a medical reason for the choice. Those to whom tutories were awarded were supposed to be male agnates. Thus, a doctor's relationship to the idiot or lunatic may have been based on kinship rather than professional capacity, and he may simply have been holding the fort until a brother could take over. This is certainly true in one case. Christian Graeme lodged for over 16 years with James Maxtone of Cultoquhey, a sexagenarian widower. Maxtone told the court that he had served a three year apprenticeship to the late Dr James Smyth, physician in Perth, and had also studied physic at Edinburgh university for two or three years after his apprenticeship was out. Prior to that Christian had lived with her mother. She was running short of male agnates by the time of the court case as she was then in her mid sixties and had been showing signs of insanity for more than 30 years. Her condition had begun after the death of her brother Alexander when she had 'shut herself up from society'; her other surviving brother Charles was himself cognosced in 1779 (having been deranged for 20 years) and may always have been felt to be unsuitable as a tutor; in the end she came under the care of her nephew.[78] Yet, even this example is open to a different interpretation. The Maxtones of Cultoquhey and the Graemes of Balgowan were closely linked both by marriage and business ties.[79] In the mid-nineteenth century the families merged. In the light of other cases and of this evidence, it is as likely that Christian was cared for by a relative as by a doctor.

Even when a doctor or minister with the correct skills was on hand he was not necessarily chosen. During the six months from July 1781 when George Henderson, portioner of Abernethy, was mentally incapacitated by a fall, a local clergyman was on hand. This was no ordinary priest for Alexander Pirie described himself as minister of the gospel and practitioner of physic at Newburgh. Pirie spoke authoritatively about Henderson, pronouncing him 'disordered in his senses'. By August the wound on George's head was said to have healed, but his senses had altered little. Pirie was also able to add that those with such disorders usually have lucid intervals.[80] Pirie occasionally visited George Henderson for short periods in his own home, but did not accommodate him. The apparent absence of a tradition of residential medical care for the insane in Scotland is underlined when we read part of the history of Duncan Campbell of Kildallaig. Neill McNeill of Macrahanish told how in the early 1720s Campbell barricaded himself in his house and was only extracted after careful negotiation followed by a violent struggle. He was sent to a Dr Smith in Ireland for cure.[81] Ireland was but 13 miles away across the sea from the Mull of Kintyre but it would have been as easy to send him by boat to Glasgow. The choice is telling. Indeed other sufferers were sent out of Scotland for specialist care. Charles Irvine was sent to Newcastle and others like Sir John Murray found themselves in English asylums under the specialist care of men like Dr Battie.[82] At first sight, it might seem that families were trying to conceal an embarrassing relative, yet such actions can be interpreted differently when set in their proper context for Scotland. Thomas Wood and James Bryce's private asylum at Saughtonhall was described as exemplary by the Sheriff's visitors and 'also possesses the peculiar advantage of being under the care of gentlemen of the medical profession.'.[83] That was true, but only up to a point. Bryce was a surgeon but admitted to an 1818 inquest that his partner Dr Wood 'takes no charge of the patients', and that the only other medical person who ever saw them was Dr Spence on the twice yearly Sheriff's visits required by Act of Parliament.[84]

Other examples indicate that England led the way not only in residential medical care but also in the 'moral treatment' which was at the cutting edge of the care of mental cases from the late eighteenth century. When in January 1813 the managers of the Morningside Asylum (later the Royal Edinburgh Hospital) were looking for a superintendent they minuted that in their search they were: 'particularly endeavouring to obtain a proper keeper who has been educated in one of the best institutions in England for the treatment of insanity'.[85] There were 19 applicants. John Hughes from London was minuted as the strongest candidate since he had had 12 years experience at St Luke's Hospital. He was duly appointed with his sister as matron.[86] Two years later the keeper of Aberdeen Asylum and his wife (the matron) were sent to York Retreat to learn about the care of patients and the management of an asylum.[87] The traffic was not all from Scotland to England. Patients and staff made the journey north and even the English had something to learn from Scottish developments. In July 1815 Mr Hughes visited the Glasgow Asylum to study management of the insane there. However, the precedence of English practice was acknowledged.

The families of those who might be subject to a civil court inquest were generally well able to afford specialist residential medical care. That they did not choose to do so shows they preferred a different regime. This contrasts with England. The late eighteenth and early nineteenth century saw the gradual replacement of non-medical by medical proprietors in England. For most of the eighteenth century no more than two-thirds of private asylums had medical proprietors. To a degree, comparisons depend on what one describes as an asylum, but there were apparently many more run by doctors in England than in Scotland.[88] Scottish lunatics might be visited occasionally by medical men, but they were only rarely entrusted to their constant care.

In fact, mad and idiotic Scots were almost always cared for by lay men and women who had no professional qualification (or pretension). Where medical practitioners learned from their training and from consultations, most keepers and under-keepers were essentially amateurs or empirics. They performed a role which blended the abilities of school teachers, jailers, and lodging-house managers. Keepers in the main hospitals might be sent away for training at prestige establishments elsewhere but most licensed private madhouses, and indeed most care of any kind, was provided by those whose only qualification was a real or imagined aptitude for dealing with the insane or idiotic.[89]

Those who ran or worked in madhouses came from a wide range of backgrounds. David Veitch, the allegedly spendthrift husband of the woman who kept the largest private madhouse in Midlothian in 1816, said that he 'was bred a farmer'. Others came to running madhouses via that route. Warrick Smith at Stonedykehead was one example as was William Lindsay, gardener in Inveresk, earlier in the century. Lindsay told how, during the 1720s, Robert Porteous came to stay with him. At first he lodged in another house, Lindsay 'several times coming and going, paying him visits in the way of his trade as a doctor to people in the distemper that Robert Porteous was under'.[90] The keeper of the Edinburgh Bedlam in 1750 was another gardener called Robert Dickie, while at Dumfries Infirmary in 1785 'the gardener of the house was appointed to be attendant upon the cells, whenever his assistance was wanted'.[91]

The word 'keeper' could be used as a description of the deponent's functional relationship to the sufferer or patient, secondary to his or her principal occupation and unfolding in the course of the testimony. Alternatively, it could mean an overseer or working owner who gave that as his occupation: similarly, the warden of a prison was 'keeper of the tolbooth'. Keepers were there to attend to and contain the potentially dangerous rather than to administer medicine. The dual use of the word (overseer and attendant) is shown in the testimony of John MacVicar, who gave his occupation as one of the soldiers of Edinburgh city guard. On 21 July 1762:

> he was appointed by Mr Kerr of Abbotrule by directions of Mr Rae surgeon to be keeper of John Rutherford . . . he has been calm at certain periods for a fortnight or three weeks but that he has often been suddenly seized with fits of violent madness and which sometimes continued for three days and that during these fits of madness he durst not come near him unless Robert Lauder, keeper of the house, [Bedlam]

had been along with him ... depones that he has been in use to attend several people disordered in their mind.[92]

James Arbuthnot went through periods of lucidity and calm between bouts of suicidal furiosity and delusions. From February 1751 to the date of the inquest on him in February 1752 he always had someone attending him and was confined to his room. During lucid moments his 'keeper' only attended him during the day but while insane (as in March 1751) he 'had a soldier constantly set over him to watch him'.[93] In the 1754 case of Robert Gordon, Margaret Miln, servant to Mrs Swinton, indweller in Edinburgh, (he lodged with her at the foot of Forrester's Wynd) described herself as his 'keeper' ever since October 1752.[94] Duncan Ferguson, a carrier of sedan chairs in his thirties, was employed to care for Charles Irvine for 26 weeks in Edinburgh and at Bankhead, 'a place of retirement', eight miles from Edinburgh.[95] Other depo-nents described him as Irvine's keeper. One meaning of the word was as a function, the other as an occupation or vocation. George Steill was keeper of the Edinburgh Bedlam from 1776 until at least 1784.[96] For at least 11 years from 1800 Thomas Hughes was 'principal keeper of the lunatic establishment at Saughtonhall'.[97] There were at least two further 'under-keepers' who looked after approximately 24 patients.[98]

Except in the case of the larger private madhouses, those who took in the mentally incapable seem to have practised lodging or supervising them as a by-employment. They only occasionally gave their occupation as 'keeper', preferring a more conventional agri-cultural or artisanal label. Females too may have regarded caring for non-family members as either a full- or part-time job, providing all or just some of their income. Women ran 10 of the 25 private Midlothian madhouses in 1816.[99] Most of these had only one or two inmates but the largest of all, with 27 patients, was owned and administered by a Mrs Veitch, while a Mrs Bourhill had 11. Some women may have been widows but others were clearly married. Women who specialised in lodging the insane, or who ran mad-houses with their husbands, had a certain authority lacking in other female deponents. Christian Thomson wife of Thomas Henderson at Stonedykehead, told how John Cunningham had been confined 'on account of mental derangement. That he was at first somewhat violent particularly when restrained from going out' but has quietened down while becoming more 'stupid'. Speaking with a matter-of-fact and competent air: 'She manages him without necessity of putting on the strait waistcoat by putting on an iron upon his leg in the night time which prevents him getting out.'[100] This private madhouse was known by Henderson's name rather than his wife's. For example, 'The character of Mr Henderson, for attention and humanity to the unhappy objects committed to his care, has for many years been well known.'[101] Beatrix Smith ran the Stonedyke-head madhouse with her husband Warrick Smith before Henderson took it over and was similarly able to give evidence about inmates on her own.[102] The quasi-professional standing of female madhouse keepers gave them an authority which transcended the normal limitations of their sex and social status.

Providers of such facilities began to advertise in newspapers in the age of George III, as in the case of this Edinburgh woman in 1785.

Mrs Stoddart, near the foot of Leith Walk, north side: Begs leave to acquaint the public that, for these sixteen years past, she has been in the practice of keeping persons *troubled in their minds*. From her experience, she hopes she may say that such as are in this unhappy state can be no where better attended to than with her. The friends of those who have been entrusted to her care bear ample testimony in her favours. Her house being at present fully occupied, she has been induced to take the one immediately contiguous and therefore has it in her power to accommodate a greater number than formerly, and from her unremitting assiduity, she hopes she will continue to deserve the public favour. The terms, which are moderate, and other particulars, may be learnt by applying at her house.[103]

The medical and legal officials who wrote pamphlets and reports implicitly or explicitly described lay keepers as inferior to doctors. A similar assumption pervades documents which describe those cared for in families. The implication is that carers could not comprehend their charge, and that one family was as good as another for dumping an idiot or imbecile. In contrast with medical professionals, men and women like Warrick Smith and his wife Beatrix, William Lindsay, or John Troup and his wife spent all their time with their lodgers or patients, variously described.[104] In giving evidence, such people had an interest in building up an image of a person who required attention (but was perhaps improving) and who was tended sympathetically (however difficult he or she may have been). Yet, their relationships with patients appear to have been based on at least a degree of accommodation and understanding. Descriptions of relationships between placid patients and staff in Glasgow Asylum or in the private madhouses of Saughtonhall or Stonedykehead have a feeling of quotidian inwardness where visiting physicians or surgeons were disruptive, authoritarian intruders.[105] From medical practitioners we derive a picture of interrogation and of gentle but insistent (sometimes impatient) confrontation with the lunatic. This was not merely a crude exercise of power, but was designed to help the patient to regain his or her standing as an independent moral agent rather than an involuntary actor. However, when the mad expressed gratitude it was not to the doctors but to those who looked after them on a day to day basis.[106] In a letter to her sister Clementine, the melancholic Jean Bannerman told how she was occasionally mistreated, yet she also went out of her way to state her attachment to her keeper's wife and to understand the family's situation. 'I am much in with Mrs Troup. It has been so cold but if the room you saw me in had a bit glass in the windows and I could get a little fire and light of any kind I would choose to be more in it for it is not convenient for any of us as they have so little room and so many young babies'.[107]

After her father's death in 1810 the imbecilic Ann Blair was moved to Alyth where she stayed with a Miss Ann Ogilvy, 'a near relation of the family', who also lodged another woman 'who was occasionally subject to low spirits'.[108] Unsurprising as it is to find women looking after other women like Ann or Jean, this is not the whole story of the nature of caring. The fullest detail about James Arbuthnot's behaviour came from Margaret Wilkie, spouse to William Watson, weaver in Edinburgh. Her husband was only aware of the most violent and destructive aspects of his lodger, suggesting that the day to day care of Arbuthnot was left to Margaret and the soldier employed to control him when he was furious.[109] Margaret lodged James in her house for a year and a half. Once, he was so delirious he had to be bound 'to prevent doing mischief to himself and others'. That was a standard justification for restraining lunatics, but there was specific meaning to what she had to say. In February 1751 she recalled how she 'came into his room and saw a part of his cravat fixed upon the top of the closet door by a knot and two pieces of it lying upon the tea table.

That at that time he told the deponent if his cravat had been strong enough he would have been hanging where the knot was'.[110] On another occasion the deponent and her servant accidentally came in and found James bleeding a great deal. He had just been bled by a surgeon, but had torn off the dressing and re-opened the wound. Refusing to allow Margaret or her servant to bind up his arm he 'begged of them to let him bleed to death for he was dying easily'.[111] Male attendants were required for their strength but much of the routine care we can document seems to have been carried out by women.

CONCLUSION

Decisions about where to care for a mentally-impaired person depended on need, entitlement, and contingency. Factors included the availability of institutional facilities, the pool of relatives available to care for sufferers, their financial situation and that of their family of origin, and the nature of their 'medical' condition. If there was little choice in the first half of our period, it is misleading to see 'care in the community' as a discrete option for Scots from the later eighteenth-century. Being looked after in the family of origin or in another household, and staying for a period in a private madhouse or public facility were bands within a spectrum of care. There was a stated preference for family care and institutional facilities were limited. The changing location of care is impossible to quantify but the sources we have suggest that a sojourn in some form of private or public madhouse was regarded by relatives as potentially desirable for lunatics, rich or poor, and was indeed tried where possible. By the 1810s, most of those cognosced before Sheriff Courts in Edinburgh or Glasgow were in a private or public madhouse. Entrants came from classes able to afford domestic care, suggesting that it is an over-simplification to claim that 'the larger the resources, the better the chance of containing the problem within the family sphere'.[112]

If being cognosced before a civil court jury was principally a matter of circumstances or contingencies, entry to an asylum or madhouse was based partly on both need and contingency but also on entitlement. A person is entitled to something if it is his or her due under a system of rules regarded as legitimate. For all this, even institutions were conceived of in familial terms. In jail, infirmary, or asylum those with money or nearby relatives might be able to recreate a family environment of sorts. Having one's own live-in servant was one way of achieving this,[113] as was having a family member provide food and clothes on a daily basis; dining with the owner or keeper and his family was another.[114] For this period, it is unlikely that we can see care in simple dichotomous terms as public or private, family- or institutionally-based. It is further inappropriate to assume that crossing the 'institutional threshold' was necessarily a sign of the *failure* of domestic and private provision: it can be construed more positively as a search for something better.[115] What we have tried to do is to understand both the complex reasons for chosing one form over another and the relationships between the different components over time.

Early-nineteenth-century advocates of asylums argued that public, institutional provision was necessarily more successful than private, domestic or commercial care and that those 'at large' were by definition neglected. This chapter has shown that their contentions remain to be tested. There are further issues which have emerged from this brief study. It seems likely that we have neglected the role of women in the care of the mentally incapacitated, privileging instead the males who wrote pamphlets on the care of the insane, who were generally the owners (and publicists) of private madhouses, and whose evidence was preferred in court.[116] For their part, public asylums had both a principal keeper and a matron whose task was not exclusively looking after females. While this may have been an extension of women's conventional roles as nurturers and healers, further research is needed. Other avenues may also be worth exploring. There were similarities with England. Idiocy remained a domestic problem, while private madhouses clustered in and around the respective capital cities. Yet, there were also intriguing differences. One is the absence of a tradition of doctors and clergy accommodating fatuous or furious people. Scottish carers and keepers were overwhelmingly empirics from non-professional backgrounds. Scotland's private madhouses were few and far between compared with England, even in the mid-nineteenth century, and the development of early nineteenth-century asylums took place against the background of 'a much more effectively organised and numerically more significant public-charitable subscription sector'.[117]

CHAPTER THREE

At home with puerperal mania: the domestic treatment of the insanity of childbirth in the nineteenth century[1]

Hilary Marland

Attacks of insanity preceding, during or following childbirth became a subject of inquiry and a source of great interest during the first decades of the nineteenth century. In the 1820s and 1830s 'puerperal insanity' was propelled into the medical arena. Both alienists, the emerging psychiatric profession, and obstetric practitioners added significantly to the brief remarks and observations of men-midwives, midwives and other medical observers[2] on the depression, disorientation, occasional craziness and violent tendencies of women post-partum described in previous centuries.[3] Publications on the topic proliferated, the condition was divided into two categories of mania and melancholia, efforts made to explain its occurrence, and advice offered on treatment. By the mid-nineteenth century puerperal insanity had a firmly secured place in the insanity literature. Yet knowledge was also claimed in understanding and treating this form of insanity by obstetric practitioners, who at least until mid-century appear to have led the way as the most frequently cited authorities on the disorder. Strong arguments were put forward by these practitioners for treating such cases in a domestic setting rather than the asylum. Although more guardedly, alienists too rejected the asylum as being the only appropriate site of treatment, particularly in milder cases.

For the majority of the insane in nineteenth-century England the committal procedure involved the handing over of the patient from one practitioner to another, a shift in authority, most often from the family doctor or Poor Law medical officer to the asylum superintendent. Puerperal insanity differed in that its origins were most frequently located in the lying-in period, when the patient was still being attended and visited on a regular basis by the midwifery practitioner who had attended at the delivery. During the nineteenth century childbirth came to be seen as increasingly marked by danger and risk, and birth attendants came to view puerperal insanity as one of the many unfavourable medical occurrences which could take place during a period of intense strain on women's reproductive organs and nervous systems. As alienists wrote up puerperal insanity in their textbooks as a discrete expression of 'moral insanity', authors on midwifery and the diseases of women placed it in the category of complications of childbirth, grouped with puerperal fever, puerperal phrenitis, diseases of the breast and other organic disturbances. When describing women's susceptibility to reproductive disorders, they were not referring to mental illness alone, but also to a range of physical problems.[4] Both groups – obstetric doctors and alienists – claimed puerperal insanity as their own, not necessarily in a blunt or decisive way, but implicitly as they wrote up their case studies and outlined their treatment regimes. Thus a discrepancy developed between alienists claiming medical authority based in the asylum and midwifery practitioners who pressed for the maintenance of their authority to supervise the lying-in period and recovery of the patient in a domestic setting.

This led to distinctions in ways of explaining puerperal insanity, although these were more of emphasis than hard and fast divisions. Midwifery practitioners associated the condition closely with the reproductive process and the strain this put on women, while alienists, dealing with a quite different grouping of patients, were more likely to emphasize the more pragmatic explanations of poverty and need. If links with physiology were made by asylum superintendents, this was more likely to be in association with weariness and physical decline as a product of having too many children and suckling them too long when the mother herself was malnourished and exhausted.[5] Midwifery practitioners tended to deal with 'nervous' and delicate well-to-do women, alienists with women worn down by hardship.

The focus here will be on the initial phase of interest in puerperal insanity, dating from the 1820s through to the mid-nineteenth century, tracing the development of ideas on the management of puerperal insanity, by whom it should be carried out – though again this is usually implicit rather than explicit – and the setting where treatment should occur. Certainly in this early phase obstetricians played a key role in treating the disorder as part of their strategy of easing the midwife out of better off practice, and as they sought to extend their remit to carry out midwifery work, to include the management of pregnancy, delivery and the lying-in period.

In 1820 Robert Gooch became the first British writer to publish on puerperal insanity. By the time he wrote his treatise, *Observations on Puerperal Insanity*,[6] in 1820 Gooch had built up a flourishing London practice, based largely on midwifery work, was lecturer in midwifery at St Bartholomew's Hospital and physician to the Westminster Lying-in Hospital.[7] Despite his premature death in 1830, his publications on midwifery, the nervous diseases of women, and puerperal insanity, were regarded as seminal.[8] Gooch was remembered in the decades following his death not merely as being the first to carefully outline puerperal insanity and for the power of his description, but also for the sympathetic and philosophical approach which he brought to his practice, his patients and writings. His book on *Some of the Most Important Diseases Peculiar to Women* was claimed by Henry Southey to be the most valuable work on that subject in any language, with the chapters on puerperal fever and puerperal madness 'the most important additions to practical medicine of the present age'.[9] In the decades to follow, Gooch's studies were succeeded by the publications of other midwifery practitioners and authors on women's diseases, including many well-known individuals: Fleetwood Churchill, Marshall Hall, James Reid, Robert Lee, William Tyler Smith, and J.Y. Simpson. Alienists too, including the most prominent representatives of this emerging field, John Conolly, J.C. Bucknill, T.S. Clouston and the John B. Tuke, were producing a literature on the condition, but it was obstetric practitioners who were largely responsible for building up knowledge on the recognition, prognosis and treatment of puerperal insanity.

THE AMBIGUOUS NATURE OF PUERPERAL INSANITY

Though a body of knowledge was being built up by mid-century on puerperal insanity, in many respects – not least because two distinct groups of specialists were generating the literature – it remained a poorly co-ordinated body. Puerperal insanity was and has remained an ambiguous category despite its strong and 'obvious' link with childbirth, in part because it is still not clear who the condition belongs to in terms of knowledge and treatment.[10] There was, however, a firm degree of commitment to the legitimacy of the condition. By the middle of the nineteenth century few obstetricians or alienists doubted the existence of puerperal insanity, or that of its sister disorders of insanity of pregnancy and lactation. However, by the closing decades of the century increased scepticism was being expressed about its distinctiveness from other forms of mania or depression, and psychiatrists were searching harder for links with predisposition, previous mental disorders and hereditary indications.[11]

Puerperal insanity was broadly depicted as a category of moral, usually temporary, insanity, 'which was usually manic, often severe and occasionally fatal'.[12] It was typically seen as being a short-term disorder, and for the most part the prognosis for the patient was good, with a cure or significant improvement being expected within a few months. The division of the condition into two categories was also adhered to even if the categories were far from rigid, 'the one attended with great excitement and furious delirium, the other characterized by the features of low melancholy'.[13] It was agreed that mania was more frequent, and showed itself earlier than the gradual, more insidious melancholia. It was also agreed that, although mania was more flamboyant and disturbing, the melancholic form was most difficult to cure.

Fleetwood Churchill, professor of midwifery in Dublin, described how, though 'the premonitory symptoms vary a good deal', puerperal mania developed from 'a degree of exhaustion, conjoined with great excitability, headache, and want of sleep; or the attack may accompany or follow convulsions, . . .'.[14] Sleeplessness, rapid pulse, pallor or flushed skin, vivid eyes, furred tongue, constipation and delirium were all marked down as features of the condition, as was in many cases great excitability, expressed through constant chattering, delusions, singing, swearing, tearing clothes and lewd sexual displays. In the worst case scenario the mother became 'forgetful of her child', or expressed murderous intent toward the infant, her husband or herself. James Reid, physician to London's General Lying-in Hospital, described how talking becomes almost incessant, and generally on one particular subject, such as imaginary wrongs done to her by her dearest friends; a total negligence of, and often strong aversion to her child and husband are evinced; explosions of anger occur, with vociferations and violent gesticulations; and although the patient may have been remarkable previously for her correct, modest demeanour, and attention to her religious duties, most awful oaths and imprecations are uttered, and language used which astonishes her friends.[15]

The final stimulus could be located in some threatening event, often minor or irritating. Robert Gooch talked of the 'interruption of mental tranquillity required during the susceptible puerperal state', or the admission of boisterous persons into the lying-in room, officious, eager or irritable nurses or relatives, or domestic anxieties.[16] Shock too played an important role in precipitating women into a state of mania: a death in the family, financial disasters, a fire in the neighbourhood.

Contemporaries, however, were uncertain as to the actual causality of puerperal insanity, whether it was moral, organic or hereditary, or some combination of these factors. The stakes in claiming competence and ability to treat appear to have been high, which is why many medical practitioners worked up their own theories from the starting point of the specialties of obstetrics, psychiatry or general medicine. F.W. Mackenzie, Physician to the Paddington Free Dispensary for the Diseases of Women, concluded that 'much diversity of opinion prevails' with regard to puerperal insanity. It was variously attributed to the suppression of the lochia, metastasis of the milk, the 'peculiar condition of the sexual system which occurs after delivery', local irritation of the mammae, uterus and 'other parts', disturbances of the vascular system occasioned by delivery, the combined effects of irritation and loss of blood, nervous irritability and excitement, etc., all, Mackenzie surmised, conditions occurring fairly frequently after delivery set against the 'comparative rarity' of puerperal insanity.[17] MacKenzie's own contention that puerperal insanity was related to anaemia was not put forward in a particularly convincing or rigorous way.[18] Like Mackenzie, many practitioners by mid-century began to be increasingly concerned with defining organic causality, but had great difficulty in doing so. The end result as regarded treatment tended, however, to be similar: gentle purging, tonics, calming medicines, nutritious diet, careful nursing, and rest. Hefty drug regimes, including the use of opiates, bleeding, and stimulants were generally disapproved of. John B. Tuke was highly critical of 'heroic' medicine; 'the patient has a better chance of sleep after a dose of beef-tea than after a dose of morphia'.[19] Such recommendations could also serve to undermine arguments outlining the necessity of removing patients to an asylum; beef tea could after all just as easily be administered at home.

As to the precise trigger of childbirth, for many the six week puerperal period marked the time within which insanity of child-birth could develop, but it was also suggested that melancholia could take much longer to make itself evident and cases were cited where women became insane months or even years after giving birth. Some authors claimed that puerperal insanity was most likely to occur amongst *primiparae*; others linked it to frequent childbear-ing. Rather than stressing the neglect of maternal responsibility which followed on from the condition, many authors referred to the overly maternal tendencies shown by the women sufferers as a precipitating cause, particularly prolonged breast-feeding when they themselves were depleted. For many women the build up over the years of the strains of repeated pregnancies, often painful labours and raising children in poverty proved too much, as in the case of Mrs Q, who by the age of 26 had already borne seven children. The final difficult delivery of twins, one of whom was stillborn, propelled her into insanity.[20]

Many observers were distressed to observe patients becoming manic following a 'normal' delivery. The disorder seemed less perverse when it was related, as it was by many, to difficult births, excessively painful, protracted, attended in an inept way ('particu-larly' by a midwife), or following the delivery of twins or a stillborn child. Some obstetric practitioners argued, bringing into service the tools of their trade, that the use of forceps to speed delivery could prevent the woman from becoming insane, describing the transient form of puerperal mania which occurred at the actual moment of birth caused by exhaustion or intense pain. After mid-century chloroform began to be advocated as a preventative. This was an era of intense debate concerning the efficacy and ethics of admin-istering chloroform in childbirth, with some midwifery practitioners citing chloroform as an actual cause of mania. It placed women, they argued, in a detached state unable to experience pain and thus retain their link to the real world of feeling and experiencing childbirth.[21] For the majority, however, chloroform represented escape from agony and even insanity produced by intense pain and shock. Charles Kidd, physician to the Metropolitan Dispensary in London, praised chloroform's good results, citing a woman who had been attacked five times by puerperal mania in the same number of confinements. On the occasion of her sixth confinement, chloroform was administered for the first time, and she showed no signs of insanity.

> The poor lady herself said that the extreme intensity of her suffering in the first labours drove her out of her mind, and 'she attributed, perhaps quite correctly, *her escape on this occasion from the horrors of a lunatic asylum* to the use of chloroform during her labour' [my emphasis].[22]

The use of chloroform in the asylum context to treat mental disorders, including puerperal insanity, detracted from the monopoly of midwifery practitioners to administer relief in this way, although they retained an edge by advocating its use as a preventative during delivery.[23]

Statements concerning the prevalence of puerperal insanity vary considerably, as do asylum admissions under this category. The proportion of female admissions listed as 'puerperal' in nineteenth-century asylums could vary from less than 5 per cent to around 20 per cent; at Abington Abbey, Northampton it was 6 per cent, at the Warwick and Hanwell Asylums 11 per cent, and over 12 per cent at Bethlem Hospital.[24] Though cases were recorded and treated in lying-in hospitals, the numbers were small: at the General Lying-in Hospital, Westminster, London only 9 cases of puerperal insanity were reported out of 3,500 deliveries, 11 out of 2,000 cases at Queen Charlotte's Lying-in Hospital.[25] A number of asylums claimed around 10 per cent of their female patients as cases of puerperal insanity, but these figures could fluctuate dramatically from year to year. The delirium accompanying puerperal fever could be misdiagnosed as insanity, yet the likelihood of large numbers of women suffering from puerperal fever finding their way into asylums seems slim. More likely is that asylum medical officers needed to make an entry under 'causes' in their admissions ledgers, and opted for a label which was appearing more frequently in the literature.

The discrepancies appearing in reports and admission records are confusing. In 1845, for example, the 'apparent and assigned causes of disease' of women admitted to Bethlem Hospital included 'physical': puerperal, prolonged lactation, weaning, and parturition, and 'moral': the birth of an illegitimate child and 'dread of approaching confinement'.[26] No cases of puerperal insanity were recorded in the West Riding Lunatic Asylum in Wakefield in the early 1860s, and only a handful of admissions due to insanity of pregnancy, yet in 1866 9 cases of childbirth as the alleged cause of insanity were listed, together with one case of insanity of pregnancy and one of 'cold after confinement'. The abrupt increase was built upon in 1867 with 19 cases of puerperal insanity being admitted, accounting for just over 10 per cent of female admissions in that year.[27] It is doubtful that the women of Wakefield developed a sudden propensity to fall victim to puerperal insanity; much more likely is that the medical superintendent was in some way alerted to the 'existence' of the condition and its potential as a category of admission, particularly if the women had given birth during the last few weeks or months. Similarly, the non-existence of the disorder in admissions records before the late 1860s suggests that these women were simply described as suffering from mania or melancholia, and the fact of their having recently given birth was not deemed important enough to warrant a separate classification.[28] One of the things we can be sure about with respect to puerperal insanity in this period is that no hard evidence can be produced on its prevalence, nor on whether it was most often treated at home or in the asylum, although we do know that it attracted much attention, as did the discussion on how to treat such patients.

THE LOCUS OF CARE, TREATMENT AND CLASS

The events surrounding a woman's decline into insanity were linked closely to her recent delivery and in the first instance were physically located in the lying-in room. However, once diagnosed, decisions needed to be made about what to do with the patient, whether she should be moved, and how she should be treated. Although considerable numbers of patients suffering from puerperal insanity were placed in asylums, many others appear to have remained under domestic management. This could be by default, where the woman and her attendants – medical or otherwise – simply struggled on until she recovered. Or, chiefly in the case of better-off women, a considered decision may have been reached to keep the patient at home, or to remove her to a private residence or to a private asylum. Case notes fall into two categories. Those cases recorded by midwifery practitioners discuss treatment in a domestic setting, while those written up by alienists describe women brought at some stage of the condition to the asylum, frequently after being ill for some time. The first category tend to be well-to-do; the latter poor, but this dividing line is by no means hard and fast. It is not clear whether being assisted by a doctor at the delivery rather than a midwife would slow or speed the process of referral to an asylum; it would depend on the family circumstances and the view of the practitioner involved, but it would seem likely that poorer women attended by midwives would have fewer buffers delaying their removal to an institution of some kind, be it a workhouse or pauper asylum.

Although reports of cases of puerperal insanity occurring as part and parcel of general practice are rare, this is probably due to the fact that few full records of such practices survive. General practitioners, however, appear to have been aware of the condition and occasionally wrote up their cases and methods of treatment and had these accounts published in medical journals. They were neither surprised nor baffled by the disorder, and took it on board as they would other complications of childbirth. It was general practitioners or surgeons who often became key witnesses in infanticide trials, and again they seem to have been knowledgeable about the disorder, although they presumably encountered it rarely. The evidence also shows that, because this form of insanity was considered 'temporary', even women who had murdered their infants were not necessarily removed to an asylum. By the time of their trial they were recorded as 'recovered' and restored to sanity.[29]

A handful of surgeons and general practitioners kept more extensive records, as did John Thomson, a surgeon who worked in Kilmarnock in Scotland, who summed up his midwifery work extending over a 15-year period in the *Glasgow Medical Journal* in 1855.[30] He recorded 3,300 cases of 'obstetricy', and a table breaking down his 'preternatural and instrumental cases' included two cases of puerperal mania. One of these women became disturbed several days after she suffered from severe bleeding and delivered a stillborn child. Thomson promptly labelled her condition 'puerperal mania' and treated it with purgatives, opiates, medicines to induce vomiting, and cold douches. He soon decided that such remedies were not proving particularly efficacious, and he abandoned them, recommending in their place a 'nourishing diet and kind and gentle treatment'. The woman recovered though she remained pale and emaciated, and occasionally her mind wandered.[31] Thomson presumably had little expert help to call on, but neither did he seem to require it. He managed the case calmly, trying different regimes until he hit on one which produced an improvement. He seems to have regarded puerperal mania as one of the preternatural occurrences he would occasionally encounter in the course of his midwifery work.

While puerperal insanity had powerful links with poverty and illegitimacy, women of the highest rank also fell prey to mania and depression. Queen Victoria suffered from severe depression following the birth of her second child, the Prince of Wales, in November 1841, when Prince Albert's secretary remarked how the Queen was 'troubled with lowness ... I should say that Her Majesty interests herself less and less about politics'.[32] Queen Victoria's decision to have chloroform administered when she gave birth in 1853 not only swung support behind childbirth anaesthesia; it was also surely a response to her belief that childbearing 'is indeed too hard and dreadful'.[33] Judith Schneid Lewis in her study of childbirth and the British aristocracy plays down the place of puerperal insanity and depression claiming that nervous complaints post-partum were not recognized by the nineteenth-century medical profession. Yet she goes on to give examples of depression caused by painful deliveries, or anxieties about babies being born in too rapid succession, or even of having too many children of the same sex, which plagued the aristocracy.[34]

The treatment of 'nervousness' following aristocratic births would take place in the country house or London residence where the birth had been attended; seclusion, quiet and a cluster of attendants were available to tend to the woman's needs and take care of the baby. But it is also hard to believe that obstetricians delivering middle-class women would be willing to hand them over to an asylum, even a private one. Part of their task in managing a delivery was to ensure that the woman traversed pregnancy safely, paying careful attention to diet and regimen, and recovered from the labour, fully enough to continue with her domestic duties.[35] The emphasis was on restoration of the woman, a theme also developed in stories of how women suffering from puerperal insanity were 'redeemed' through caring treatment and placed back in their accustomed and natural setting as wives and mothers.

The claim was advanced with increasing conviction during the nineteenth century that civilized women were likely to undergo many forms of trauma during pregnancy, birth and breast feeding – their comfortable lives and tendency to nervous behaviour had ill-prepared them for strain and physical effort. In 1841, Michael Ryan, author on midwifery and medical jurisprudence, declared that for

> all classes in civilized society in which these laws [of nature] are frequently violated or forgotten, or when the constitution is impaired by the luxury or dissipation of modern times, the process of child-bearing is attended with more or less danger, both before and after it is completed ... It is, however, fortunate for suffering humanity, that the process of parturition may now be greatly accelerated, and the greatest of mortal suffering relieved by the advice and skilful exertions of the obstetrician or medical attendant, and with the most perfect safety to the parent and offspring ... [36]

Ryan warned too of the dangers of puerperal mania which could occur soon after delivery or during lactation when the system was 'exhausted', but believed it 'rarely incurable'.[37] Like other authors, Ryan stressed mild treatment, careful handling and removal of the patient from her home and its associated distress. Preventative action took the form of the employment of a doctor trained in obstetrics.

The task of the attendant became pre-emptive in the sense that they were to guard against and if possible prevent a recurrence of the disorder in future confinements. In emphasising this aspect of their work stress was placed on the importance of opting for a male midwifery practitioner rather than a midwife to attend at deliveries. The physician who had attended the woman in childbirth also had a vested interest in treating the condition; it was he who had witnessed the slippage into insanity and it was his task to cure it and to take care that it would not reoccur in future confinements, at the same time taking care to preserve the custom of the woman's family.

The question of whether it was possible to prevent future attacks of puerperal mania once the woman had been afflicted was put by

Robert Gooch in his essays on the subject. He set down in some detail the case of a lady who a few days after labour became maniacal. Her symptoms subsided in about five weeks, and she made a good recovery. When she became pregnant again, Gooch was called to attend her, without being aware of the previous episode, until the nurse informed him of it during labour. Gooch was apprehensive. As he put it, if hereditary predisposition had anything to do with disease, the woman was an 'emphatic instance' as nearly all her relatives were mad, or had died mad, and the lady had married a gentleman whose family were equally mad. Following her first labour Gooch heard how her friends thought it a time of merriment, 'footing it about the house, which resembled a rabbit warren'. Gooch determined that this time it should be otherwise, and kept the house quiet. Gooch described the delivery as being an easy one, and the woman did well for ten days until a fire broke out near the house where she lived; in the evening she caught sight of some sparks flying about outside her window. When Gooch visited, she looked and talked 'oddly', and a paroxysm was evidently coming on. Gooch slept in the house that night, and was summoned at 2.00 a.m. The woman then asked him to look at her forehead: 'do you see anything?' This he denied, and then clasping her hands, with a whining methodistical tone, she exclaimed, "Then I was presumptuous; I am deceived; I thought a glorious light issued from my temples, and that I was the Virgin Mary". Gooch bled the woman, but with little benefit. However, with careful attendance to her bowels, after three weeks she recovered, 'without seeming to have been cured by any thing that was done'.

The next time the woman became pregnant, Gooch called to see her three weeks before the delivery. He recognized a 'derangement of her hepatic functions'; she had white stools, yellow eyes, a jaundiced face and yellow urine. Gooch prescribed calomel and aloes, 'which produced two or three evacuations daily'. The prescription was continued after delivery and she suffered no maniacal affection. Gooch's advice to midwifery attendants was to be aware of any disposition to the complaint and to endeavour to prevent it by administering a purgative before and after delivery to keep up the regular action of the bowels.[38] Gooch was in many ways combining his treatment of puerperal mania with his notion of how a midwifery attendant should deport himself. This included being generally alert and watching for potential complications. It was, according to his contemporaries, this sensitivity and great care which pervaded all Gooch's midwifery work and his sick room manners: natural, quiet, impressive, kind, and ready to sympathize with the feelings of others, 'he rarely failed to attach his patients strongly'.[39] Not all midwifery practitioners would be as attentive one assumes, yet most would be attentive to their reputations, fees and clientele. They were also seeking to establish a gentlemanly approach to midwifery which they contrasted with the rough and ready ways of the midwife.

The scope and value of treating women in a domestic setting was flagged up by many midwifery practitioners. W.S. Playfair explained that 'only the worst and most confirmed cases' found their way into asylums.[40] Domestic management of cases was advocated because of the special therapeutic regime required, but also because of the 'specificity' of the condition – it not being like other forms of madness – and the generally good prognosis. Treatment should not, many argued, be linked to incarceration, but to separation from the specific domestic circumstances which so distressed the patient.

Obstetric doctors if not unanimous were fairly certain in expressing their opposition to asylum treatment, encouraging private seclusion and proper nursing. William Tyler Smith, Physician-Accoucheur to St Mary's Hospital, Lecturer at St Mary's Hospital Medical School and President of the Obstetrical Society of London, well-known for his conservatism and resistance to chloroform anaesthesia in childbirth, opposed institutionalization on the grounds that women suffering from puerperal mania were not like other insane patients, and should be protected from the stigma of the asylum. Such cases should always be treated as if they would recover fully as, Smith emphasized, it was temporary conditions which produced the insanity. Smith believed 'that great mischief is frequently done by placing puerperal patients in public and private lunatic asylums'. He cited the example of Bethlem, where some of the women incarcerated had killed children while suffering from puerperal mania:

> Some of these poor creatures have passed the childbearing age, are perfectly clear in intellect, conscious of what they have done, and suffer intense misery therefrom, while they have their desolation enhanced by mixing constantly with confirmed lunatics.[41]

Thus even in the worst case scenario, the asylum could be rejected.

James Reid, one of the foremost authorities on puerperal disorders, maintained that 'general opinion' was against the removal of patients labouring under puerperal insanity to the asylum, unless the case lapsed into a 'chronic and lingering form'. Rather

> If change of scene be deemed requisite, it is better that the patient should be removed at first to a quiet country village, or to the sea-side, under the care of an experienced nurse, but the frequent visits of the medical attendant will here be advisable, . . . The friends of the patient should also pay occasional visits, to examine into the domestic arrangements and comforts of the place, without, however, seeing the patient herself, . . .[42]

In his *Principles and Practice of Obstetric Medicine and Surgery*, Francis Ramsbotham considered the propriety of removing the patient from home. He recommended a change to another residence, particularly from 'confined to a purer air, and from a noisy to a quiet situation', yet not to placement amongst 'permanent maniacs, because of the great hope we entertain of a restoration, the uncertainty how long the affection may continue, and the chance of her recovery being sudden'. The best option was to have a whole or part of a house devoted to the patient; failing that placement in a smaller, presumably private, establishment was recommended.[43]

Thinking laterally, for not all patients could not afford the luxury of secluded care with suitable nurses, some physicians recommended, that if it proved impossible to remove the patient from her home, then her husband and family should move out, leaving her in rest and quiet. Gooch recommended the removal of husbands and relations, particularly if the disorder threatened to be 'lasting'.[44] William Tyler Smith suggested that philanthropy should offer a remedy for treating such cases in a humane, home-based setting when family means were limited.[45] The infant in all of these discussions gets short shrift; it seems to be simply assumed that someone will take care of the newborn in the mother's absence.

Alienists were more guarded in making recommendations about where treatment should take place, weighing up the good rates of recovery and cure from puerperal insanity against the need to incarcerate such women in the first place. But overall they were of the view that in mild cases the asylum was no place for the puerperal maniac. Thomas Clouston, reporting on the activities of the Cumberland and Westmorland Lunatic Asylum which he superintended in the 1860s, remarked that cases of insanity occurring after childbirth helped 'keep up the standard of curability', at the same time suggesting that when symptoms were mild and manageable, there was really no need for such women to be in the asylum at all.[46] John B. Tuke, writing up cases treated in the Royal Edinburgh Asylum, Morningside, again in the 1860s, referred to puerperal mania as '*the* most curable form of insanity', to be placed under asylum treatment 'as a *dernier ressort*'.[47] Yet of course the *dernier ressort* patients would also be those most likely to lapse into incurability, dementia, imbecility, or to be liable to attempt suicide. And while alienists professed that milder cases need not be admitted to asylums, at the same time stress was placed on treating puerperal insanity quickly, on catching cases before they became serious and entrenched. Cases which developed slowly or some weeks after delivery could become the most intractable, such as the extreme example cited by A. Campbell Clark of a woman who had become insane three months after the birth of her first child, who, after four years of illness, 'had ultimately to be sent to an asylum'.[48]

Some features of the asylum were retained in a domestic setting, even strengthened. The need for close watching was stressed, on a one to one, or even two to one basis, with nurses working shifts. Although those suffering from puerperal mania were regarded as 'helpless' they were also endlessly crafty, testified to by their ceaseless efforts to trick their attendants into leaving them, giving them the opportunity to either do away with themselves or their infants.

> It is scarcely necessary that I should insist on the patient's never being left a moment alone in any of the forms of mental aberration, nor in the removal from her reach of whatever can be canverted [*sic*] into instruments of self-injury; such as knives, cords, garters, or any articles of dress by which strangulation could possibly be effected. The door should be kept locked, and the windows tightly nailed down, or so secured as to be only capable of being opened to the extent of admitting the requisite quantity of fresh air. If the case is likely to be of long standing, her nurse and other domestic servants should be removed; two females accustomed to the charge of insane patients must be substituted; and they should take their rest alternately.[49]

Seclusion was to be matched by restraint, and 'general moral management'. A particular type of nurse should be sought out, which re-affirmed the patient's isolation from loved ones:

> the *attendants* should be *peculiarly adapted* for their duty; the usual domestics, and even the experienced monthly nurse, are not so valuable as one who is accustomed to the care of this class of patients, and it is advisable, therefore, to replace them. A vigilant, firm, though kind superintendence, soothing violence, encouraging and cheering despondency, soon produces its effect; and a nurse who is skilful and experienced in these cases, will have much more moral control . . .[50]

The role of family members was typically minimized to inspecting the arrangements concerning treatment. Husbands, often the butt of hatred on the part of the women sufferers, come out poorly in case notes. The wealthy variant is rarely criticized but he is decisively pushed out of the therapeutic regime, his wife being removed from his presence and authority, taken from her home and separated from her 'dearest' connections, visits being severely restricted. One almost amusing German account of the husband being 'cuckolded' by the doctor was reported by Prof. Berndt in the *Lancet* in 1829. The usually mild-tempered Madam D, aged 23, became agitated and indisposed six days after giving birth. She talked incessantly and lay in provocative postures in bed. 'She told her husband, who was rather an old man, that she did not want him any more, because she had other lovers; and when M. Berndt came to see her, she made him a formal declaration of love, etc.'[51] In most cases usurpation of authority is less blatant, but the doctor strove to put himself in a position where he, and he alone, would manage the case. In poor families, if the husband is mentioned at all, he is often blamed for the woman's condition; he was a poor provider, the woman had married 'beneath her', he was violent, a drinker, a womanizer or a deserter. The authority of the doctor in attendance, who replaced the husband, and insisted on removing friends, relatives, familiar nurses and servants reigned supreme, and he gained the time and space needed to effect a cure: 'It is necessary to gain, by firmness, a mastery over such patients. They recover more quickly when not allowed to see their husbands, infants or immediate relatives, and they are most easily managed by nurses whom they have not previously known'.[52]

DOCTORS, PATIENTS AND THE ROUTE TO REDEMPTION

Yet this authority was worn with a velvet glove, and, in a doctor-patient relationship where the two parties potentially had much to gain from a period of respite, the bearing of the doctor was often guided by sympathy and great patience. Both patient and doctor won time. The way case histories are written up and the patient's story as told by the doctor, with the usually 'happy ending' variant of conclusion, together with an epilogue of future confinements unmarred by insanity, reveal that these, albeit unequal, partners could expect 'benefit' from the diagnosis of puerperal insanity. We could take this further and talk of puerperal insanity in terms not of protest and rebellion, but of alliance and respite, not of deviation and defiance, but of shared interests. Part of this shared interest could be to keep the patient out of the asylum.

Of the British puerperal insanity writers, again the earliest, Robert Gooch, gives us insight through his detailed case notes, of the intimate sphere which evolved between doctor and patient. His 1820 essay *Observations on Puerperal Insanity* set the pattern by giving detailed accounts of cases he had encountered. He outlined both moral and physical treatment as we would expect, listing five essentials: to protect the patient from injuring herself; to evacuate impurities by occasional purgatives; to watch circulation and guard against congestion or inflammation of the brain; to procure sleep at night; and 'to manage the mind of the patient, soothing it during irritation, encouraging it during depression, never to attempt the removal of her delusions by argument'.[53] 'I would rather allow a patient to think her legs were made of straw, and her body of glass, than dispute either proposition.'[54]

What is striking is the sympathy with which Gooch regards his patients and a sense of co-operation between doctor and patient, though Gooch too referred to the rumbustious behaviour which could go with the condition: 'the patient swears, bellows, recites poetry, talks bawdry, and kicks up such a row that there is the devil to play in the house'.[55] He also on occasion put his patients into a straightjacket. But for the most part stress is on rest, quiet, separation from 'loved' ones; Gooch's role is protective, not only of the patient from herself, but also of her from her responsibilities. Yet it is more than patronizing and enfeebling. The cases required extreme care and patience, 'moral treatment' at first often having little effect. Gooch described one case precipitated by a near relation having had a 'frightful incident', followed by sleepless nights and a fear on the part of the woman that she would lose her reason. The woman nursed the child for three to four months 'without feeding it'. She was persuaded to 'wean the child', given light tonics and gentle laxatives, and sent to the seaside. Yet the treatment had little benefit. After great fluctuation the woman worsened, becoming more violent. She was moved again to the countryside 'under the care of an experienced attendant, separated entirely from her husband, children and friends, placed in a neat cottage surrounded by agreeable country'. Still there was no improvement; she was preoccupied and disillusioned, believing she was to be executed, and that her infamy had caused the death of her husband and children. An ill-advised visit from her husband had the potential to make matters worse. The woman initially believed that he had returned from the dead to haunt her, yet gradually she became calm and interested in what he was saying, and the cure came as if by 'magic'.[56] Gooch, explaining himself out of the need to keep the husband at a distance, claimed that the patient had been approaching convalescence 'in which the bodily disease is loosening its hold over the mental faculties, and in which the latter are capable of being drawn out of the former by judicious appeals to the mind'.[57]

Doctors' patient treatment was usually well-rewarded. As both alienists and obstetricians laid claim to professional expertise in treating the disorder, they could point to good, often excellent, rates of cure. In this respect too the stakes were high. Thomas More Madden cited several sources, all of whom claimed good rates of recovery: Gooch in private practice and Johnston and Sinclair at the Rotunda both had rates of almost 70 per cent.[58] Richard Gundry, in his analysis of 56 cases of puerperal insanity, described 63 per cent as either recovered or improved.[59] James Reid described in a nutshell the typical development and progression of puerperal mania, the form of preferred treatment and the anticipated good outcome:

Mrs—, aged 20, had been distressed by some family occurrences which caused her much anxiety. Four days after her first confinement, she became much excited, and at length exceedingly violent, swearing and using most obscene language, although at other times a lady of most correct demeanour. As the usual treatment seemed to produce no good effect, and she had taken an inveterate dislike to her husband and child, it was thought advisable to remove her to a cottage in the country in the charge of two experienced nurses. In about five months she was restored to perfect health, and on asking to see her husband, he was immediately allowed to visit her. She has since this period borne several children, but although of a nervous temperament, has had no return of the complaint.[60]

The woman needed to be protected from herself, but also her reputation needed to be preserved; this was best done by continuing to treat her in a domestic environment, be it her own home or another well-suited location. The advice to move patients to country cottages and the seaside was also a way of masking the nature of the 'convalescence' taking place. This also served to protect the practice of the obstetric attendant who kept such cases under his control and out of sight. Ramsbotham even emphasized the need for great care in alerting the family to the affliction, which was such a dreadful calamity following delivery.[61] Such cases were to be treated with the greatest tact. Husbands and families too could show great reluctance to hand over women, particularly when they had recently given birth, to an asylum; it was a particularly sad and shocking conclusion to what should have been a happy event. Isabella, the wife of the author William Thackeray, developed puerperal mania and attempted suicide after the birth of her third child, but Thackeray felt himself unable to entrust her to an asylum, finding even the well-reputed York Retreat too austere. Finally Isabella was left, ultimately until her death, in the care of a nurse in Camberwell.[62]

For alienists, their early ambiguity about whether puerperal insanity should be treated in the asylum was replaced increasingly by certainty that it should as the century progressed. Puerperal insanity became less a condition to be watched for and guarded against, but something to be actively treated and cured once it had developed. The more expectant approach of obstetricians who perceived the condition holistically as a potential part of the cycle of giving birth and recovery was to some extent lost; women suffering puerperal insanity were only admitted to the asylum once the condition had made itself known, and perhaps reached an alarming state. The subsuming of such cases into asylum regimes along with other forms of mental illness, including mania and melancholia, may help explain why puerperal insanity came to be treated less and less as something different, special, requiring specific treatment in a specific environment.

Yet some fluidity remained. Many patients were retained at home for lengthy periods before removal to an asylum, and even toward the end of the century psychiatrists were still questioning whether such patients should be institutionalized. The psychiatrist George Savage, writing in 1884, explained that the question 'as to which class of patients should be sent to asylums, and when' remained a pertinent one. There was strong feeling, for example, against sending a young married woman to an asylum when insanity developed after the birth of the first child, because the child might suffer socially, and the mother would learn to dread future confinements:

> If the friends have ample means, if their home is in a healthy district, and if the doctor can see the patient twice daily at least for the first few weeks, it is possible to treat almost the most serious case as home, . . .[63]

Even if it was found necessary to send women to asylums, 'they must not be kept under control too long, but should be sent home as soon as symptoms of danger have passed'.[64]

During the second half of the century, however, it seems likely that more cases of puerperal insanity, or purported cases, were finding their way into the asylum. Even taking into account recording anomalies and the difficulties already referred to in making sense of the figures, admission figures for women suffering from puerperal insanity appear to have been rising. In 1860 admissions to Bethlem under the category of puerperal insanity accounted for one-eighth of the total female intake over the previous five years.[65] By 1886–88 some 18 per cent of female admissions to the Warwick County Asylum of childbearing age were assigned a puerperal cause (over 11 per cent of all female admissions).[66] Between 1889 and 1891 over 14 per cent of the women admitted to the Rainhill Asylum, Liverpool were said to be suffering from puerperal insanity.[67]

Accumulating numbers represent a shift away from treatment by individual practitioners, the family doctor or obstetrician who had attended the delivery, to a situation where puerperal insanity became absorbed into general asylum regimes and therapeutics.

Writing in 1883 Campbell Clark describes frequent resort to forced feeding with a pump, the administration of morphine, the use of powerful emetics, vaginal injections with carbolic.[68] He also illustrates another shift, when he talks of women of 'good social condition' being admitted to the asylum. Women suffering from puerperal insanity seem to have been fed into the expanding asylums, run by an increasingly confident psychiatric profession, as they provided a more acceptable locus of care. Middle-class families, finding it difficult to continue to pay for private medical care, allowed their female relatives to slip into the large public asylums. At the same time, though some aspects of the gentle, painstaking regimes were retained, open air, quiet and careful nursing, associated with the darker aspects of heredity and predisposition, puerperal insanity towards the close of the century takes on a gloomy and frightening aspect.

CHAPTER FOUR

Family, community and the lunatic in mid-nineteenth-century North Wales[1]

David Hirst and Pamela Michael

INTRODUCTION

> With regard to the other class of Insane Paupers, not in Asylums, those, namely, who are living with their relatives or with strangers on a parish allowance, our information is comparatively scanty. The insane of that class very seldom fall within our personal observation, and for our knowledge of their numbers and condition, as well as the peculiar form of their malady, we depend almost entirely on the annual returns from the clerks of the Board of Guardians or Overseers ... At present, however, these returns are still very defective; and although they have latterly exhibited a manifest improvement in the diligence of those whose duty it is to prepare them, they are not yet sufficiently regular and complete to enable us to found any confident or very definite conclusions to their contents.[2]

The observations of the Lunacy Commissioners in their Ninth Report could have been written by a twentieth century historian, for the twin influences of Foucauldian theory and the availability of institutional records has led to an emphasis on study of the growth of institutional confinement. For those in asylums, and to a lesser but increasing extent those in workhouses, the administrative records of admission books, case books, visiting committee records, and the centralised bureaucracy of the Lunacy Commission have all been used to identify the minutiae of their existence.

For the 'single' lunatic, those living with relatives or boarded out in the community, the situation is different. The treatment of lunatics in the community before the nineteenth century has been explored by Rushton and Suzuki, using Quarter Sessions records, though both authors acknowledge that these are more likely to identify those for whom the community found it difficult to care adequately.[3] More recently, David Wright has suggested that the history of the nineteenth century asylum must be seen as only a part of a continuum of care for the nineteenth century lunatic, and the role of the family as carers and as agents of committal needs further exploration.[4] This observation is particularly relevant in the Welsh context, as many lunatics and idiots remained in the community when those in England were largely confined. Even in 1860, 988 of the 1754 cases in Wales remained outside institutions, compared with just 44 out of 3686 in Middlesex.[5] In north Wales, the majority of idiots remained with their families, or were boarded out in the community, at this date.

It is the identification of lunatics and their treatment in the community which creates difficulty for the researcher. Parish or poor law union records may not explicitly name paupers as lunatics, or may do so once in a long series of data. This article seeks to use the lunacy return as a means to first identify those lunatics living in the Denbighshire community during the period 1828 to 1858, and then to explore their treatment and the basis for decisions on their care.

SOURCES AND METHODOLOGY

From 1828 parishes were required to submit an annual list of 'Lunatics and Dangerous Idiots' resident in the area.[6] From 1842, responsibility for compiling the return passed to the Clerk to the poor law union.[7] The returns were submitted to the Clerk to the Quarter Sessions for onward transmission to the central authorities. The Poor Law Commissioners thought the change in 1842 produced more comprehensive lists, enabling them 'to inquire into any cases which apparently are improperly retained in the workhouse, or which should have been sent to an asylum.'[8] Only with the Thirteenth Report of the Lunacy Commissioners in 1859, however, was it considered possible to publish figures from a complete series of the annual return, as previously many unions had neglected to reply.[9] Even those replying were considered to contain incomplete details. Noting that the numbers of lunatics in the several Workhouses which have been visited, as taken from the Parliamentary Returns, often differ widely from the numbers in the same Workhouses, as given by the Visiting Commissioners, and are generally, though not invariably, less

the Lunacy Commissioners suggested that the numbers of lunatics in workhouses had been understated by one third. Without producing any supporting evidence, they then argued that this underenumeration must also apply to the numbers of those residing with family or boarded out.[10] Reports from visiting Commissioners also stressed the incompleteness of the annual lunacy return. In one instance in north Wales

I learned that Clerks to Boards of Guardians are very negligent in making the statutory returns. The Annual Return does not contain an accurate account of all the cases belonging to the Union. For instance, the quarterly returns made for the Union of Holyhead and Anglesey, show an excess of 21 patients over the annual.[11]

Nevertheless, for those cases recorded, the lunacy return provides the names of lunatics and idiots, the parish or poor law union to which they were chargeable, whether they were in an asylum, licensed house, or workhouse, or were boarded out, or living at home or with friends or relatives, the cost of their maintenance, whether idiot or lunatic, whether dangerous or otherwise, whether possessed of 'Dirty Habits' and, often, additional remarks by the officer making the return. The statutory declaration by a doctor, usually the local poor law medical officer, may also survive, though these only rarely depart from a formula. The lunacy returns thus provide an annual list of names, and, however defective the data, it can be used by historians, as the Lunacy Commissioners sought to use it, as an aid to 'knowing the condition' of lunatics in the community. Using the returns for a number of years permits the reconstruction of longitudinal histories, illustrating the experiences of lunatics and idiots who remained in the community for at least part of the time they were afflicted. The names recorded also serve as an index to the surviving parish and union records, so lunatics and idiots may be traced in these records even when not specifically named as such. The sources can then be linked together to see how lunatic and idiot paupers were treated by the parish and union authorities.

The Quarter Sessions papers for Denbighshire, in north Wales, contain an incomplete set of returns for the period 1828 to 1858.[12] After 1858 there is a six year gap in the records. During this period, the returns list lunatics and idiots chargeable to 57 out of 59 parishes. Generally, coverage is more complete for agricultural parishes in the Vale of Clwyd than for the more industrialised north east of the county.

The approach adopted was to link records in the lunacy returns considered to relate to the same person. In the context of mid nineteenth century Denbighshire, this poses problems. The patronymic basis of many Welsh surnames meant that a high proportion of the population shared a small number of names. On one estimate, the ten most common surnames in mid nineteenth century Wales covered 55.85 per cent of the population, the ten most common surnames in England, by comparison, only 5.15 per cent. For most of north Wales in the period 1812 to 1837, the ten most common names would cover more than 70 per cent of the population, while in the hundred of Penllyn, Merionethshire, over 30 per cent of the population bore the surname Jones.[13] With some records, moreover, individuals might be referred to by both patronymic and parental surname over a span of years. While some work has been done on computer linkage of historical data in areas with a high proportion of patronymics, this has not embraced records where patronymic variations for the same person may exist, so matching of records was performed manually.[14]

RESULTS

Entering the surviving records for the period 1828 to 1858 gave 1975 entries, of which 49 were excluded as coming from parishes bordering Denbighshire. From the remaining entries, 572 individuals were identified, 248 of whom were recorded only once. In contrast, 69 lunatics or idiots had eight or more entries. More than 20 per cent of the single entries appear in the last year for which the individual union returns are available. Non-response by local officers when parishes and, in the more populous north eastern area of Denbighshire, townships within parishes, were individually responsible for making the return, explains other cases.[15] The difficulties of positively identifying individuals amidst the patronymics is another contributory factor, while some confusion is evident in the early years between recording those pauper lunatics

Table 4.1 *Consistency of records, 1842–58*

Union	All cases with 1+ record	Of which, 1 possible entry missing	More than 1 possible entry missing
Wrexham	8	1	1
Ruthin	49	4	1
Llanrwst	28	4	1
St Asaph	29	4	0

and idiots dependent on the parish, or only those resident in it,[16] and recording all idiots, or only those considered 'dangerous'.

After 1842, when responsibility for making the return passed to the clerk to the poor law union, cases were generally recorded in the lunacy return every year, irrespective of whether the named person was in an institution or the community. The table below (Table 4.1), for the four main poor law unions in the area, shows how consistently cases with more than one entry in the returns were recorded between the date of first entry, and the last entry.

The question is whether the returns contain all the names they should. The evidence here suggests they do not. While there is consistent recording of names, the average period they appear in the records is short. There is some evidence from both the comments and the time affected columns in the returns that many cases had been afflicted for some time before the first entry. Their eventual incorporation into the return might thus reflect a change of circumstance, a move from family support to pauper status, or both. This may be confirmed by a look at those names newly recorded some years into the sequence. In 1843, 34 were recorded for the first time, 26 were idiots from birth, with ages between 9 and 72 years, of whom two had entered the workhouse, the remainder were with family or boarded out. The eight lunatics had been afflicted for various periods, ranging 'from birth' to 'three months'. Four were with relatives, the others boarded out. For some, it is clearly the transition to the institution, rather than the onset of the disease, which results in their appearance in the returns. Thomas Williams of Llanrhydd had been of unsound mind for 13 years, but is first recorded in 1843, after entering the Chester Asylum in April 1841.[17]

By definition, the returns are confined to pauper lunatics and

idiots, and exclude those whose families supported them independently of parish relief. There is some evidence from other sources
that a number of lunatics were being cared for in the community
by their families, without recourse to the poor law. Only when
faced with the expense of asylum care do they appear in the
statistics as pauper lunatics.

In 1844 the Metropolitan Commissioners in Lunacy visited North
Wales, and a number of the cases they saw in Denbighshire were
not then being recorded in the lunacy return, in some instances
specifically because they were not then paupers. Two of these were
subsequently reported as living in the community, while one,
possibly two, later entered Denbigh Asylum, and thus contributed
to the 'increase in lunacy'. Ann Storey was 'first affected with
Insanity after the death of her husband, who was drowned while
bathing about four years ago. For a short time in Gloucester
Asylum'.[18] This would suggest her family were not paupers, for
according to Samuel Hitch, the Medical Superintendent of the
Gloucester Asylum 'We do not receive any Pauper Lunatics but
the Paupers of our own County. We have had several Welsh
Insane, but they were people above, just above, the condition of
pauperism, whom we placed in our charity wards.'[19] Ann Storey
appears in the lunacy returns between 1851 and 1853 (the last year
for which the St Asaph Union returns are extant). Still living with
her parents, she received one shilling relief, and 'two shillings
weekly from club', presumably a benefit on the death of her
husband. She was recorded as a harmless idiot or imbecile, rather
than a lunatic.[20]

Robert Jones was specifically recorded as not being a pauper
when the Commissioners visited. A 'dangerous idiot' who drew
complaints from the neighbours when at large, he was 'kept low by
medicine', or sometimes 'fettered and bound while wandering'.[21] A
Robert Jones, described as a harmless lunatic, entered the Denbigh
Asylum in 1852, funded by the Ruthin Union. There is no conclu-
sive evidence that this is the same person.[22] The Commissioners
were assisted during their visit by, among others, the Dean of St
Asaph, Charles Scott Luxmoore, and Dr Richard Lloyd Williams
of Denbigh, two prominent advocates of an asylum for Denbigh.
Also visited, though not then in the Lunacy Return, was Lucy
Lloyd, who was 'Formerly a servant to Dr Lloyd Williams.' Lucy
Lloyd lived with her daughter, until admitted to Denbigh Asylum

in 1849.[23] A fourth case, Anne Davies of Betws-yn-Rhos, had been drawn to the attention of the Guardians by the union surgeon as requiring medical attention if she were not to be a permanent burden on the parish. Although judged by the Commissioners to be 'evidently insane', the Guardians took no action. Two years after the Commissioners visit, Anne Davies is recorded in the Returns as a harmless lunatic, 'subject to fits'. She was living with her parents, and receiving 1/6d weekly relief.[24]

Concerned by the continuing under-recording of single lunatics, the Commissioners called in 1858 for stricter regulations for the local officials:

> As a means of securing due attention to single pauper patients I submit that the Clerk to the Board of Guardians should require from the Relieving Officer the names of all parties for whom money is advanced on account of the mental infirmity, and that he should transmit the names of those patients to the Medical Officer of the District in which they reside and receive from him the required return four times annually and in cases of neglect that he should report to the Board of Guardians, Poor Law Board and Commissioners in Lunacy.[25]

They recognised, however, that the greatest influence was a pecuniary one. The reluctance to act of the poor law medical officer might be due to 'a wish to avoid trouble in the performance of a duty for which the statute has provided no specific remuneration.' The 1853 Lunatic Asylums Act provided some incentive to the medical officers to visit pauper lunatics in the community by specifying a fee of 2/6d for each quarterly visit.[26] In scattered rural areas it was suggested even this was insufficient incentive:

> The great distance from the residence of the Medical Officer who receives only 2/6d for one visit is doubtless one obstacle to a satisfactory compliance with the Act in remote and thinly populated districts. Hence it becomes a question how far it might be advisable in certain localities to increase the remuneration and in certain cases to require more frequent visits – such as, for instance, where patients affected with insanity are placed under the care of strangers and to diminish the visits in others as for instance in cases of idiots and imbecile persons residing with relatives.[27]

Costs were a key issue for smaller parishes, and one which the Lunacy Commissioners recognised when they referred to the problem of small, impoverished parishes, where even one chargeable pauper in an asylum would be costly. Here, the temptation was to keep pauper lunatics within the locality, preferring not to send them even to the workhouse, as there they would 'fall under the observation of the whole of the Board of Guardians'.[28] A number of examples in the lunacy returns hint at this form of concealment. In Llanrwst the Metropolitan Commissioners visited David Williams, who was boarded with his mother, having been

> first affected in mind upon his father's death, fifteen years ago. [He] Has been at times very violent, and a source of alarm to his family; the neighbours have been sometimes called in to protect the mother from his violence. Once seized a knife, and was disarmed by his brother. Apparently treated with kindness. His family were very anxious that he should be sent to an Asylum, for which Mr W. Hughes, Union Surgeon, thinks him still a proper object.[29]

Williams appears in the lunacy returns between 1841 and 1856. Apart from the money from the parish, he also received 3/- weekly from a club. He remained with his mother until 1850, after which he was boarded out in 1851, and subsequently entered Denbigh Asylum in 1853. In this, he is among a minority of the non-institutionalised cases visited by the Commissioners. Williams' status as a lunatic is largely concealed from official records. Apart from the first year, when he is recorded as a dangerous lunatic, he is regularly recorded as a harmless idiot during his time in the community.[30] This was not the only such example. Thomas Williams was described in the lunacy returns for the parish of Aberchwiler as an idiot on all but one of the nine returns made. Only in 1836 is he declared to be a lunatic. In the surviving Overseers Accounts for the period, however, his madness is always acknowledged; for example, in March 1836 they record: 'Dr Roberts, examination of Thos. Williams a Lunatic by order of the Justices 11/-; Dr Ellis, on a/c sundries Thos Williams, 12/9d.'[31] Aberchwiler was a small rural parish of 500 people, and the cost of his transfer to an asylum would have been considerable. The visit of the Metropolitan Commissioners revealed similar considerations prevailing elsewhere in north Wales. With John Jones of Ceidio, near Nefyn, the 'case had been discussed at the Board of Guardians, and the sole objection urged against sending him to an asylum was the expense, Ceidio being a small parish.'[32] It was not until 1862 that the cost of sending a pauper lunatic to an asylum ceased to

Table 4.2   *Cost to Poor Law by type of placement, 1828–58*

Placement	Average Cost per month (expressed in pence)			
	Idiots	Lunatics	Dangerous	Harmless
Asylum	175.8	187.3	187.4	186.0
Licensed House	150.0	152.7	153.3	150.0
Workhouse	49.2	51.6	48.6	49.3
Lodged or Boarded Out	43.9	80.3	82.5	46.2
At Home	45.7	78.4	89.0	48.9
Relations or Friends	45.8	69.9	67.5	48.7
Placement not shown	42.8	77.1	93.5	45.0

have some direct effect on the finances of a parish, for then the 1861 Paupers Removal Act specified the cost was to be met from a common fund, the contributions to which were to be calculated in proportion to the rateable value of the parishes in the union.[33] Previously, any common fund contributions had been 'apportioned to each parish according to the average expenditure on account of its paupers.'[34] That the financial consequences of institutionalisation no longer bore directly on the parish after 1862 may explain the decision in 1865 of the Eglwysbach Vestry that 'The Guardians were recommended to consult the Medical Officer regarding Marg[are]t Wynne, Mary Jones, Pwllterfyn and Alice Williams, Brynrhyd, the Vestry being of opinion that they ought to be sent to the Asylum.'[35] Despite these financial changes, however, the Lunacy Commissioners continued to complain about the incompleteness of the returns.[36]

COSTS AND CARE

Recording individual cases allows a breakdown of costs beyond those in the published returns. The differential costs of lunatics and idiots, dangerous and harmless, can be seen in Table 4.2:

A cross-tabulation of the costs of those persons in the community rather than in institutional care, in Table 4.3, shows that lunacy produced a cost premium over idiocy, and that those deemed dangerous cost more than those considered harmless.

In a study of the Old Poor Law in Anglesey, which also shows

Table 4.3   *Costs to Poor Law, non-institutionalised cases, 1828–58*

	Average Cost per Month (expressed in pence)	
	Harmless	Dangerous
Idiots	44.4	68.6
Lunatics	71.8	96.0

that lunatics were liable to receive a higher rate than idiots even when the carer was a family member, it is argued that this is because the mad needed full-time attention which prevented the carer from undertaking other paid work.[37] An alternative explanation is that it is an indication that a premium had to be paid to persuade people to undertake the care of more volatile cases.

'Dangerousness' is an ambiguous term in the returns, which asked whether the individual was dangerous to himself or others. A minority of the entries in the lunacy returns specify 'to self', 'to others', or 'both'. Only 43 records of 'dangerous' idiots can be found, covering 26 individuals, against 1393 records of harmless idiots. For idiots, dangerousness might be defined as inability to perceive danger, or as boisterousness which threatened physical violence on others. William Whitehill, an idiot in the Wrexham Workhouse, was 'in danger of injuring himself.'[38] A similar concern was expressed over epileptics. Edward Davies of Ruabon was dangerous to himself as he was 'liable to fits.'.[39] In 158 records, lunatics were considered dangerous, either to themselves or others, against 312 instances where the case was regarded as harmless. Again, dangerousness might embrace both the suicidally depressive, dangerous only to themselves, or people suffering from mania who might threaten others. The preponderance of records for idiots in the lunacy returns reflects the position of north Wales as having the highest proportion of idiots to the insane in the country.[40]

FAMILY AND CARING

Some lunatics were living independently, in sometimes even when considered unsuitable to be in the community. Mary Williams, 53, of Llandrillo yn Rhos, considered a dangerous lunatic, was 'at her own home in Colwyn', though 'not fit to be at large.'[41] Sisters Ruth

Table 4.4   *Main carer, lunatics and idiots living 'at home' or with relatives, 1828–58*

	Lunatics	Idiots
Immediate Family		
Parents	6	37
Father	3	24
Mother	6	33
Wife	5	1
Husband	1	
Children	4	2
Grandmother		1
Total, Immediate Family	25	98
Extended Family		
Sister	2	15
Aunt		2
Brother		2
Niece		1
Uncle		2
Cousin		1
Total, Extended Family	2	23

and Catherine Hughes, variously described as lunatics or idiots, but not idiots from birth, shared a house in Wrexham.[42] Mary Allen, a dangerous lunatic, was 'in her own residence in Denbigh since she became a lunatic.'[43] Lunatics were more likely than idiots to be married, or to have dependants, and this is probably one reason why the number of lunatics in their own home is larger than the apparent number of idiots. Where individuals were living with family or friends, the returns sometimes specify the relationship, as indicated in Table 4.4:

Table 4.4 shows the preponderance of female carers. While no different from contemporary family relationships[44] the evidence is significant, given that poor law records may tend to emphasise the male as head of household and recipient of payments. Under the legislation in England and Wales 'the Poor Law had imposed an obligation not only on parents to support children, husbands to support wives, and adults to support their aged parents, but grand-parents to support grandchildren.' There was no duty to care for siblings.[45] As Table 4.4 indicates, where a lunatic was in the care of his or her family, that caring role was almost exclusively undertaken by those who had some legal obligation. Parents, jointly or individually, were overwhelmingly the main carers, perhaps indicating long-term health problems for many classed as lunatic, but the presence of more spouses and children shows that mental illness could strike at any time of life. The extended family played a lesser role in the primary care of the mentally ill, only two sisters being listed. This suggests that if the immediate family was unable or unavailable to care for the individual, boarding out, the workhouse or institutional care were the only options. For idiots, the pattern is somewhat different. Close relatives, particularly parents, still formed overwhelmingly the largest single group of carers, but there is more evidence of the extended family, particularly female siblings, undertaking the caring role.[46] The number of sisters involved in caring suggests that the familial responsibility invariably passed from mother to daughter. Welsh kinship systems were often intricately woven, and were reinforced by the fact that obligation and reciprocity passed through the female line.[47]

LUNATICS IN THE COMMUNITY

The existence of these legal obligations raises questions about the willingness with which these family members undertook their duties. One case which suggests that family members consented to care for potentially dangerous relatives is that of Margaret Jones of Denbigh. She was visited by the Commissioners in 1844. As they noted, she had been described in the 1843 Lunacy Return as a lunatic, and 'very unruly at times, and requiring much attendance.' She was boarded with her sister, the proprietress of a cake shop in Denbigh, whom she had 'violently assaulted' two years previously. On the union surgeon's testimony, Margaret Jones had on occasions been dangerous. When her sister applied to the local Guardians for an increased allowance the surgeon, with Richard Lloyd Williams' support, reported that she was not a fit subject for the workhouse, and recommended that she be sent to an asylum. The Guardians then arranged for the sister to continue to care for her, though the allowance increased from the previous 2/6d to 6/- weekly. This was a case which would seem suitable for the asylum at Denbigh when it opened in 1849, but the lunacy returns covering the years 1840 to 1853 show that Margaret Jones, always described in them as a harmless lunatic, remained with her sister even after its opening, though in 1850 her weekly allowance was reduced to 4/- weekly.[48] Other examples suggest that pressure from the Guardians resulted in dangerous cases being sent back to unwilling relatives, even though additional help might be offered. Richard Evans had been in Chester Asylum, but was taken out by the Overseers. He was now living with his wife and children at Bersham, though considered dangerous to others.[49] William Griffiths, a 68 year old lunatic from Ruabon, was 'with his wife at Bangor' [probably Bangor Monachorum in Flintshire]. The threat of violence was such that the Parish was paying 14/- a week for day and night attendance, more than the cost of asylum care, and the total cost of the family was 16/6d per week.[50] Hannah Edwards, of Llanfair Dyffryn Clwyd, was 'dangerous at times to her children' and the parish paid 5/- each week to have a woman in attendance.[51]

Sometimes, the problems of caring for a lunatic relative proved too much for the family. Ellen Evans of Betws-yn-Rhos appears in the records between 1828 and 1849. In the earlier years she is living at home with David, her spouse. Later, though, she was 'deserted by her husband' and was lodged with a woman farmer, with whom she remained.[52]

In an area bereft of an asylum of its own, a complex set of factors influenced the decision to retain most cases in the community. One was geographical distance; Chris Philo has explored the 'distance decay' factor in asylum admissions.[53] Community concerns for the fate of the Welsh speaking lunatic sent to English asylums, and traditions of family care were also important,[54] as was the difficulty of surveillance by monoglot English speaking agents of the central bureaucracy. One official visitor to Anglesey

> endeavoured to seek out the Patients returned in the quarterly lists of the Medical Officers. Owing, however, to the remoteness of the localities and the inability of the inhabitants to speak English, I soon found the task a very difficult one. Subsequently I obtained from the Medical Officers the exact addresses of their Patients, but even with this additional help I was only able to visit a small number of cases.[55]

Many of those who remained in the community were free to roam, but could be subject to the attention of the curious and taunts from those intolerant of difference. Dr Lloyd Williams rescued 'a poor woman who was under great excitement from the mischievous teasings of a crowd of boys and girls.'[56] Danger to the lunatic, or the threat of the lunatic to the family, could lead to a more restrictive approach. Edward Lloyd, boarded with his father, was reported to have had his first attack of insanity in 1840, and to have been sent to Chester Asylum for nine months. He was 'subject to frequent fits of passion, during which he seizes knives, and requires to be disarmed.' He had sometimes been confined at night 'by a belt and muffs in order to keep him quiet, and for the protection of his family. The father, mother, two sisters and a brother, sleep in the same room with him, which contains three beds, and is crowded and close. We found the poor mother in bed, sinking from phthisis.' The lunacy returns show Edward Lloyd, chargeable to Derwen, as a dangerous lunatic between 1840 'from May last' to 1846, when there is no further record. His time at Chester is not revealed.[57]

Such confinement could become permanent, aided by an actual or contrived ignorance by the wider community which helped to avoid official surveillance, particularly by the central government. When the visiting Metropolitan Commissioners were led to confined lunatics by local officials or others with local knowledge, they highlighted the discovery to emphasise the need for reform. By far the longest section of the Commissioners 1844 Report devoted to any individual was that concerning Mary Jones, boarded with her mother at Llanrhaeadr yng Nghinmerch. The case had been mentioned by the union relieving officer and union surgeon while the Commissioners were at Ruthin. With Richard Lloyd Williams, who acted as an interpreter, the Commissioners went to the cottage and 'In a dark and offensive room, over a blacksmith's forge, upon opening a bolted door, we discovered the miserable object of our search. The only window was closed up by boards, between which little air could find admission, and only a feeble glimmering of light.'

The description of Mary Jones, and the subsequent activity by Charles Scott Luxmoore, Dr Lloyd Williams and others, covers six pages of the report.[58] Despite the obvious acquaintance with the details, denial seems to have been prevalent:

Close to a public road, within ten yards of the Church, in a cottage belonging to the Squire of the Parish, a really humane man as his

conduct today showed, if I had not otherwise known it; within a quarter
of a mile of the Clergyman's home, who, with his wife and family, take
an active interest in all that concerns the poor, but who had never heard
of her until this morning, although the mother was well known to them
– this wretched woman is confined without their knowledge. If the
neighbours did know her state, they thought nothing of it.[59]

A witness, however, recalled seeing Mary Jones at the window
calling for food. 'After that the boards were more closely made
up.'[60] For the Commissioners, Mary Jones was a prime example,
illustrating the argument for an asylum to be provided for Welsh
speaking lunatics. At the time of the visitation, Luxmoore and
Lloyd Williams decided that

> as we have no Asylum, and as it would be dreadful either to leave her
> where she is, or to send her to an English Asylum, where the poor
> object could not express her wants, [we] agreed that she was not insane,
> but a fit object for the Denbigh Dispensary, where there may be some
> hopes of restoring her, in some degree, to the use of her limbs.[61]

In our study of the lunacy returns, it is clear that Mary Jones never
entered Denbigh Asylum. The first record of her is in 1833, when
she is recorded as having been a harmless lunatic for eight months,
with 'friends' [i.e. family] in Llanrhaeadr yng Nghinmerch. There
is no subsequent record until 1841. Between 1843 and 1846 Mary
Jones appears three more times, now chargeable to Ruthin, though
still said to be with friends in Llanrhaeadr. Still a harmless lunatic,
she is said to possess 'dirty habits'. Mary Jones appears never to
have entered an asylum. In 1850, the last record which can reliably
be linked to this case, she had entered the Ruthin Workhouse, and
was now recorded as a harmless idiot.[62]

LEAVING AND RETURNING TO COMMUNITY CARE

In his study of Lancaster Asylum, John Walton refers to the
removal of lunatics from the community, and their eventual return,
as 'casting out and bringing back' cases.[63] In an environment where
the retention of lunatics within their family or the local community
remained the norm, the factors influencing decisions to cast out or
bring back are particularly relevant.

Those who were 'cast out' were those whose behaviour provoked
the community beyond endurance and those who became visible to

the squirearchy familiar with the new views of moral treatment. In a letter to the *North Wales Chronicle* the anonymous author, subsequently identified as Luxmoore, wrote of seeing a lunatic 'fettered and manacled, and basking in the public street, exposed to the rude gaze of the thoughtless passers by. [Another] I have seen led about the streets, and even to Church, in the restraint of a strait waistcoat.'[64] From the lunacy returns and other evidence, the first of these can be identified as Evan Lewis of Abergele. A former soldier, Lewis had spent some time in the Liverpool Asylum, but the Abergele Vestry had consistently sought to keep him in the community with his father or, when that proved impossible, with others who would 'look after' him for a fee. His presence in a busy market town was noted by Luxmoore, and the Guardians received a letter from William Day, the Assistant Poor Law Commissioner, saying that 'The Commissioners have received complaint that a Lunatic Pauper at Abergele in the St Asaph Union is brought out to bask in the sun in the streets chained.'[65] After threatening the Guardians with legal sanctions if they did not act, Day wrote to the Poor Law Commissioner, George Cornewall Lewis, saying he knew about this 'insane pauper of Abergele Union [sic]' personally, for he

> came to my notice in consequence of having followed Mrs Day into a shop in that town, and abused her exceedingly. Great objection was made to the *Parish* Guardians to sending him to the Chester Asylum in consequence of the increased expense which would attend such a step but at length the Guardians at large overruled it, and an order was made to have him taken before the magistrates for the purpose of placing him there. The man is at all times insane, and periodically violent at *known* intervals. . . . I sent a letter to the Clerk of the Union on the subject, but if it were to come officially from you instead of myself it would have more effect . . .[66]

The financial imperatives influencing the reluctance of local overseers and vestries to send even the most unruly to asylums, and their desire to limit the time for which expensive asylum fees would have to be paid, is evident in the reconstructed history of another lunatic who alternated between asylum and community. Martin Smith was an attorney's clerk from Denbigh, whose case indicates that lunacy could pauperise families who would not normally be classed among those in need; clearly an educated man in a position requiring verbal and literary fluency, the family's descent into pauperism indicates that his wealth was as yet insubstantial. Diagnosed by the Parish Surgeon as suffering from monomania,[67] by 1827, he had been sent to Liverpool Asylum, and the Denbigh Vestry agreed to the charge of 12/- weekly.[68] This was paid by Mr Sankey, a local banker and member of the Vestry, on its behalf. The next year 'Mr Sankey having produced a bill amounting to £41–10–7d paid by him to the Governors of Liverpool Infirmary [sic] on behalf of Martin Smith', the Vestry was asked for reimbursement. As the Overseers did not have the money available, it was resolved to pay Sankey 'the balance in hand from the last year's accounts and also £10 out of the next until the . . . claim is liquidated.'[69]

When Sankey asked for reimbursement again the next year, the Vestry tried another approach, it 'appearing that Mr Lloyd of Tros y Park's rates applicable to the discharging of this debt and arrears, ordered that Mr Lloyd be reminded of this account.'[70] Smith returned home at some time in 1829, but was subsequently sent to the newly opened asylum at Chester.[71] While Smith was confined, his family needed support, and it was ordered 'that Martin Smith's wife have a weekly allowance of 2/6d.' With the continuing expense, the Vestry at the same time decided to investigate whether Smith could be removed, and asked the Overseer to 'look out for a house in the country to place the family in.' In the hope of transferring the expense another way, it was also decided to conduct an examination of Smith's place of settlement.[72]

The evident pressures on the Vestry's resources are confirmed by subsequent entries in the minutes. Two years later, it resolved to

> immediately borrow from Messrs Sankey or other person willing to advance the same, a sufficient sum of money to procure the release of Martin Smith . . . from the Chester Lunatic Asylum, . . . and that the sum borrowed, as aforesaid, be reimbursed out of the rates.[73]

Smith remained in the asylum, with increasingly severe consequences for the finances of the Parish. By May 1833 the situation was very serious, as the Vestry minutes record:

> That it is the unanimous opinion of the Vestry that the Debt owing to the Cheshire Lunatic Asylum amounting to £210 and others making an aggregate of nearly £500 ought to be immediately paid to prevent the

consequences of legal proceedings which are threatened. That notice of a Special Vestry be given for Monday 24th instant to devise a means of raising a sufficient sum for the purpose of discharging the same by borrowing a sum of money on the responsibility of the Parish or otherwise That the continuing of Martin Smith a Lunatic in the above asylum or having him sent home be at the same vestry taken into consideration, and if it be decided to continue him there that the guarantee required by Act of Parliament be forwarded to the proper officer of the Asylum.[74]

Although the cost made it imperative to remove Smith from the asylum, anxiety about his behaviour made his accommodation a matter of equal concern. By December, when he remained in the asylum, the Vestry considered the matter again, proposing:

> That the question of the removal of Martin Smith from the Lunatic Asylum be taken into consideration at the next Vestry, and that in the meantime Mr Simon [Assistant Overseer] enquire into his present state of mind and look out for a suitable place for his being kept distantly removed from Denbigh.[75]

By February, the Vestry was again considering Smith's removal from the asylum, though not until much of the debt had been discharged:

> Ordered that additional rates be raised on the Parish, one to be raised immediately and the other at the end of six months for the purpose of liquidating the debt owing to the Cheshire Lunatic Asylum. That Martin Smith is to be brought from the Cheshire Lunatic Asylum when the first one hundred pounds of the debt due from this Parish to the asylum is paid, and a house to be taken for him and his family to live together.[76]

Not until 1836, however, was the Vestry able to secure Smith's removal, discharging the asylum invoice and giving the necessary notice at the same time.[77] Smith was evidently less unwell, for after a year on parish relief, he began working for Mr Horne, a local attorney, in May 1837, and thence disappears from the record.[78]

Again, many of the same themes emerge from this case history; the crippling cost to the individual parish, the desire to reduce costs by taking patients out of the asylum, the transference of the problem, in this instance not so much to the family as to some neighbourhood outside of Denbigh, and in the face of all these countervailing pressures, the necessity of keeping a troublesome lunatic away from the community. Smith's madness does not, however, seem to have stigmatised the family. His son enjoyed a successful public career as churchwarden and managing clerk to T. Gold Edwards, solicitor and leading member of the Denbigh Asylum committee.[79] In 1881 the widow of Martin Smith [senior] is still living in Park Road, Denbigh, one of the most desirable areas of the town, two doors away from her now widowed daughter-in-law.[80]

CONCLUSIONS

Until the opening of the North Wales Lunatic Asylum at Denbigh in 1848, most lunatics in north Wales lived in their own communities, many cared for by their own close family. This much is documented by the lunacy returns. More difficult to trace, but probably significant in facilitating the continuance of this pattern of caring, was the practical backing provided by kinship links and community support. Extended families were still an important social institution in mid-nineteenth century Wales. Indeed the strength of kinship ties, bound together by intricate social and economic linkages, and by arrangements of mutual reciprocity, was still a distinguishing feature of Welsh rural communities when investigated by anthropological researchers in the mid-twentieth century.[81] The extent to which wider family networks could help support the immediate carer of an insane relative remains, however, elusive. It is not revealed by the lunacy returns, and can probably only ever be a matter of speculation, or at most supposition. Occasionally, fragments of evidence surface, as for instance when relatives and neighbours actively intervene during an outbreak of violence. The records of patients admitted to the North Wales Lunatic Asylum also indicate many were admitted following the breakdown of long-standing family arrangements for care – arrangements which previously had gone completely unrecorded.

The prolongation of an agriculturally based rural economy, and of relative poverty, further help to explain the perpetuation of community care of the insane in Wales. Poverty affected arrangements at two levels. Firstly, as documented here, it influenced small parishes burdened by the heavy cost of placing a lunatic in long-term care, to seek the cheapest alternative. Secondly, the lack of alternative employment opportunities, and the low standard of living, made the small cash payments offered for the care of a lunatic or idiot an inducement likely to entice carers to shoulder the burden.

Reconstructing the lives of the 'single lunatics' or idiots in the community is a difficult task. Reconstructing the lives of the carers is even more so. This article has shown that the Lunacy Commissioners were correct in their belief that the lunacy returns on which they relied for details of these cases were both incomplete and inaccurate. They do, however, have a contemporary value as a tool both for exploring longitudinal histories of lunatics, and in providing a key for identifying relevant records in other sources. As the cases in this article show they can provide an insight, partial though it might be, into the detail of community care for the insane, the burdens born by the families of lunatics, and the financial pressures placed on small communities by the decision to send their lunatics on the journey to asylum.

CHAPTER FIVE

Boarding-out insane patients: the significance of the Scottish system 1857–1913

Harriet Sturdy and William Parry-Jones

INTRODUCTION

The pioneering policy of boarding-out harmless, chronic insane patients in the community was implemented formally by the Scottish Board of Lunacy in 1858, following the passage of the Lunacy (Scotland) Act, 1857. Up to 25 per cent of registered pauper and private patients were boarded-out under the terms of this Act, offering the benefits of increased freedom in a domestic setting, while vacating space in overcrowded asylums. This chapter offers a brief assessment of the nature, growth and influence of the system in nineteenth and early-twentieth century Scotland, locating the Scottish practice in a broad, comparative context.

During the last 20 years, the study of the history of psychiatry has become increasingly popular. Historians of nineteenth-century provision for the insane have focused largely on the growth of asylums and the general move towards the 'incarceration' of the insane. Recent work on lunacy provision in Scotland has focused on the prestigious royal asylums; either as a group,[1] or in profiles of individual institutions.[2] However, the contribution of district asylums, with one exception[3] and private madhouses has not received detailed assessment.[4] Further, the influential system of boarding-out has been almost wholly neglected. Boarding-out was an important component of lunacy provision, particularly in Scotland. The prominent psychiatric journals of the time, not just British but German, French, Italian, and American are full of lengthy descriptions and assessments of the Scottish system, and doctors came from around the world to see boarding-out in practice. Despite its innovative nature, the number of patients involved, and the implications for the late-twentieth century attempts at community care, the policy has received little systematic attention this century. The few recent articles which acknowledge the existence of an official system of non-institutional provision do little more than refer readers to the work of Parry-Jones[5] and McCandless.[6] Both of the latter studies offer a brief and tantalising introduction to the system, but neither are, or were intended to be, comprehensive.

Although this chapter explores the growth of a system of non-institutional care, it is helpful to be aware of the availability of asylum provision during the period. The Lunacy (Scotland) Act, 1857, led to marked growth in the number of asylums, on a similar scale to that implemented over a decade earlier in England and Wales. Before this legislation, provision for the insane in Scotland had been wholly inadequate for the growing demands of the population. Within ten years, available repositories for the insane comprised royal asylums, a steadily developing network of district asylums, a small number of parochial asylums, licensed wards in poorhouses, a proliferation of private madhouses, two schools for the training of imbecile children and the Lunatic Department at Perth prison.[7] By 1913, there were seven royal asylums, 21 district asylums, one parochial asylum and three private madhouses. Further, there were 14 poorhouses licensed to receive lunatics. It was, therefore, in a period of growth in institutional provision for both pauper and private patients that an active system of community care was developing. Thus, boarding-out needs to be seen in the context of an increasing trend, nationally and internationally, towards institutionalisation of the insane.

Insane patients resided in the community in Scotland long before any legislation was passed formalising their status, but there was no official centralised provision before the mid-nineteenth century. The investigations of the Royal Commission, established in 1855,[8] exposed 'deplorable' instances of what was regarded to be neglect, cruelty and insanitary living conditions. Countless patients were in need of asylum provision, others, who were harmless and quiet, required accommodation in a closely supervised home, far removed from the filth and neglect in which they lived. Members of the Commission concluded that 'an appalling amount of misery prevails throughout Scotland' in the lives of single patients.[9]

DEVELOPMENT OF POLICY

It was not until the Lunacy (Scotland) Act, 1857 that boarding-out was instituted as a legally controlled system of providing for the insane. Under the terms of the Act, all insane patients were ordered to be admitted to an asylum or other institution for the insane. However, it was recognised that many could be provided for more appropriately in domestic surroundings, if properly regulated by officials. Therefore patients who were certified as incurable and harmless could be kept in a private house with the sanction of the Board of Lunacy. As the newly appointed Commissioners in Lunacy asserted:

> the features of insanity are so variable and so dependent for their expression on the circumstances in which the patients may be placed, that it is extremely desirable that the law should afford every reasonable facility for varying the manner of their disposal.[10]

Patients categorised as idiots and imbeciles, as well as those suffering from 'acquired forms of insanity' (the term adopted by the Commissioners to describe persons who had become insane since reaching adulthood), were boarded-out. The Lunacy (Scotland) Act, 1857, defined lunacy in such a way that it included every person certified by two physicians to be a 'lunatic, an insane person, an idiot, or a person of unsound mind.'[11] However, the Commissioners were aware that the term lunacy, which included 'any mad or furious or fatuous person, or person so diseased or affected in mind as to render him unfit ... to be at large',[12] was not strictly applicable to the majority of idiot and imbecile patients deemed suitable for residence in private dwellings.[13] The broader term insane, therefore, was utilised frequently as an alternative in describing boarded-out patients. The Commissioners recognised two broad divisions of insanity, the first comprising idiot and imbecile patients, and the second, embracing all acquired forms of insanity, including dementia, chronic mania and melancholia. A distinction between these divisions was not made on a daily basis. The terms lunatic and insane were used interchangeably in annual reports, and no clear distinction was made in articles discussing boarding-out. In view of this terminological and nosological ambiguity, and reflecting the practice of the Lunacy Commissioners, the generic term 'insane' is used here to describe all persons of unsound mind.[14]

Boarding-out, while administered locally by parish officials, was regulated by a centralised administration based in Edinburgh, namely the General Board of Lunacy. Commissioners appointed to the Board were entrusted with the management and supervision of all registered insane patients in Scotland, private and pauper, in institutions and private dwellings. They instituted instructions and regulations for the guidance of parochial officials, and directions to guardians regarding the acceptable standards for accommodation, clothing, food and general treatment.

Patients were placed in private dwellings, generally comprising the cottage of a suitable guardian, in either a town, or, more usually, a farming or village community. Insane persons could be admitted to the roll of boarded-out patients either having received 'dispensation from removal to an asylum' by the Commissioners, thereby remaining in their own homes, or having been transferred from institutions for the insane. In light of the unsatisfactory nature of prevailing conditions in private dwellings, Commissioners determined that existing arrangements should be formally controlled and supervised. No attempt was made to introduce any special system and instead, the Board:

> allowed the mode of administration to shape itself; and the form which it actually took grew naturally out of the Board's efforts to obtain the correction of what was bad and to encourage the development of what was good.[15]

Patients were boarded with relatives or unrelated persons (generally described by the Commissioners as strangers) 'in their own condition of life', either singly or in numbers not exceeding four. Sanction for residence outside an asylum could be withdrawn at any time by the Board of Lunacy. To the Commissioners, the essence of the system lay in:

> an attempt to place all quiet and harmless insane people who no longer require asylum care ... under home conditions as ideal as can be obtained.[16]

A number of factors contributed to the general consolidation and endorsement of the boarding-out system, including increased efforts by asylum superintendents to discharge chronic patients in order to relieve overcrowding; greater enthusiasm among parish officials to co-operate with the Board of Lunacy, and the steadily rising costs of maintenance in asylums. The initial practice of placing patients with strangers had demonstrated to parish officials that there was a plentiful supply of suitable, willing guardians to receive patients. Growing confidence among the public also contributed to its development. Further, in the early years of the system, re-admission to an asylum, if a patient proved unsuitable, necessitated new medical certificates and a fresh order by the sheriff, thereby entailing considerable expense and trouble for parochial authorities. The introduction of probation as a preliminary to boarding-out from asylums therefore served to encourage asylum and parochial officials to select suitable patients for discharge for a six month trial period. During this time, the original order and certificates remained in force. Patients were returned, when necessary, to the asylum with comparatively little effort or expense. This resulted in the number of patients boarded-out from asylums rising steadily, connected closely with a growing flexibility regarding the mental characteristics of those thought to be suitable for such provision. By 1890, the Commissioners were convinced that, despite sustained international interest, the system was no longer a novelty, but, rather, had

> reached the stage of maturity at which its successful working is best shown by its unobtrusiveness and by routine performance of its functions.[17]

The majority of large parishes practised the policy, the selection of suitable patients and guardians becoming an integral part of the duties of the inspector of poor. In certain districts, generations of children grew up with an insane patient in their household. In this way, boarding-out was in many places 'an institution associated with the earliest impressions of a very large number of the inhabitants'.[18] To such persons it was entirely natural to share a house with a harmless lunatic. The familiarity with which the system was viewed, its economic benefits, and the gradual breaking down of prejudices against the insane, assisted its steady development.

Concerted pressure and encouragement by the Board of Lunacy further ensured its growth throughout Scotland.

Boarding-out was marked by continual fluctuation in numbers. In 1859, two years after the passage of the Lunacy (Scotland) Act, 1804 single patients were boarded-out, but by 1875, the number had fallen to 1472.[19] The initial decline was evidently due to the gradual elimination of unsatisfactory cases and to the establishment of new district asylums, in areas previously deficient in accommodation. Access to asylums became easier, facilitated by the improvements in travel across the country. Further, some asylum superintendents were reluctant to discharge unrecovered patients to the care of untrained guardians. From 1876, the proportion of patients boarded-out rose. Relative causative factors were the introduction of a government grant the previous year, prompting an increase in registration of paupers as insane[20] and overcrowding in all district, and most royal, asylums. A new generation of parochial officials were less suspicious of the system and more willing to co-operate in the selection and placement of suitable patients.[21] However, although the general trend was one of increase, there continued to be a degree of fluctuation in the number of patients boarded-out annually. This was attributed to the fact that many parochial authorities and asylum superintendents acted only when asylums became severely overcrowded. Further, it would have unrealistic to expect that the same number of suitable patients could be found each year.

The most notable trend in lunacy administration in the late-nineteenth century was, in fact, a continued increase in asylum admissions.[22] Even though boarding-out was adopted by parishes across Scotland from the 1860s, and in spite of the assertion by Commissioners that there was no increase in insanity, admissions to asylums rose annually. Nevertheless, over 20 per cent of registered pauper insane were boarded-out from the 1880s up to the first decade of the twentieth century. In 1888, for example, out of 11,609 registered insane patients, 2402 (20.6 per cent) were in private dwellings, albeit with substantial variation among districts.[23] Private patients only ever comprised a small proportion of boarded-out cases. In 1858, 20 were officially boarded-out, and although 35 years later, this number had increased to 115 out of 2,034 (5.6 per cent) this was only a tiny proportion of those actually residing in private care, the majority of whom remained undetected and therefore, unsupervised.[24] Although there remained a small number of officials who were unconvinced of its merits it is evident that the benefits of the system were accepted gradually throughout Scotland, with the number boarded-out almost doubling between 1876 and 1908, from 1,492 to 2,907 patients.[25]

Boarding-out remained a useful alternative to asylum provision throughout the early decades of the twentieth century, although the number provided for in this way declined during World War 1 and failed to achieve pre-war levels in the following years. As a result of the Mental Deficiency and Lunacy Act (1913), changes in classification led to many patients previously boarded-out as lunatics being certified as mental defectives, and so, although still boarded-out, not appearing in Lunacy Board statistics for lunatics in private dwellings. Decline was not precipitated by any tangible dissatisfaction, rather the continued development of lunacy provision, and the changing conditions brought about by World War 1 led to an unspoken, but ultimately irrevocable challenge to its status.

SPECIAL LICENSED HOUSES

Following legislation passed in 1862, patients were not only placed singly in private dwellings, but also boarded with unrelated guardians in houses licensed for the reception of up to four patients of the same sex. Provision in these specially licensed houses became an increasingly important component of the boarding-out system as the century progressed and within thirty years of their introduction, more patients were placed in such houses than boarded singly. Special licensed houses were distributed across Scotland, but, while many districts contained only one or two such houses, certain parishes became notable for the large presence of patients. The growth of such aggregations was most marked in the 1870s, in Fifeshire, Stirlingshire and Perthshire, until the Board of Lunacy was compelled to limit their development, forcing parish officials to adopt new localities.[26]

One characteristic feature of the location of aggregations was their tendency to occur in places which had once been active areas of industry, for example, centres of hand-loom weaving, which from the mid-century underwent a rapid decline with the introduction of power looms. The population in these districts had decreased, with the exodus of younger people to urban centres in search of employment. In turn, their departure created superfluous accommodation. Although the positive effect of the presence of patients in certain locations was perhaps exaggerated by the Commissioners, their comments throughout annual reports from the 1870s indicate their conviction that the development of special licensed houses had saved certain villages in Central Scotland from extinction.

Reports in medical journals, particularly those from overseas observers, indicate a tendency to focus on these specific districts when discussing boarding-out. The existence of aggregations of the insane in these small villages was attributed initially to the success that ensued from Edinburgh parish officials boarding-out pauper children in the village of Kennoway, Fifeshire. From 1862, they began to send pauper lunatics as well.[27] Several neighbouring parishes were also deemed suitable for the reception of lunatics, and, in this way, an aggregation of patients developed rapidly, facilitated by a steady supply of guardians and suitable accommodation. The aggregation in the village of Kennoway became the most well-known. Physicians and administrators from overseas were taken, almost invariably to this village, thereby creating the false impression that the grouping together of lunatics in small areas was the archetypal feature of the Scottish boarding-out system. While this was misleading, its importance cannot be disputed. These villages became well-known for the presence of insane residents and the memory of this remains strong in Kennoway today.[28]

Although remarkably few objections were raised against the aggregations, there was concern by the Commissioners and the general public that the presence of large numbers of insane persons would make them appear too prominent and that public feeling might become unfavourable. The aim, expressed repeatedly by the Board of Lunacy, was to restore patients as far as possible to the circumstances of ordinary life and to expose them to contact with sane persons. If they were in a village where the insane were 'so numerous as to form an appreciable element of the population',[29] patients could lose the benefits of domestic life and be treated as a class apart from the rest of the community. Such a distinction would then lessen the likelihood of patients being regarded and treated as ordinary members of the family.

One of the most important purposes of special licensed houses lay in accommodating patients who could not be provided for otherwise, having either no suitable relatives, or relatives living in large cities, where residence for patients was not encouraged. Without the opportunity of discharging patients to quiet, rural villages, city parishes would have been severely restricted in finding suitable homes. Although theoretically attainable in any rural location, in practice it was villages in Central Scotland which provided a steady supply of houses for patients from urban locations, most notably Glasgow and Edinburgh, thereby minimising the initial work of inspectors of poor in searching for satisfactory accommodation. There was the added advantage that the development of such houses in rural settings was considered beneficial to the health of patients.

The continued endorsement of the Board of Lunacy for the accommodation of insane patients in special licensed houses is evident in the steady increase in the number of licenses issued during the 1880s and 1890s. During the eight years after the 1862 Amendment Act, 96 licenses were granted, while between 1885 and 1890, 357 were issued.[30] The possibility that aggregations of the insane could overwhelm certain areas was taken seriously by the Commissioners, who were forced to limit the number of licenses granted in specific districts.[31] Nevertheless, the number of patients boarded-out in specially licensed dwellings continued to rise during the early years of the twentieth century, through the utilisation of new locations. Although the Board of Lunacy never overtly encouraged the expansion of special licensed houses, it was consistently enthusiastic about the advantages of such a system. With the growing proportion of patients being discharged from asylums as incurable, the existence of experienced guardians in locations where other patients had been boarded successfully, was welcomed and by 1913, 55 per cent of pauper lunatics were boarded-out in special licensed houses.[32]

CHARACTERISTICS OF PATIENTS

The Board of Lunacy had a clear perception of what constituted suitability for boarding-out. Exemption from removal to an asylum was granted to any patient who was apparently incurable, harmless and not suffering from any bodily or mental disorder requiring specialised treatment. The Commissioners were firm in their conviction that such patients did not need the discipline or treatment available in asylums and instead took up valuable space that could be better utilised by more recent cases of acute insanity. In the most suitable cases, the mental state was a well established condition of defect rather than disease where, 'so far as mind goes, their condition should as much as possible be one of simply of loss, or want, or void . . .'[33]

Those suffering from epilepsy or progressive brain disease were generally considered unsuitable for boarding-out. If restraint or confinement was necessary, or if patients were dirty, troublesome, 'offensive to public decency,' or a possible danger to themselves or other people, they were equally unsuitable. Any who were liable to erotic tendencies, or likely to refuse food were also disqualified. Patients with delusions of grandeur were usually rejected, because they were thought to be irritating to their guardians and difficult to manage. Further, any patients who were potentially curable were to be provided for in an asylum. As one physician contended, from a psychiatric standpoint boarded-out patients did not present many interesting features.[34] The most frequent disorders included mild and chronic mania, harmless delusions, dementia, congenital insanity, idiocy and, though less often, dipsomania. Patients suffering from severe delusions and active insanity were rarely found in private dwellings.

The majority of patients boarded-out between 1858 and 1880 had never been admitted to an asylum, resided with relatives and suffered from congenital forms of insanity, in particular, imbecility and idiocy. The gradual transformation in the classification of patients was one of the most notable developments. In 1858, two-thirds of those in private dwellings suffered from imbecility and idiocy. As the system expanded, the diagnostic profiles underwent marked transformation resulting from the sharp rise in patients being discharged unrecovered from asylums suffering from mania, melancholia and epilepsy, if quiescent. Increasing numbers were discharged in a state of chronic insanity, or 'passive mania', a manic condition having passed into a quiescent stage. Experience had shown that if such patients were quiet and harmless, they were as suitable as those suffering from congenital forms of insanity. The putative success of boarding-out certain potentially problematic patients each year led to the inclusion as 'suitable' of a 'greater variety of cases from a pathological point of view'.[35]

Nevertheless, proliferation of acute cases in private dwellings was never actively encouraged by the Board of Lunacy. One of the major tenets adhered to by the Commissioners was the early removal of patients to asylums, following a period of acute insanity, since it was assumed that the potential for cure was higher when patients were in immediate receipt of asylum treatment. The gradual rise in the proportion of those classified as suffering from acquired forms of insanity led to the balance between the two forms of disorder being almost equal by 1900, when it was estimated that 47 per cent of boarded-out patients were classified as congenitally defective, while 53 per cent were reported to suffer from various forms of acquired insanity, predominantly dementia.[36]

The transformation in the classification of boarded-out patients was a result of the sharp rise in those discharged unrecovered from asylums, usually to special licensed houses. In the first twenty years, patients certified insane and granted 'dispensation from removal' to an asylum made up over 80 per cent of the total number. However, by the late 1870s, the increase in former asylum patients was marked. For example, in 1873, among patients visited by one Commissioner, only 29 per cent (200) of patients had previously been in an asylum, while 71 per cent (482) had received dispensation from removal and remained in their homes.[37] Less than ten years later, in 1881, 43 per cent (324) of 758 patients visited by him were ex-asylum patients.[38] The disparity continued to widen as the system developed (Figure 5.1) and between 1885 and 1900, 65 per cent of patients had been discharged from an asylum, almost always to unrelated guardians.[39]

Imbalance in the distribution of male and female patients was a marked feature of boarding-out. Females predominated, especially in houses licensed for three or four patients. Only very rarely were four male patients boarded together in one house, the Commissioners maintaining that physically active males were too demanding for a single guardian. The ratio of males to females was approximately 100:134 among single patients and 100:187 in licensed houses. Female patients were thought to be more easily provided for, and to have less unmanageable habits, manifesting 'few or none of the propensities which would render the presence of the insane objectionable'.[41] The Board of Lunacy thus main-

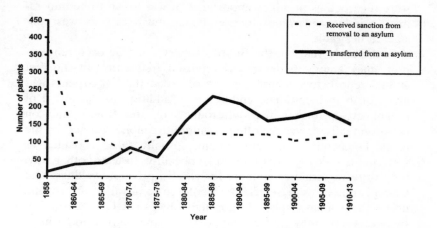

Figure 5.1   *Mode of admission to the roll of patients in private dwellings, 1858–1913*[40]

tained, with confidence, that the number of female boarders could safely be double that of male patients.

Specific risks relating to younger patients often prevented their residence in private dwellings receiving endorsement. Not only were young men considered harder to occupy, but there was greater apprehension among potential guardians regarding the safety and suitability of such patients. There were enduring concerns that young women could be sexually assaulted or become pregnant. Where there was a risk of pregnancy, or where the patient was sexually disinhibited, sanction to reside in a private dwelling was not granted. Nevertheless, one of the major criticisms levelled against the system was the risk incurred in placing vulnerable females in a community where they could be sexually assaulted. The Board of Lunacy shared the preoccupation of critics and the general public regarding the threat of hereditary degeneracy and instructed the Commissioners to warn guardians, at every visit, to keep close watch on their charges. However, the Commissioners maintained that the low tone of morality in certain districts in Scotland, particularly in the Highlands and Islands, where males and females often shared a bed, rendered the protection of imbecile or weak-minded young women a difficult task.[42] Where this was so, and such accidents

were regarded as of minor importance, it was found to be impossible to induce guardians to exercise as much care as was considered desirable.

In the early years of the Board's supervision, the occurrence of
pregnancy among patients was reported frequently. In the first
annual report, for example, it was recorded that 18 patients had
given birth to illegitimate children.[43] In addition to the threat of
pregnancy, a further fear entertained by the Board, and on
occasion realised, was the offence caused to 'public decency' by the
erotic behaviour of certain patients, usually those classified as
suffering from congenital idiocy or imbecility. In every other way,
they were regarded as suitable for care in private dwellings. The
Commissioners were reluctant to enforce removal to an asylum,
unless the women displayed 'thoroughly bad sexual propensities'.[44]
In cases where they showed 'no grossness and no talk about men,
but, rather a modest coyness, and a general bearing'[45] it was
difficult to justify their forcible removal to an asylum. Beds were
always at a premium and such patients were rarely able to benefit
from treatment in an institution. Further, the expense of providing
for them all in asylums would be prohibitive. In reference to 669
potentially vulnerable women aged between 15 and 49 years, the
Board of Lunacy announced that:

> to relegate all such imbecile women to confinement in an asylum ...
> would be nothing short of cruelty, besides entailing a waste of public
> money, since experience has shown that such persons may be cared for
> in private dwellings in such a way as to keep them safe.[46]

The occurrence both of pregnancies and manifestations of sexually active behaviour declined as local inspectors became more
familiar with the selection and supervision of patients and, by the
1890s, reports of sexual assaults were rare. While critics of boarding-out received new ammunition each time a pregnancy was
recorded, supporters maintained that incidents of assault, illegitimate pregnancy and offensive behaviour were an inherent feature
of life among the sane population and, therefore, impossible to
eradicate.

It is evident, therefore, that although imbeciles and idiots were
recognised as particularly suitable for care in private dwellings,
there was substantial variation in mental condition. The Board of
Lunacy emphasised the importance of treating each case individ-

ually, maintaining that it was impossible to define scientifically what constituted a chronic, harmless case. A number of such patients in fact proved ultimately unsuitable for domestic care. It was recommended instead that officials:

> must not attach too much importance to the terms dementia, melancholia etc as per se they do not afford any absolute or reliable indication of the suitability or otherwise of placing persons in private dwellings, because it is not so much the form of insanity which determines the propriety of boarding-out but considerations such as physical infirmities, defective habits, temper and conduct.[47]

Care and treatment of patients was held to be more important and influential than specific mental classification, which was not always possible. The Commissioners were clear about this, emphasising that the degree of success in boarding-out patients classified as suffering from similar forms of insanity varied markedly, depending upon the suitability of the guardian, the nature of accommodation, and the individual personality of each patient. To the Commissioners:

> the whole matter of boarding-out is essentially a practical one, and therefore its merits and demerits can only be ascertained by the actual boarding-out of patients who seem suitable.[48]

PROFILE OF GUARDIANS

Patients were placed under the care of relatives or strangers who were paid a weekly sum for maintenance. Although the Board of Lunacy did not undertake the selection of guardians, it laid down strict guidelines for parish officials regarding the type of person most suited to take on the guardianship of insane persons.[49] Many applications for licenses were rejected annually, either on the grounds of unsuitability of the dwelling, or incompetence of the potential guardian. Inspectors of Poor had to ascertain that applicants were of good moral character, that they were not motivated solely by the prospect of financial gain and that they were capable of providing a comfortable home. When contrasted to the attributes of guardians before the system was regulated, who might include the 'retired or bankrupt butcher or baker,'[50] it is evident that most guardians receiving approval by the Board were far superior.

The opinion of local officials, the clergyman, doctor and school-teacher was sought frequently since inspectors from distant parishes had no knowledge of the characteristics of each applicant. The possession of particular qualifications or experience was not deemed necessary; kindness and honesty were considered enough. Among those regarded as unsuitable, former asylum attendants were thought to be unsatisfactory, because, the Commissioners maintained, they were often too regimented and official in their approach to patients. In the early years of boarding-out, when inspectors of poor had only a limited number of applicants to choose from, difficulties had been encountered in the selection of guardians. The Commissioners recognised that the majority of labouring people were deterred from receiving insane patients out of fear of their behaviour and characteristics.[51] Notwithstanding this hesitancy, once the practice had become widespread, applications for patients were made by neighbours of existing guardians. The ease with which patients were accommodated, and the affectionate relationship which developed in many cases, encouraged others to make applications as people became 'educated . . . as to the practicability of caring for the insane in their homes.'[52] Thus, by the 1880s, the number of applications for patients in certain locations exceeded the number of available patients. To the Commissioners, it seemed to be 'only necessary to plant the boarding-out system in some suitable spot, for it to grow until it requires pruning at the hands of the Board'.[53]

When patients had been granted exemption from removal to an asylum, they habitually remained in their own homes. A minority, however, were removed to the care of a stranger, if their relatives were considered unsuitable, or unable, to take charge of them. The gradual decline in the proportion of patients boarded with relatives is one of the most notable developments in the system. Although not a designated part of official policy, the increase of unrelated guardians was welcomed by the Board of Lunacy, which contended that the quality of care offered was superior. Where they proved incompetent, Commissioners could intervene, and remove the patient. This was less straightforward among related guardians. If the interference of the Board was resented, and recommended improvements not forthcoming, the threat of Commissioners to remove the patient carried little weight. Relatives could remove their insane patient from the poor roll, and thus from the Board's jurisdiction.

From the mid-1870s, the trend towards placing patients with

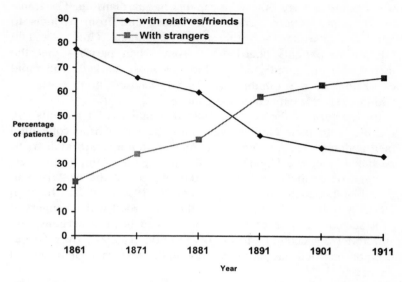

Figure 5.2   *Percentage of patients boarded with related and unrelated guardians (strangers), 1861–1911*[54]

strangers was established (Figure 5.2). In 1861, 1384 patients were in the care of relatives, representing 75 per cent of the total number in private dwellings. Among them were most of the cases regarded as unsuitable for home care. By 1875, the number boarded in this way had declined by approximately 40 per cent, to 843 patients. One explanation for this was the introduction of the parliamentary grant-in-aid in that year, which led to a rise in the numbers of weak-minded persons being classified as insane, registered as pauper lunatics and removed to asylums. Thus, while in 1861, 23 per cent (403) of patients were boarded with strangers, twenty years later, the proportion had doubled to 46 per cent (777). The extent of the transformation is further indicated by noting that of the 228 patients admitted to the roll of boarded-out patients for the first time in 1881, nearly three-quarters were committed to the care of strangers.

The transition is also explained by the unsuitability of living conditions in many urban areas where patients were often confined in small crowded rooms, without fresh air or exercise. These restrictions were thought to make their homes unsuitable even

when relatives were otherwise capable of guardianship. The transfer of many patients from their homes and from asylums to
unrelated guardians was therefore encouraged. Thus it was in
relation to patients boarded-out from urban parishes that the
increase in unrelated guardianship was most marked. The rapid
expansion in the number of special licensed houses was an
additional factor explaining the change.

By the turn of the century, the great majority of patients still
residing with their families were those suffering from congenital
mental defect. They were more numerous in poorer, rural districts,
particularly in the Highlands and Islands; for example, the percentage of insane boarded with relatives along the western sea-
board of the mainland was the same in 1900 as it had been in
1862. In contrast, the majority of those boarded with strangers in
central and southern parts of Scotland had been in asylums, and
suffered from acquired forms of insanity. By 1900, over 60 per
cent of boarded-out patients were under the care of unrelated
guardians.

DAILY LIFE

Lunacy Commissioners determined what was an acceptable level
of care for boarded-out patients. The standards of treatment and
living conditions tolerated were often adjudged to be lower than
those demanded in asylums. However, the benefits of living in a
domestic setting and the lack of confinement were held, by proponents, to be sufficient compensation. Regulations were detailed and
extensive; sufficient space for personal belongings had to be provided and it was generally recommended that patients were given
a separate bed. Much emphasis was placed on the importance of
sharing mealtimes with the guardian, who was also expected to
encourage patients in suitable occupation and exercise and in
attendance at church. Such strictures were laid down to ensure that
patients were treated, as much as possible, as members of the host
family. A major objective of boarding-out was to secure a degree
of freedom and contentment for patients, without the constraints
and discipline imposed in an institution. The relationship between
patient and host family was, therefore, of utmost importance. The
emphasis placed on this was fully justified, because:

upon this question of admission to the family life hinges the whole success of the Scottish system; where it is neglected, however perfect in other respects the guardianship may be, the results are disappointing.[55]

Nevertheless, the extent to which insane boarders could ever be wholly assimilated into the lives and homes of strangers must be questioned. Even protagonists of the system accepted that there would always be disappointing cases, where patients were regarded merely as paying residents or where they were treated cruelly. However, by the 1890s, cases of abuse were reported only rarely. In most years, less than 3 per cent of patients were returned to an asylum, for any reason, and under 1 per cent of guardians were reported to be unsatisfactory.[56] Facilitating the achievement of an increasingly high standard of care was the unbroken connection with patients experienced by a number of families. This was recognised as one of the most encouraging features of the system, particularly when contrasted with the limited and tenuous relationship between patient and asylum attendant. The experience and expertise accumulated in such cases was sometimes thought to be the determining factor in seemingly intractable patients becoming easily managed and helpful. Thus, the notable successes attained by generations of guardians were highlighted:

> it is not uncommon to find guardians who have ... when ill health and other circumstances made it impossible for them to carry on ... , handed it over to younger members of the family trained by long experience to the ways and peculiarities of patients and to the methods of dealing with them practised so successfully by their parents.[57]

The devotion and proficiency demonstrated by many guardians was a source of pleasure to Commissioners and parochial officials alike and cases outlined in annual reports testify to the generally high standards of care bestowed on those in private dwellings.

REASONS FOR THE IMPLEMENTATION OF BOARDING-OUT

Boarding-out developed rapidly throughout Scotland, facilitated by only minor legislative enactment.[58] The system was held by its proponents to offer the most convenient, natural, and most economical means of treating the chronic insane. Improvements in the physical and, on occasion, mental health of patients were reported regularly and the mortality of the boarded-out insane was always the lowest of all classes of insane.[59] The number of patients provided for in this way between 1858–1913 highlights its significance, and the amelioration it brought to recurrent difficulties created by the steady increase in asylum admissions from the 1860s, and the resulting overcrowding.

The relative costs of institutional and domestic provision were stressed without fail in discussions on the various merits of boarding-out. Foreign alienists reiterated the traditional belief that Scotsmen were preoccupied with mercenary concerns and that they accepted the system with enthusiasm for that very reason. The economic advantages certainly appeared to increase the impetus to remove patients from asylums wherever possible. This is illustrated by the following figures. In 1890, 70 per cent of registered insane patients were located in asylums, 2 per cent were in private madhouses, 7 per cent in poorhouse lunatic wards and 21 per cent in private dwellings.[60] If the latter two classes had been placed in asylums, it would have forced the erection of new buildings, at an estimated cost of £700,000.[61] This provides an indication of the economic value of the boarding-out system, with its utilisation of existing accommodation. At its peak almost 25 per cent of registered patients were boarded-out. Had they been retained in institutions, it was estimated that they would have filled six asylums. Such calculations led the Commissioners to insist that the system had become 'permanent and established ... which could not be superseded without enormous expense'.[62]

Allied to this was an increasing preoccupation with the role of the asylum, although its effect in encouraging boarding-out was varied. Physicians and lunacy administrators faced real dilemmas in their attempts to define and to clarify the appropriate function of the asylum. One important incentive to boarding-out arose from the move towards the 'hospitalisation' of asylums, manifest in a determination to adopt, where possible, the methods employed in hospitals, for investigating and treating disease. However, progress towards this was hampered by the concentration of incurable dements and idiots in asylums, demanding intensive care and attention, yet unable to benefit from any advances in hospital treatment. Their presence was seen to detract from the status of the asylum as an establishment concerned with the cure of insanity. There was, therefore, widespread enthusiasm for a policy which, in relieving overcrowded asylums, facilitated the management of curable cases. Protagonists emphasised that the reduction of pressure on accommodation allowed asylums 'to turn more to their proper purpose of acting as hospitals for the cure of the insane' instead of being 'mere lodging-houses for [those] who happen to be of unsound mind.'[63]

Advocates of the system declared, with an accuracy that was never fully tested, that an active policy of boarding-out would be 'virtually a death-blow to the existence of monster establishments' seen in England, such as Colney Hatch and Wakefield, each with populations in the mid-nineteenth century of over 1500 patients. Lindsay, for example, was confident that boarding-out 'would effectually prevent the further development of the monastic or barrack asylum system.'[64] In practice, asylum growth was never prevented; admissions continued to rise throughout the century and additions to asylum buildings were extensive. But this does not negate the impact of boarding-out in reducing the rate and extent of asylum expansion. It would be unrealistic to expect domestic provision to accommodate more than a comparatively small proportion of the insane, leaving large numbers every year to remain in confinement. Boarding-out was perceived only as a complement to asylum provision, being one of many methods of accommodation. As one Commissioner explained when questioned as to which system he preferred: 'you cannot separate the systems, the boarding-out system is purely supplementary to asylums ... you cannot do without asylums'.[65]

Boarding-out was seen to offer numerous advantages, and if its main recommendation, in the eyes of many observers, lay in its financial benefits, the fact that it also offered the potential for greater well-being for as many as 2500 patients annually cannot be overlooked. The major reasons for developing the system stand up to rigorous criticism. Nevertheless, Morel's warning should be remembered:

> in our disposition to deprecate monumental asylums, let us not be carried to the opposite extreme. Neither colonisation, or family treatment can be applied indifferently to all the insane. Many will be unsuitable at all times ... I do not reject family treatment, but the system to overrule all systems is the clinical one.[66]

CRITICISMS AND SHORTCOMINGS

A system of provision which catered for up to 25 per cent of registered insane patients attracted considerable comment from those concerned with lunacy administration, throughout the United Kingdom and worldwide. While criticisms were forthcoming, and enduring, many were easily refuted or dismissed, and as the system expanded, a decline in the ferocity and validity of attacks is evident. Complaints in the early years focused on potential neglect and injudicious treatment of often severely disturbed and vulnerable patients, by uneducated, untrained and, possibly, mercenary guardians. However, although the rate of maintenance paid allowed for a small profit, guardians were usually from the 'respectable poor', and while appreciative of the money, did not depend on it for survival. Far from reflecting the image portrayed by critics, and even though they were neither learned or affluent, the majority, in fact belonged to the respectable working class, often occupied as crofters, small farmers, carpenters, weavers, labourers and shoemakers and of the same, or higher, social class than asylum attendants. Instances of abuse or neglect recorded in the annual reports of the Board of Lunacy were, after the first few years, isolated occurrences. By the 1880s, the Commissioners were confident that, with close official supervision, such abuses could not remain undetected. Increasingly favourable reports from parish visitors give credence to their claim and indicate that detailed recommendations for improvement were largely implemented. Concurrently, criticisms by commentators that patients were received only for financial gain, and were generally neglected or exploited by poverty-stricken, uneducated crofters, declined in urgency, prompting claims that guardians were 'as a rule, faithful and intelligent, and often found to devote themselves to the discharge of duties exceptionally burdensome.'[67]

Although the nature and extent of supervision of patients was commented on adversely by critics, the Commissioners were confident that the number of official visits ensured that persistent abuse or neglect could not remain undetected. In conjunction with visits from Commissioners, patients were visited officially by inspectors of poor twice annually, but in practice with greater frequency. In smaller parishes, inspectors lived in close proximity to many of the patients, thereby facilitating frequent, surprise visits. Their official visits were often made in the company of deputations from the parochial board of origin. The parochial medical officer made four visits annually, advising on the management and control of the patients. His duties included ensuring that patients received sufficient outdoor exercise and suitable employment. The food was inspected and recommendations for dietary improvements made. It was also recognised that the most effective safeguard against abuse was the unofficial supervision of neighbours. Patients wandered freely about their village, and were well known to local residents. It was considered likely that instances of neglect would soon be brought to the attention of an official, prompting one Commissioner to declare that:

> [it is] a distinct advantage that most of the aggregations ... are in villages or hamlets where there are many residents not directly concerned with the boarding-out system, and where the everyday life of all the inhabitants is seen and freely commented on by the community at large.[68]

Critics also maintained that only very limited types of patients were suitable for such provision; that there were few opportunities for therapeutic intervention; that patients lacked stimulation and were resented by the local community and that the few official annual visits could do little to ameliorate their quality of life. It was argued, too, that 'even the romance of rurality' and the 'associations of country life which have been cast around this scheme, must be sorely invaded, if not dispelled.'[69] Not only were some patients boarded in and around towns, but conditions in many villages were hardly comparable to the pictures of rustic charm so widely propagated in romantic Victorian literature. The lack of modern amenities such as lighting, heating, adequate nutrition and organised recreation, all available in asylums, was deplored by critics. Even the most enthusiastic supporters recognised certain inherent disadvantages to a system which placed insane people at a distance from the control and discipline of an institution. Despite the validity of some of these claims, there was consensus among Commissioners and medical observers alike that the advantages of home life and personal liberty could be sufficient compensation. This recognition of balance, that boarding-out had a role to play in lunacy administration, although not necessarily any greater than other forms of provision, contributed to the success of the system.

Particular concerns were expressed regarding personal safety, the destruction of property by potentially violent lunatics, offences against public morals and the reduction in house prices. Tuke, for example, observed the apprehension among some villagers towards patients in Kennoway and reported complaints against the constant presence of 'such depressing and melancholy objects.'[70] In view of the number of patients boarded-out, often closely congregated in small communities, there were, in fact, remarkably few objections against their presence, and those reaching the Board were investigated thoroughly. On no occasion was the complaint regarded with such gravity as to warrant a change in policy.

There was sustained anxiety regarding the possible production and perpetuation of hereditary degeneracy and fear that the presence of the insane could have a detrimental effect on the host family. This concern was considered in depth by the Commissioners, who contended that:

> the influence of the lunatics on their associates cannot be entertained as one of the primary considerations determining the disposal of them. The law requires that if he is dangerous or offensive, he must be sent to an asylum, but it does not recognise the existence of any other disagreeable :accompaniments of lunacy which would entitle society to isolate the lunatic. If sanctioned by the Board for a private dwelling, it shows that he is not offensive to public decency or dangerous . . .[71]

Nevertheless, the potential threat to the well-being of host families was of sufficient importance to merit inclusion on the agenda of successive Home Relief Congresses between 1901 and 1904.[72] Although there was agreement among delegates that the companionship of the insane in institutions could be prejudicial to the mental well-being of staff, they did not consider that this was necessarily true of those living in private dwellings, where the illness of patients was less severe. Further, the freedom available to patients meant that guardians did not have the same unremittingly close contact with them throughout the day. One Commissioner estimated that, by 1908, 10,000 people had had some form of contact with the 2,780 patients in private dwellings in Scotland.[73] However, he claimed that in 14 years of inspections, only five cases of insanity had occurred in the families of unrelated guardians, and these, he held, were unlikely to be attributable to the presence of the patients.[74]

Concern for the well-being of the family was linked with the specific fear that children were affected adversely by growing up with an insane person in the household and several alienists questioned the long term effects on children. One physician remarked:

> I remember with horror even now, a single day spent in a home in Scotland where two defective members of the family were being cared for. It was days before I could think of it at all calmly ... Am I wrong? My thought is for the children.[75]

Hack Tuke, a consistent critic of certain aspects of boarding-out, was convinced of the unsuitability of boarding-out the insane in houses containing children or young women. In his opinion, the risk of moral injury to the family, especially to younger members, was often overlooked.[76] Despite their enthusiasm for boarding-out, the Commissioners did not dismiss these fears, rather they acknowledged that the selection of patients for the special circumstances in which they were placed, determined the success of the system. Patients who were irritable, unsympathetic to children, or likely to use offensive language in houses where there were young families, clearly jeopardised outcome. In a few cases, therefore, the removal of a patient was recommended due to these perceived risks, although such occurrences proved rare.[77] When one Commissioner, Macpherson, began visits to patients, he had expected to find the association of the insane to be unhealthy to children. In fact, thorough inquiries among doctors, schoolmasters and parents had removed his doubts. He reported that guardians found such an idea amusing, and that many insisted that the presence of the insane in their homes was beneficial to their children, making them more considerate and kindly. In addition, it was observed that no doctor had ever come across any ill-effects on guardians or their children.[78] Commissioners remained confident, therefore, that under a carefully supervised and controlled administration, no adverse influence on children or adults could be traced to the presence of insane boarders. Citing 'many pleasing instances of great solicitude and devotion,' they concluded that, 'the care of the weak produces a healthy altruism'[79] and that caring for insane patients could produce an elevating effect on guardians and their surroundings, as it raised the standard of household order and cleanliness.

Supporters argued that the moral and social objections were more sentimental and imaginary than sustainable. The limited number of severe accidents and assaults against patients were emphasised by proponents. Among even the most vocal of critics was a recognition that carefully supervised and controlled, the policy could provide some relief to overcrowded asylums. For this reason, it was generally accepted as a useful component of lunacy administration where the inherent advantages outweighed any potential risks to the patient and the community in which they were placed.

CONCLUSIONS

Foucault's argument that tolerance for the deviant within the community was diminishing throughout the nineteenth century has little to support it when applied to the boarding-out system in Scotland.[80] Public concern about the presence of the insane, although clearly apparent initially, declined steadily as it became evident that they were, in general, neither dangerous nor offensive to public decency. The actual expansion of boarding-out in any district indicates a gradual acceptance of the insane, with applications for boarders often in excess of the number of available placements. In addition, the educative effect the presence of the insane had upon the community was emphasised. The Board of Lunacy maintained that mental defect became regarded less to be feared, and more deserving of sympathy and understanding. This may indicate undue optimism on the part of certain observers. Such an outlook has not been attained even today, but it is apparent that, historically, some local populations were increasingly willing to accept insane boarders. Towards the end of the century, the editors of the *Journal of Mental Science* were able to announce that boarding-out had become an approved and integral part of lunacy administration in Scotland and that:

> every good Scot accepts it as ... an eminently satisfactory solution of difficulties with which a nation is brought face to face in dealing with the mass of chronic lunacy.[81]

The extent to which boarding-out created the opportunity for asylums to represent themselves as places of cure, rather than of confinement, should be assessed further, particularly in view of Scull's insistence that the asylum in the nineteenth century was merely 'a dumping ground . . . for a heterogeneous mass of physical and mental wrecks'.[82] This brief study provides concrete evidence challenging Scull's thesis. The very existence of a system in Scotland, if not elsewhere, which endeavoured to remove such patients from the constraints of asylums, counters his claim. Boarding-out offered the benefits of domestic life for selected patients, while removing the accumulation of chronic cases from asylums. In turn, this enabled greater concentration on the development and implementation of methods of cure for asylum patients potentially receptive to such treatment.

The sustained attention and attempts to implement the 'Scotch system' remain one of the most remarkable aspects of the boarding-out policy. The number and frequency of references to boarding-out in Scotland in European and American journals is exceptional. Notwithstanding the greater age and fame of Gheel, it is rare to find an article on family care which does not refer to Scotland. The system was heralded widely as an innovative, effective, experiment which merited close replication overseas. Colonial, European and American specialists were commissioned by their Governments to visit 'in order to see the modus operandi and these have returned with such favourable accounts that other nations are following suit'.[83] American observers, for example, were, almost without exception, enthusiastic proponents, advocating its adoption in their country and convinced that 'nowhere else has boarding-out been so extensively and so successfully tried as in Scotland'.[84] It is certain that the Scottish system had an enduring and far-reaching impact upon the development of family care throughout the world. Even where it was not imitated directly, it was closely assessed and widely referred to. The pride of Scottish Commissioners in their development and control of such a pioneering system was justified by the scale of interest provoked. The declaration of the German alienist, Jolly, was echoed internationally, with his belief that 'in the Scottish family system there lies an advance in lunacy administration . . . the fundamental principles may be adopted with confidence from Scotland'.[85] By 1900, similar systems were in place worldwide.

However, despite the activity in Scotland, a cohesive, centrally-organised system of domestic provision failed to flourish in England, Wales or Ireland. Although similar concerns about overcrowded asylums were voiced throughout the United Kingdom, the option of accommodating patients in private dwellings was rarely advocated. With the exception of Chancery lunatics, those in the community received little systematic supervision or regulation.[86] While there was considerable support for boarding-out by a number of prominent physicians, including Maudsley, Stallard and Bucknill, lunacy administrators proved unable, or unwilling to implement this potentially valuable adjunct to institutional care. In 1867, for example, the proportion of patients boarded-out in Scotland was well over twice that in England, prompting the suggestion that, 'one or other of the systems must be wrong, if 27 per cent of pauper lunatics of Scotland can be treated at home, so must they in England.'[87] In Wales, large numbers of patients were accommodated in the community throughout the nineteenth century. Some reports suggest that the proportion was comparable to that in Scotland; throughout the 1880s, approximately 25 per cent of all insane patients were in private dwellings.[88] However, such patients were, as in England, under no official control or regulation and, therefore, not formally boarded-out. Patients who remained outside the constraints of asylum provision went unsupervised and unreported.

The scepticism and apathy surrounding any attempt to introduce a formally controlled policy of boarding-out south of the Border was remarkable, in view of the widely heralded success in Scotland. While Scottish Comissioners promoted the policy with great enthusiasm and dedication, boarding-out was met with ambivalence by many physicians and widespread rejection from Commissioners in the rest of Britain.

A number of questions are prompted about the reasons underlying the particular and striking success of the policy in Scotland. The ease with which the policy was adopted was attributed by some to the philanthropy of the Scots and the 'staid, unostentatiously affectionate character of the people, traditionally noted for their attachment to the weak.'[89] A further explanation could lie in the comparative poverty of the nation and the resulting willingness of an impoverished population to receive insane boarders, but this does not stand up to rigorous appraisal. Wealthier countries, most notably Germany, implemented a similar policy of boarding-out with marked success in the late-nineteenth century. Clouston suggested that the smallness of the country, which enabled Commissioners to know each asylum and its local circumstances in some detail, and the lack of any prominent scandal or lunacy law suit, contributed to the extension of a policy which was dependent upon extensive supervision and the acceptance of the insane in the community.[90] In fact, the most convincing explanation relates to the nature, extent and effectiveness of the supervisory control exercised by the Board of Lunacy, and its unwavering endorsement of the principle of domiciliary care. Boarding-out flourished in Scotland not because of any particular differences between Scotland and other countries, or specific characteristics of its indigenous population, but because of the enduring enthusiasm and control exercised by the Commissioners. Without their consistent encouragement and pressure, it is certain that boarding-out in Scotland would have remained little more than an *ad hoc*, uncontrolled, way of providing for the insane.

Despite increasing recourse to organised systems of family care across the world, Scottish lunacy administrators were accurate in claiming that no other country had such large numbers of insane patients residing in private dwellings under such extensive control and protection from the State. Nevertheless the policy never attained the prominence of the open-door system or of ideals of moral management. Although the Board of Lunacy endorsed it wholeheartedly, only a limited number of asylum superintendents championed boarding-out, even if the majority put it into practice. By contrast, the earlier movement towards abolishing the employment of mechanical restraint, popularised by Conolly, although widely criticised initially, was almost universally adopted. Increasing freedom within asylums was implemented across the United Kingdom, usually with enthusiasm.[91] Despite its more circumscribed appeal, the system of boarding-out can be seen as a natural progression of a lunacy administration which, recognising the advantages of more humanitarian treatment of the insane in asylums, also acknowledged an active policy of non-institutional provision as a valuable supplement.

A system which catered for almost a quarter of registered insane patients warrants greater research attention than it has so far been awarded. Boarding-out offered an early form of care in the com-

munity, closely regulated and supervised, or, to echo the assessment of Henderson, was 'the first medico-social experiment in the
community care of the mentally afflicted'.[92] As a contribution to
the on-going debate regarding the best mode of provision for the
mentally ill, it is maintained that the innovative system of boarding-
out in Scotland in the nineteenth century had much to recommend
it. Johnson's declaration regarding the role of history appears
particularly apposite when set in the context of current concerns:

> to judge rightly of the present, we must oppose it to the past; for all
> judgement is comparative, and of the future nothing can be known . . .
> The present state of things is the consequence of the former; and it is
> natural to inquire what were the sources of the good that we enjoy, or
> the evils that we suffer. If we act only for ourselves, to neglect the study
> of history is not prudent. If we are entrusted with the care of others, it
> is not just.

CHAPTER SIX

Enclosing and disclosing lunatics within the family walls: domestic psychiatric regime and the public sphere in early nineteenth-century England

Akihito Suzuki

At the outset, in order to put the concept of psychiatry and community in a historiographical context, it seems helpful to distinguish two interpretive models in the present scholarship in the history of psychiatry from the early modern period to the nineteenth century. One is centred around the psychiatric institution; the other lays emphasis on what happened within family. In the institutional model, the sinew of the development of psychiatry was incarcerating institutions (asylums and psychiatric hospitals, as well as General Hospitals of the *ancien régime*, houses of correction under the Old Poor Law, and workhouses under the Old and New Poor Laws), with their medical, legal, political, and ideological apparatuses. The most forceful and well-known advocate of this view is Michel Foucault.[1] In his *Histoire de la folie*, Foucault identified the starting point of the prototype of modern psychiatry in the creation of public institutions for confining lunatics with petty criminals and vagabonds by the French absolutist state. The subsequent unfolding of psychiatry was, according to Foucault, the development of different techniques to cope with the incarcerated insane within institutional walls. Similarly, Andrew Scull's account of the making of English psychiatry is framed around the creation of the nation-wide system of publicly-funded county asylums, which emerging 'psychiatrists' or 'mad-doctors' appropriated as the power-base to consolidate their professional status.[2]

The 'domestic' approach, on the other hand, emphasizes the importance of the family's private need to cope with the problem of the lunacy of their family member. The work of Michael MacDonald best represents this direction of investigation.[3] In his examination of the psychiatric practice of Richard Napier, Mac-Donald has clarified that Napier's psychiatric encounters were initiated by the clients, rather than being imposed by an authoritarian and disciplinarian figure. The patients and their families disclosed their personal and domestic problems, and the sympathetic clergyman attentively listened to them, tried to console the patients, soothed their personal agony, and sometimes forced them into behaving in socially acceptable ways. One of Roy Porter's arguments on psychiatry in eighteenth-century England follows a somewhat similar line, stressing the role played by the family in the development of profit-making institutions for the insane.[4]

There are several recent attempts at integrating the two models by self-consciously examining the interaction of the institutional and the domestic. Robert Castel views French asylum committal as the post-Revolutionary replacement of *lettres de cachet*, which had been a powerful means for a patriarch to punish wayward family members. From this, Yannick Ripa argues that the way in which domestic problems were settled was influenced by the presence of public asylums in the day-to-day landscape of late nineteenth-century French society.[5] Ripa maintains that alongside recourse to police, the 'voluntary' committal of lunatics gave the family another means to settle the family discord by mobilizing public authority's intervention, and asylums served the purpose of suppressing juvenile and female domestic rebellion as well as silencing political and social protest. In her article on committal to a late-nineteenth-century Parisian asylum, Patricia Prestwich shows that the family's increasing demand for institutional psychiatric service created a new role for the asylum and its doctors: the asylum and alienists were unexpectedly seen as a convenient and temporary access-point for settling or relieving domestic problems.[6] In her study of Boston Psychopathic Hospital, Elizabeth Lunbeck has perceptively pointed out that family did not necessarily protect its members from society's oppressions, surveillance, and control; rather, family became a powerful vehicle of 'domination, management, and regulation of individuals' that were functions of the hospital and medical authority.[7] These recent works have shown that psychiatry in the past was shaped by a multitude of complex bilateral interactions between the family's need and the institution's power and authority. On the one hand, the power of psychiatrist and public authority embodied in institutions penetrated into domestic realm, sometimes reinforcing the patriarchal power over wives and children, sometimes transforming the power-structure within the family.[8] On the other hand, the psychiatric apparatus designed, established and maintained by the state or other public authorities was under constant improvisation by the clients, to which doctors had to respond by inventing – sometimes unwillingly – new roles for themselves.

These sophisticated analyses, however, tend to bypass the intermediary area between the family and the institution, a vast realm which lies outside the immediate family, and at the same time, outside the institutional walls. Only marginal attention has been paid by historians of psychiatry to the role played by agents in this middle area, namely, extra-familial relatives and kin, neighbours, men and women on the street, except in studies of 'care in community' as an alternative to or antithesis of asylum.[9] Although organized provision for the insane outside the institution is an important phenomenon, there existed other aspects in the extra-familial or 'public' sphere, which were crucial in moulding the culture of psychiatry in nineteenth-century England.[10] The aim of this paper is to fill the historiographical lacuna and to examine the influence exercised by community, neighbourhood, and public space in general on the general outlook of Victorian attitude to the insane. The family with an insane member attempted to construct a barrier of surveillance, control, and management between private and public spheres, and between the domestic realm and the world outside in their attempt to *contain* the patients within the private sphere. At the same time, the barrier was under constant threat, and vulnerability was intrinsic to its nature. This was largely because of particularly strong interest which people outside took in lunatics in the private sphere. Motivated by kindness, sense of justice, interested concern, and, of course, nosy curiosity, neighbours, friends, the crowd on the street forced their way into the closed domestic world in which the family tried hard to enclose the patient. In other words, the existence of a lunatic in a family itself destabilized the boundary between the public and private spheres and invited forceful intervention from the outside world.

A few words are necessary about the sources used herein to explore this somewhat nebulous area. In many ways, the records of the court of commission *de lunatico inquirendo* or commission of lunacy by inquisition provide extremely rich material. The Commission of Lunacy (not to be confused with the Lunacy Commission or Commissioners *in* Lunacy) was a legal mechanism, allowing any person to ask the Lord Chancellor to examine whether a person in question was a lunatic or an idiot, and, if so, to deprive him or her of some of his or her civil rights, and to appoint a person (usually the next of kin) to take care of his or her property.[11] In order to prove the insanity or sanity of the alleged lunatic, the petitioner or the respondent produced witnesses. These were often family friends or neighbours, whose experience with the alleged lunatic was reported in detail. The family's difficulty with coping with the alleged lunatic was also fully described (usually by servants and keepers, who were directly responsible for taking care of him or her), with strong emphasis being laid on the embarrassment caused by their odd behaviour in the public spaces such as the street, church, places for business and so on. These commissions took place in an open court before a jury and large audience. Most importantly, the Commission of Lunacy was attended by a host of shorthand reporters for national newspapers, whose fully detailed accounts of the examination appeared in the paper the next day. Between 1825 and 1845, there are about 150 reports of the Commission of Lunacy in *The Times*. Those trial reports usually filled several columns, occasionally more than an entire page for a week or even longer period. These newspaper reports, which have been utilized only partially in the history of psychiatry, form the core material of the argument below.[12]

There are, however, two limitations in this source material. Firstly, the Commission of Lunacy had a very large bias toward the wealthy sector of the society, and the practice discussed below seems to have been limited to the upper- and middle-classes. The emphasise on the code of respectable behaviour and on the sacrilization of family were disproportionately found among the upper sections of the society, if not specific to them. The second limitation is that of periodization. For unknown reasons, regular coverage of Commission of Lunacy trials in *The Times* was restricted in the two decades between 1825 and 1845, and the number of the cases reported declined sharply after the period. It is thus difficult to tell whether the patterns presented below were common features found throughout the long history of the legal practice. This chapter concentrates on the structure of the private and public sphere framed around the issue of insanity in the wealthy section of the English society at a given time, largely leaving the question of the class-specificity and periodization open to further investigation.

The word 'community', with its implications of shared values, toleration, and the spirit of co-operation, now often carries positive meanings and associations. The resonance in discussion over modern psychiatric care is no exception: with all its shortcomings, care in community is something to be defended and developed. In the nineteenth century, which was the heyday of asylum, people thought otherwise, many equating the growth of public institutional provision for the insane with the march of enlightened humanitarianism, Christianity, and medical science.[13] Moreover, the Victorian period was also the pinnacle of family and domestic values, and well-off families who had to take care of mental patient must have seen the idea of 'community care' as out-and-out anathema. From what was reported in detail at the trials of Commissions of Lunacy, one can see how hard families tried keep their insane members out of the *notice* of the public. To be brief, their basic strategy was to contain and enclose the lunatic in the private sphere and to prevent his or her lunacy becoming a public problem.

It is proverbial that insanity was a great stigma to the family, who tried hard to conceal the existence of insanity in the family blood.[14] To conceal and hide the physical presence of their insane members, the family had several options. Committal to a licensed house and boarding them at a private lodging attended by keepers were usual choices, while secretly shutting the lunatic up in the attic in one's own house, immortalized in *Jane Eyre*, seems to have been relatively uncommon.[15] Besides these radical means, which uprooted the patients from their ordinary lifestyle, there were more unstable makeshift means, achieved at their own houses, to prevent the lunatic from 'exposing' his or her lunacy in a public space--on the street, at church, at public dinner-table, at a place of business, and so on. Without removing the patient into an abode designed to detain inmates, the family continued to live with the patient and could persuade, influence, or intimidate the lunatic into behaving well in public places, avoiding public attention and keeping up ordinary appearances.

The most prominent concern within this makeshift domestic regime, reported in court, was to control property transactions of the lunatic in question, from minor purchase and signing a cheque for a small amount to transactions to an entire estate. There were a variety of means to achieve this end. The most simple but effective one was not to give any pocket money to the lunatic. Before Mather R. Ebbing, formerly a merchant with extensive business, was put in Kensington House, he temporarily lived with his sister. A servant testified: 'His sister took his purse. He used not to pay his own bills when I knew him, but his sister discharged them.' The fourth Earl of Portsmouth, who had an annual income of £20,000, did not have the command of money and had to sometimes borrow money from his gardener.[16] Another simple and crude solution was to deprive the lunatic of access to shops. Lady Charlotte Sherard was kept in a private asylum but does not seem to be particularly violent or dangerous. When she wished to walk about, the medical attendant did not allow her to do so, 'as she was so extravagantly disposed of money', and 'her trustee, aware of this improvident expenditure of money, desired her to draw no more draughts on Messrs. Goslings.'[17] Similarly, personal vigilance over the lunatic at a shop was sometimes necessary. Rosa Bagster, a weak-minded heiress of a wealthy London printer and a subject of a Commission of Lunacy in 1832, was said to have 'never made a single purchase' during the whole course of her life. One of the governesses recalled that she was so ignorant of the value of money that she would have paid a shilling or a sovereign for a yard of two-penny riband at a shop, if the governess had not been with her.[18] When Barbara White, whose obsessional grief over her deceased mother and some bizarre delusions alarmed her relatives, went to an ironmonger's shop in Oxford Street and wanted to purchase an iron bath to prevent people from seeing her, her clerk prevented the purchase in a discreet way, without making his control too overt: he 'motioned to the shopman not to serve her.'[19] Although these examples sound minor, these disruptions signalled for the family and other people a potential danger of more serious damage to property. When Miss Louisa Ridge, of a wealthy family near Yarmouth, was found to have paid her poulterer's bill without inquiring the price of articles, her relative expressed her fear: 'she was very imprudent in her domestic concerns, and it is my opinion that any designing person could have easily duped her out of property.'[20] Outside the protected domestic sphere, the family feared, lunatics would be easy prey to unscrupulous wretches. The public sphere, with its relatively free contact between people, meant danger to the lunatic and his or her property.

The surveillance of female behaviour, especially those acts related with the sexuality of young single women, was particularly tight, partly because large amounts of property were often at stake. The family of Princess Bariatinski, a weak-minded daughter between an English mother and a Russian nobleman, finally petitioned a commission of lunacy when they found that the Princess wrote a letter to one Mr. Newman:

> Since I have had the pleasure of seeing you I have thought of a pleasant scheme. I think I should like to go to Walmer [sic]. I dare say Mrs. Brooks will let me go with you any day, and I should like to have a child very much.[21]

The family had to prevent the Princess's pleasant scheme of having a child with Mr Newman before it was too late, to protect the family reputation and to prevent the unwanted property transaction through marriage.

Likewise, the sexuality of weak-minded Rosa Bagster, who also successfully ran away with and married a man, was constantly subject to subtle and almost invisible vigilance. One Mr. Windus, a family friend, recollected that at a public dinner held at the Mansion House, he took his seat next to Rosa. He did not know her before, and he paid her the usual courtesy of inviting her to take wine. At that moment, 'she turned round and looked at me very full in the face'. In a few minutes, 'she said she was in love' and then told him that 'she was going to be married to Mr Jupp'. Mr Windus was astonished at the conduct of the granddaughter of the Lord Mayor, which he communicated to Crowder's family and the chaplain. He was not only concerned with just Rosa's breach of decorum at the dinner-table, but also anxious about her over-familiarity, her over-intimate conversation, and the lack of the sense of genteel distance which a girl of her class was expected to keep between herself and members of the other sex. Mr Windus, therefore, advised that 'she ought not be sent into company without being "fenced" in ... by female friends on each side.'[22] He clearly thought that the family should create a covert and discreet gender barrier and prohibit Rosa's uncontrolled association with men, especially on public occasions.

The breach of the code of behaviour of the lunatic in public space posed serious problems and embarrassment for the family. Particularly, serious misconduct at church, one of the most important public spaces, embarrassed the family great deal.[23] The family of Lord Suffolk was so shocked when Princess Bariatinsky laughed, put out her tongue, and made faces at church, that they stopped allowing her to attend service.[24] The family of Solomon Cohen thought that his serious departure from a rule of Jewish religious ritual was 'the first positive indication of his insanity'. It is notable that the family thought this breach of public religious behaviour, which was in itself harmless (rinsing his mouth with water), was greater evidence of insanity, than the serious domestic violence threatened by him (putting his sister's baby upon the fire).[25]

Likewise, the family of Rosa Bagster were gravely concerned with her behaviour on the street, as well as at the public dinner table. One thing which particularly annoyed the family was 'the crowd' in town. Miss Clayton, one of many governesses of Rosa, remembered that Rosa's violent and strange behaviour assembled a crowd at every public place they went to:

> I accompanied, Mrs and Miss Bagster, in August last, on a tour to the West of England. . . . In the course of this tour, Miss Bagster conducted herself very violently; and at Lauceston, she tore her mother's bonnet, also Mrs. Horn's bonnet and dress, and threw the reticule, and her mother's watch, out of the carriage window. We were not got out of the town at the time, and a crowd assembled; . . . It was 9 o'clock when we got to Holdsworthy, and it was past 11 before we could get her into the inn. Miss Bagster attempted to kick a witness, but was restrained by some persons in the crowd which had assembled. Miss Bagster laughed at the crowd, and asked what they were staring at her for. . . . When we were about to leave, a great crowd of persons had assembled to see her, in consequence of her conduct on the preceding evening. . . . [In Dover], She suddenly rushed upon her mother, tore her hair, and threw her shoes and other articles out of the window into the street. On the quays also she behaved and conducted herself in a most violent manner before all the spectators. . . . At New Romney, I believe, she behaved in a most childish manner, and the passengers laughed at her, and inquired if she was in her senses.[26]

The governess was aware that outside the protected private space of the carriage and a room in the inn, there existed an open public space with curious people who would assemble into a crowd looking at and laughing at lunatics.

As is suggested in one passage in the quote above ('We were not got out of the town at the time . . .'), town was particularly full of such curious people. When John Brome insulted and struck women at York Place and Bond Street, he collected a crowd around him and Sir C. Aldis, his relative and medical attendant, had to get him into a cab and take him home.[27] The private space of a carriage or a cab was precarious, however. Princess Bariatinski was put into the carriage but 'laugh[ed] out of the windows in such a manner that people would frequently stop to look at her.'[28] Even the private house had windows to the world outside. Mrs Catherine Jennings, a lunatic widow with large property, lived in Windsor. When the castle was illuminated in honour of the marriage of Queen Victoria, she 'got out of bed, and remained an hour and a-half standing at the window looking into the street, causing a mob of 200 or 300 persons to assemble, with nothing on but her night chemise.'[29]

When there was no attempt by the family to contain the insane behaviour within the private space and curb its exhibition, things might grow wild. Such was the case with Daniel Gundry, an insane gentleman of means living in Albany. When his wife, who had been continually abused by him since marriage, finally left him, he was entirely left on his own:

> [He] sat upon the [horse] opposite the door for an hour and a quarter, making the most extraordinary gesticulations all the time. He collected a crowd of about 200 persons round him, and it was eventually found necessary to send for the police to disperse them. . . . Latterly, whenever he went out on horseback, he was followed by a mob calling after him, 'There goes mad Gundry.'[30]

Unlike most people today, who, when passing by a lunatic on the street, try their best to ignore him or her or to conceal their curiosity, the mobs and crowds mentioned in the testimonies were highly and openly interested in watching lunatics. The family had to hide the lunatic from their curious eyes.

The crowd were, however, far from just curious or searching for entertainment of freak show.[31] As the social history of 'mob' and popular movement has clarified, the crowd had their own sense of justice and morality and often acted accordingly. Especially when they believed that a wrongful confinement was going to take place, they frustrated the attempt. G.M. Burrows, a leading London alienist in the 1820s explained as follows:

It frequently happens, in removing a lunatic from one place to another, that he is very violent, or endeavours, by making artful appeals to those near him, to attract their attention, and raise a feeling to rescue him. In such a case, the populace are almost always sure to side with the lunatic, and sometimes liberate him.[32]

It seems that Burrows frequently experienced the crowd's intervention. When keepers of his asylum tried to remove Edward Davies, a neurotic tea-merchant, from Furnival's Inn Coffee House to Davies's own house at the request of Davies's mother, the coach was stopped by people at the coffee house, and it was only by the production of a faked certificate of lunacy signed by Burrows that the coach could go on.[33] In *The Mysteries of the Madhouse*, an anonymous fiction published in 1847 which dealt with the wrongful confinement of a young gentleman, a very similar scene was depicted: a coach arrived at an inn; an appeal was made by the alleged lunatic to people around him or her; people assembled, involved themselves in the situation, and showed their readiness to rescue the alleged lunatic.[34] An alleged lunatic's appeal to strangers for help at public places and the intervention on behalf of the lunatic seems to have been a commonly held idea in the mental landscape of early nineteenth-century English people. From the viewpoint of the family, therefore, there existed at a public space the danger of the disruption and frustration of the control over the lunatic: from the lunatic's viewpoint, a public space meant a greater chance to escape the family's control with the aid of strangers. Perhaps the protesting Rosa Bagster might have been vaguely aware of the existence of this culture of public place, sensing that she could embarrass the family more effectively by carrying her struggle in public places with potential enemy against the family and potential allies with her.

As well as anonymous crowds on the street, familiar faces in neighbourhood seems to have been often dreaded by the family, who attempted to limit and control the lunatic's contact with neighbours. One tactic of avoiding neighbours and removing the patient is seen in account of Nathaniel Hastings Middleton, a London banker whose mother became insane in 1816.[35] When the news of the mother's mental breakdown came to Middleton, he was first optimistic and did not take the situation seriously. Before he actually saw her, he wrote that this mother would benefit from living with his family with the children at his own house, offering kind hands of help to the afflicted mother:

> the seeing and cohabiting with our darling children might successfully tend to stimulate her depressed sensibilities, and the known disposition of the two elder gentle creatures [his wife and himself], to sympathise with, and soothe those they see in affliction, will be pleasing, & comfortable to her.[36]

The promised 'known disposition of the two elder gentle creatures', however, evaporated quickly as soon as he saw the actual state of the mother. Just after he saw her, Middleton suddenly changed his opinions, writing that no benefit could be expected from 'receiving her into our family, or even having her near us', since she was totally incapable of appreciating the tenderness and attention of his sympathetic and kind family.[37] The true motive of his was, no doubt, his fear of rumour among his neighbours. A few days later, he wrote as follows:

> With respect to an asylum for my severely-visited parent, I conceive that [his house in] Brighton should be the *last* place proposed – she would not be there twenty-four hours, before, busy slander, ever mischievously inclined, would noise throughout the whole town, that Mrs Middleton, once so provident, and highly-gifted, was under surveillance & incompetent to the management of her own affairs, and thus a stigma would be thrown upon herself and family, and a publicity given to the occurrence which would aggravate our misfortunes, and render her return to the world, and to her friends, doubly difficult . . .[38]

Instead, he proposed that the mother might be better placed in 'a small house in an open situation, on the sunny side of London, somewhere about Clapham or Stockwell'.[39] His fear of rumour and his preference for suburban anonymity made him give up living with and providing tender care to the mad mother. In this case, the power of rumour removed the patient away from the family of her immediate son to a private lodging in a comfortable but remote and anonymous place.

The Smith family near Birmingham reacted differently, but the fear of neighbours played no less significant a role in their strategy in coping with their weak-minded brother, George Smith. Isaac Smith, the father of George, was a wealthy farmer in the county of Stafford. George was born around 1785, and he had been feeble-minded from his early childhood. His parents treated him with affection and tenderness, according to the lawyer for the plaintiff, 'as was often found where infirmities had fallen upon a poor child'. The mother, who had mainly taken care of him, died in 1807, and the father's death followed in 1812. After their death, the major duty of taking care of him fell upon the shoulders of Sarah, the eldest sister of the family.[40] Perhaps Sarah was the only member of the family whom the parents could ask to play the role of a full-time house-nurse for George. Many servants and ex-servants to the Smith family testified to the almost religious self-sacrifice of Sarah in taking care of George.[41]

There is no reason to cast cynical doubt onto the devotion of Sarah and tender care of the rest of the family. The problem was that all these acts of familial love, affection and tenderness went on behind a strictly closed door. Soon after the mother's death, the father moved the family to a new farm in Mucklestone Wood and kept George in a separate room in the house. The window of the room where he was lodged was literary bricked up, on the pretence that they found the light tended to irritate George and to throw him into fits. One of the purposes of their doing so was obviously to hide George from the sight of other people. George was hidden even from the sight of visitors to the house: although Martha Haskett described herself as having 'an intimate knowledge of Mr Smith's family for the last 30 years', she testified that 'she had never seen George but once in her life.'[42] The Smith family's secrecy about George aroused curiosity and suspicion of people around, which in turn aggravated the family's nervous concern to hide him. Whether true or not, a newspaper article said that 'the brother and sister then spread a report that their house was haunted, in order to deter persons from visiting it.' Mary Hulme, the servant to the house, recalled that 'there was people (the Standwickes) always jawing her, and telling her to go to Muckle-stone Wood to see the madman.'[43]

The vicious circle of secrecy and suspicion culminated in the forceful raid on 25 January 1826 on the Smith house by two magistrates, who believed they were going to find flagellant and cruel abuse and neglect of an idiot.[44] The magistrates sent for John Garret, house surgeon to the Staffordshire County Lunatic Asylum, to which George was taken in the same evening.[45] Moreover, the magistrates later openly propagated what they saw at the house perhaps with great exaggeration, upon which William brought an action against Broughton for having propagated calumnies. Broughton responded by prosecuting the family for cruelty to their brother. While these suits were pending, *Birmingham Journal*, a Whig-radical newspaper, published two articles which included a totally fictive account of cruelty of the family toward George. William brought another legal action for libel, this time against the proprietors of the paper. After a trial which involved contradicting testimony of major protagonists, William Smith won the case and the proprietors of *Birmingham Journal* were fined £400.[46]

In this case, the influence of rumour among neighbours was crucial, both for the public authority and for the private family. As already noted, the family's secrecy fermented unfriendly curiosity and suspicion among neighbours. The counsel for the defendant argued that the magistrates took this rumour seriously – or, believed it before they examined the house.[47] When the magistrates arrived at the house, therefore, they treated the family members just as they did criminals, forbidding them to move and threatening the use of force.[48]

Most importantly, there are some signs which seem to show that the Smith family themselves felt keenly awkward about the situation. The servant admitted that she had once told a lie and denied the existence of George in the house, because she wanted to keep out people's curiosity.[49] The testimonies of both the servant (on behalf of the plaintiff) and the magistrates (for the defendants) revealed that the brother initially did not tell the magistrates in a straightforward way that they kept an idiot in the house.[50] Any firm protest from the Smith family against the forceful intervention of the magistrates at the moment was conspicuously absent, as if they had committed a crime or had something to be hidden.[51] Perhaps, at the bottom of their heart, the family was not absolutely sure about the propriety of taking care of George behind a closed door and bricked window of their own house.

The examples analyzed above are largely anecdotal, and do not lend themselves to definitive conclusions. Nevertheless, a few points seem to be worth making for future research and historiographical reflection. To begin with, it should be noted that the barrier the family tried to set up to enclose its insane member was under constant threat, not only from the inside, but also from the outside. Of course, it must never be easy to contain a mentally diseased person within the private sphere and present an ordinary outlook (or its semblance) to the world, for the inability to behave in socially acceptable ways and to act an expected 'sick role' is one of the most common features of the disease. It does not seem appropriate, however, to assume that the difficulty *felt* and *experienced* by the family has been historically constant, being independent of cultural context. The intensity of the threat from outside, or the level of readiness of outsiders to intervene into the domestic realm over the issue of insanity, seems to differ among different cultures and different ages. A crowd assembling around a mental patient on the street is, for example, no longer a familiar part of urban landscape. In the early nineteenth century, the domestic regime was not only resisted from within by the lunatic, but also threatened from outside.

The role of public authorities in undermining domestic control of lunatics was ambiguous. In some cases, they forced their way into the closed door. The case of Brent Spencer, was a relatively straight-forward case of abuse at one's own house, with the all-too-familiar story of neglect, cruelty, and filth.[52] The example of George Smith presents a more ambiguous case. The conduct of the magistrates was severely criticised by the counsel for the plaintiff: 'he [the counsel] could fearless[ly] assert their conduct on this occasion to have been indiscreet and improper'.[53] The legal power for county magistrates, or any public authority, to inspect a non-pauper lunatic in his or her private family or remove him or her from there was at best dubious.[54] The Englishman's castle was, at least in theory, legally guarded even when there was a lunatic in it. That does not mean, however, that there was no moral pressure on the family. The same counsel that criticized the magistrates did not think that the Smith family was entirely blameless: 'he was not there to say, that this family had acted wisely in not sending this poor creature so some great asylum, where he might always have had at hand the best medical aid.'[55]

Moreover, Commission of Lunacy sometimes provided relatives outside the immediate family with a means to break the domestic barrier. Anyone could petition to the Lord Chancellor for a Commission of Lunacy, although notice had to be given to spouse of the alleged lunatic if he or she was married.[56] While the family could use the state machinery to control the lunatic, that very machinery could itself be used to frustrate their interest.

There were many cases in which relatives and 'friends' outside the direct family asked for a Commission of Lunacy, to break the domestic barrier set up by the family to control the lunatic.[57] If a relative outside the immediate family was not happy at the domestic situation of his relative whose sanity was questionable, he could ask for a Commission of Lunacy to effect a drastic change in the situation so that he would benefit. The 'benefit' could mean various things: effecting direct financial gain, preventing the family reputation from being tarnished, or rescuing one's daughter from an unsuccessful marriage.[58] The cases of Robert Clement and J.P. Robinson, two cases involving rich old men whose property transactions were controlled by their wives, exemplified the private motivation of petitioners to break into the domestic barriers. The nephews of J.P. Robinson asked for the Commission of Lunacy in order to 'protect his property' and delivered barely concealed criticism against his wife for exercising undue influence on the matter of the old man's finance and property transaction.[59] In Robert Clement's case, the claim of the petitioner was that if Mr. Clement had remained capable of managing his own affairs, he would have appointed the petitioner's son as a partner in his bank. This rather shaky petition undermined all efforts of Mrs Clement to keep the lunacy of her husband within the private sphere and to present a 'normal' outlook to the world of his business, by tutoring him to sign a deed, cheque, etc.[60] Moreover, from the early 1830s, under the lead of Henry Brougham, it was designed to make it easy for people to make use of the Commission of Lunacy, by simplifying the procedure and lowering the cost.[61] The domestic barrier guarding the lunatic within the family walls was thus made more vulnerable to the extra-familial intervention.

Although there is no case in which unrelated neighbours initiated a commission, madness seems to have offered neighbours a legitimate entrée into the domestic realm. Finding or inventing a lunatic in another person's family effaced the boundary between the private and public realms and made the usually closed sphere an open one. This is exemplified in the testimony of one Mr Edward Harris, a highly respected Quaker living next door but one to George Davenport, whose religious zeal was regarded as excessive by his wife's family:

> It was not until I heard that the [psychiatric] keeper had been sent here
> that I offered my advice and assistance to Mrs. Davenport; but since
> then I have been in the daily habit of coming in and sitting with him.[62]

Apparently, the attendance of a keeper to George Davenport, indicating the existence of a lunatic, acted as a license for him to intervene. Harris felt entitled to meddle into the personal affairs of his neighbour, only when he was proven to be a lunatic.

Most importantly, the vulnerability of the domestic psychiatric regime and the threat from outside seem to have been internalized by the family member themselves. This is exemplified in the Commission of Lunacy for Major Andrew Campbell in 1842. Major Campbell suffered from a delusion that there were galvanic wire figures 'which twitched his face into various contortions, and compel him to swear against his will.' He was kept in the notorious Whitmore House at Hoxton, which seems to have aggravated his disease. The major's half-brother was responsible for the choice of the site of his care, and he rather apologetically explained his motive for putting his brother in such a madhouse:

> Only that witness and the Major's family were on bad terms, he would
> not have sent him to Whitmore-house, but would have taken a house
> and put him under the surveillance of two keepers, who should have
> complied with his whims; but he did not do so for fear his motives might
> be misrepresented.[63]

The crucial difference between a house with two keepers and Whitmore House was that the former was an essentially private and semi-domestic dealing, while the latter was sanctioned by public authority, in the form of two medical certificates and quarterly visits by the Metropolitan Commissioners in Lunacy. These procedures made the option of the Whitmore House a more public way of dealing, and reduced the chance of his being 'misrepresented'. Being without any sort of inspection by public authority, the private lodging, on the other hand, had the ample room for suspicion and doubt and perhaps smelled of secrecy and abuse. Here, the brother's fear of other people's suspicion and misrepresentation removed the patient from the private lodging with better care to the publicly sanctioned place of detention with inferior quality of care. Here, the fear of suspicion, doubt, and malicious rumour disfranchised the private sphere as the proper place to care for the patient, and the public authority provided a safeguard against the suspicion.

Although this chapter has made only tentative suggestions about the role of the public sphere in moulding the family's strategy in coping with its insane member, I hope I have thrown some light on the complex relationship between the psychiatric private and public spheres – the family, relatives, neighbours, crowd on the street, public authority, and so on. The family's strategy to contain and control the lunatic was constantly undermined by external factors. The family with a lunatic was always aware and afraid of the external forces hostile to them, penetrating through the domestic barrier, and frustrating their attempt to contain and control the lunatic. The records of Commissions of Lunacy, disclose numerous attempts by 'designing' persons to take advantage of the lunatic, outwitting the guarding family. When the lunatic behaved strangely on the street and started a struggle with the family, he or she assembled a curious crowd, who sometimes took the side of the lunatic. Gossip in the neighbourhood about a lunatic in the attic, or the 'politics of rumour' tormented the family, and the family suffered from their lack of confidence in the private dealing of their own lunatic family member. There was a constant erosion of the domestic psychiatric regime. An alleged lunatic in a family was, thus, by his or her very existence, constantly threatening to transform the domestic sphere of the family into an open field of contention.

CHAPTER SEVEN

Lunatic and criminal alliances in nineteenth-century Ireland

Oonagh Walsh

This volume of essays addresses itself to the relationship between lunatic asylums and the communities outside their walls in nine-teenth-century Britain and Ireland. Recent scholarship on this subject, and on nineteenth-century psychiatry in general, suggests that this is a complex topic. Power in the asylum was negotiated between patients, physicians, relatives, and outside the asylum through figures of authority such as poor law commissioners, workhouse masters and police. The pioneering work of scholars such as Andrew Scull, Roy Porter, Elaine Showalter and others, while forging a path through unknown territory, have been revised and expanded to a considerable extent.[1] Perhaps one of the most interesting developments has been the emergence of a significant body of work on individual asylums, which, in addition to broad-ening our knowledge of psychiatric history, has emphasised the importance of local factors in the treatment of the insane.[2] Com-munity responses to the construction of asylums differed across Britain, with local politics, customs and economics playing quite distinct roles in different areas. Thus we can now, at least partly, construct a of patchwork of asylum histories, rather than a blanket history of the insane, which considerably enriches our understand-ing of the position of the asylum in the nineteenth century.

I will be concentrating in the main in this paper on the records of the Connaught District Lunatic Asylum, established at Ballinas-loe, Co. Galway in 1833 for the care of the lunatic poor, and exploring the relationship between the asylum and the community outside its walls.[3] In the first section, I wish to discuss the relationship between the asylums, gaols and workhouses in Ireland as a whole, and raise the question of how the administrators of these bodies perceived each other's functions. I then want to focus on the issue of public perceptions of the asylum, and in particular the attitude of the relatives of the insane. Finally I wish to explore the question of how patients viewed the asylum, and examine specifically the relationships between patients and the asylum physician. For these latter sections I will be using material relating to just one year – 1893 – in order to demonstrate how an average year of admissions displays considerable complexity in terms of negotiations of power. The Ballinasloe records suggest that far from the insane finding themselves 'incarcerated in a specialized, bureaucratically organised, state-supported asylum system which isolated them both physically and symbolically from the larger society',[4] the asylum was intimately associated with the community outside its walls. In a very obvious sense, it could not have been otherwise. The movement of individuals in and out of the institution, the contact between relatives and staff, the economic importance of the asylum to local contractors and employees, in a traditionally impoverished area, meant that the sense of isolation described above could not be unproblematically sustained.

I

The Irish poor law system was significantly different from that of England, despite being largely based upon it. Ireland's economic situation, with very few ratepayers to support a nation-wide network of workhouses, had made success unlikely from the outset. The Whately Commission's Report of 1835 in fact recommended that an alternative structure be imposed on Ireland, but this cautionary advice was ignored.[5] The Act of Union of 1800 had ·created, in theory, a constitutional equality between Ireland and her sisters within the United Kingdom, yet there was a constant fear that the Irish, if offered a comprehensive poor law system, would become a continual drain on governmental resources. 'The poor law system was based on the principle of 'less eligibility': i.e. the conditions for those in receipt of poor law must be worse than those of the poorest labourer.'[6] Thus the Irish poor law was deliberately intended to deter all but the most desperate from application. Until it was seen to fail miserably during the famine, worked relatively efficiently to keep people out of the system.

The Irish asylum system also differed from the English model in so far as it operated independently of the poor law.[7] Although 'the Irish poor law placed a much greater emphasis on medical relief'[8] than the English system, this referred to a dispensary system for the treatment of physical ailments, not lunatic care. The Irish insane came under the direct control of the Lord Lieutenant, based at Dublin Castle, who also controlled the prison system. Asylums and prisons in Ireland were intimately linked, with the Inspector General of Prisons acting simultaneously as the asylums inspector.[9] From the earliest discussion on the subject, it was clear that Irish asylums were envisaged, in official quarters at least, as tailored institutions for the imprisonment of the insane. Robert Peel in 1816 'stressed the impropriety of uncontrolled lunacy: it was not right these unhappy beings should go abroad free from restraint.'[10] Moreover, under the dangerous Lunatics Act (see below), individuals admitted to Irish asylums were automatically criminalised, as they had threatened violence towards others.

The relationship between the asylums and workhouses was however more complex. The expansion of Irish district asylums was closely associated with the creation of the Irish poor law in 1838, but following debates over the purpose of asylums, nevertheless remained formally outside the control of the Poor Law Commissioners. The popular belief, as Joseph Robins points out, was that there were very small numbers of Irish lunatics, therefore building specialist institutions for their treatment was not likely to have dire financial implications.[11] In addition, 'special measures for pauper lunatics were unlikely to increase lunacy',[12] unlike the workhouses, which might encourage the shiftless to lean on the state for support. Thus from the outset, Irish asylums regarded themselves as institutions for the care and rehabilitation of those deemed insane, not merely receptacles for undesirable pauper members of the population.

Asylum administrators faced certain difficulties in moderating the intake of patients to their institutions, owing to the liberally formulated insanity legislation. The most important act regulating Irish lunacy was the so-called Dangerous Lunatics Act of 1838,[13] which allowed for the committal of an alleged lunatic to an asylum by two Justices of the Peace, acting on a sworn statement by a third party – most often, in Ireland, a relative. The Lord Lieutenant also had discretion under the act to cause 'an individual under sentence of imprisonment or transportation to be removed to a lunatic asylum.' Individuals awaiting trial could be sent to an asylum, although if subsequently convicted, they were then removed to gaol. Apart from the automatic association made under the act between criminality and lunacy, it made the committal of lunatics very easy in Ireland, and was particularly open to abuse.

Any person charged under the 1838 act was sent in the first instance to gaol, and thence to an asylum. The process could move appallingly slowly, and many patients spent considerable periods of time, up to a year, before being removed to the asylum. In 1867, the act was amended, but it failed to address the major failing of the earlier act, that is, the ease of admission of patients. Under the new act, lunatics were sent directly to the asylum, they had no right of appeal against their charge or committal, and no automatic review of their case. More worryingly, the asylums could not legally refuse to accept any patient admitted under the act, even when staff there felt that they could be better cared for in the work-houses, or indeed even if they believed them to be sane. This caused enormous difficulties for asylum administrators, as unfit cases were presented for admission, but the tension between the asylums and those outside who saw in their expansion oppor-tunities for themselves, had a longer history than the 1867 amendment.

From the opening of the various district asylums, there were differing opinions as to how these new institutions should be used most profitably. At Ballinasloe, for example, the Board of Governors believed that they were in charge of a modern, enlight-ened body, for the care of curable lunatics. This was reflected most obviously in the asylum buildings, which were fitted with wooden floors, without barred windows, and with large, open dormitories, suitable for recuperative patients, but not the violent, incontinent or immobile. At the very first meeting of the Board on 26 Novem-ber 1833, it was decreed: 'That the Manager be requested to notify to the public through one paper in each county of the province, that the Connaught District Lunatic Asylum at Ballinasloe is prepared for the reception of patients, and that printed forms of admission can be had at the Asylum, advertisement to appear in two publications of each paper.'[14]

This congenial announcement to the general public was, as it turned out, unnecessary. A flood of patients appeared, but not quite of the kind the Board had been expecting. The masters of workhouses and the managers of gaols in the counties served by the asylum welcomed the prospect, as they saw it, of clearing out all the allegedly lunatic inmates of their institutions into the asylum. Thus the first patients received at Ballinasloe were 'twenty one male and thirteen female lunatics now in the poorhouse at Castlebar (Co. Mayo).'[15] One month later, the Board agreed to accept 'twenty three lunatics at present confined in the Old Gaol in this town (Roscommon) whom we deem fit and proper subjects to be received into the Connaught District Lunatic Asylum at Ballinasloe.'[16] Within a short period of time, the majority of Ballinasloe's patients had come from the gaols, and were presenting a worrying prospect for the Board. By May 1835 the asylum was almost full. There were 146 patients, '... of this number eighty six have been admitted from the several gaols of the Province who with a few exceptions have been Incurable, Epileptic or Idiotic and are therefore likely to remain in the asylum during life.'[17]

One of the many problems associated with the transfer of lunatics from gaols was that they often came in groups, numbering between twenty and forty persons, in order to save on security and transportation costs. This meant that individual admissions to the asylum from outside these institutions were frequently blocked, as the administration struggled to cope with mass admissions. In July another twenty lunatics were sent from Sligo Gaol, causing the Board to protest that they were being swamped with already institutionalised, long-stay inmates. Their protests fell on deaf ears, however, for the simple reason that the Inspector General of Prisons, Major Woodward, who was also the Inspector of Asylums, clearly regarded the latter institutions as an adjunct to the smooth running of the gaols. He was swift to point out the legal obligations of the asylums to accept lunatics from gaols: 'The Commissioners of any lunatic asylum are empowered to receive of Idiots and Epileptics etc. a number not exceeding half of their establishment (this in Ballinasloe would be 75) and even to build additional accommodation for them.'[18] Woodward then demanded that a further forty lunatics be removed from Sligo gaol to Ballinasloe, whom the Board reluctantly accepted, on condition they were allowed funds for expansion. This officially sanctioned attitude –

that Irish asylums existed in order to facilitate the smooth operation of the prison system – served the asylum system poorly.

It should be noted however that the Board at Ballinasloe did not object in principle to the admission of lunatics from gaols. They saw themselves as playing a vital role in controlling and modernising the province of Connaught, and in this they acted in accord with the intentions of the managers of workhouses and gaols. In July 1835 they noted: 'the Governors are still of [the] opinion that it is desirable to relieve the counties from the nuisance of insane persons going about at large, and wish to continue to do so, as far as the accommodation of the asylum can meet that object without interfering with the principle [sic] end of the institution viz. the reception of curable lunatics.'[19] What distressed them was the clearly held opinion of those other institutions of control – workhouses and gaols – that the asylum should be used as a means of removing any potentially disruptive elements from their midst. In this sense, the asylum system was perceived by contemporaries as a means of control, not cure, or at least they were unconcerned whether the institutions held a curative possibility. From their perspective, the removal of lunatics left only those individuals in workhouses and gaols who would respond to a disciplinary regime.

The conflict between the administrators of these three institutions reflected a general disagreement in Ireland over the most suitable form of treatment for criminals, paupers and lunatics. Workhouses, with their deservedly bad reputation for living conditions, remained the cheapest means of support for the destitute, which included pacific pauper lunatics. Asylums were in turn cheaper than gaols, owing to the high staff costs in the latter institutions.[20] However the masters of workhouses remained the most persistent in attempting to transfer patently unsuitable cases from their institutions to the asylums. In 1866, there was a danger that all the available beds in the Castlebar asylum would be filled with workhouse cases. The Inspector's report claimed that 'within three years it [the asylum] will be congested with inmates, very many of them suited, with ordinary care, to be maintained in poorhouses, such as the imbecile, the idiotic, the aged, and tranquilly demented. Hence it would be highly advisable in all instances when admission is sought from Union workhouses, that an engagement be distinctly undertaken by the masters to take back patients when required to do so by the Board of Guardians, on the recommendation of the Resident and Visiting Physicians.'[21] However, not only did the workhouse masters refuse any such undertaking, they abused the provisions of the Dangerous Lunatics Act in order to send inmates to gaol, when they could not have them admitted direct to the asylums. The workhouse mentality reflected the true spirit of the Irish poor law system. Only those individuals who were completely destitute, and who had voluntarily or otherwise surrendered all rights to property as a tenant or owner gained admission to the workhouse. Lunatics were clearly viewed as having another resource – the asylum – and as such were unwelcome in the workhouse.[22] The government felt sufficiently anxious about the abuse of the act to order the Poor Law Commissioners to tackle it, but with little effect.

> In our last report we expressed our regret that a circular letter issued by the Poor Law Commissioners, for the purpose of preventing the committal of lunatics to gaols from poorhouses, had failed to have effect in many instances, and we are sorry to observe that such continues still to be the case; for it frequently occurs that if an insane inmate of a workhouse manifests any excitement, or is troublesome or violent, he is at once taken before the magistrates, and committed to gaol, without the least effort being made to obtain his direct admission into the asylum.[23]

The workhouse masters had a particularly strong hand in terms of removing lunatics. Diagnosis of insanity was open to interpretation at the best of times, but the Act removed even the pretence of medical corroboration, as decisions regarding the state of mental health were made by Justices of the Peace.

Lunatics were highly likely to be victimised in workhouses and gaols, principally by other inmates, but also by staff. Mark Finnane has pointed to the concern amongst prison managers that lunatics disrupted the smooth running of gaols, and acted as a disruptive influence on other prisoners.[24] In reality, it was the lunatics who suffered from prison contact, in that they were subject to physical abuse, excessive restraint, theft of their few possessions, and so on. Staff in these institutions were swift to declare known lunatics troublesome, and to punish them more severely than other inmates. 'Many of these cases are reported by the Bridewell keepers to have been violent and destructive in their dispositions, and of course means had to be used to prevent them from destroying property or injuring themselves, such as confining their limbs, or otherwise restricting their movements, which, when left to be done at the opinion of and in such a manner as an inexperienced person, without suitable appliances at hand, can at the moment accomplish must unavoidably be attended with unnecessary pain and inconvenience to the unfortunate lunatic.'[25]

The sane criminals and workhouse inmates resented their forced association with lunatics. Indeed, so strong was the criminal dislike of the tag 'lunatic' that those individuals who were deemed to have become insane whilst serving prison sentences, and were transferred to asylums, vigorously protested their sanity in order to be removed from the asylum. In 1870, it was noted that prisoners moved from Mountjoy prison to the district asylums regulated their behaviour in order to return to prison. 'However reckless on admission, and ungovernable before, after a time they become for the most part well-conditioned and amenable, but what may appear extraordinary, some of them request to be sent back to prison, asserting that they were never mad, from some sort of innate discontent – perhaps, too, from a dislike to associate with individuals whose delusions they promptly notice. But they are scarcely back in penal confinement than they break out again.'[26] Women were believed to be especially effected by the atmosphere of the asylum, and to seek transfer from it. Violent and aggressive inmates from the Richmond asylum in Dublin when transferred to the asylums 'at once become amenable and frequently useful, and as a matter of course (are) discharged at the expiration of their imprisonment.'[27] This behaviour caused the Inspector to wonder 'how far the habits of profligacy, intemperance, and depravity in its every form may be regarded as more correctly indicative of criminality or insanity'. He did not pursue the question, which cast doubt not merely on the uneasy relationship between the asylums, prisons and workhouses, but on the nature of insanity itself.

By the end of the nineteenth century, to judge by admission figures, it would appear that madness had taken a firm grip on the Irish population. From a position in the 1830s where capacity for 400 patients at Ballinasloe was considered sufficient for the whole province of Connaught, by 1904 there were 2,119 residents in the asylum, drawn from the counties of Galway and Roscommon alone, and the administrator were still calling for increased accommodation.[28] However, there were large numbers of lunatics also confined in gaols and workhouses, despite the best efforts of these institutions to have them removed. What is more, the numbers were rising steadily. In 1870 there were 2,754 lunatics in workhouses throughout Ireland: the following year, there were 2,914. This large increase in the insane would seem to offer support to the traditional Foucauldian model of the 'great confinement'. Lunatics appeared to be increasingly identified and processed, and the reach of the asylum grew steadily. But did this spread reflect an increasingly authoritarian governmental policy, or a negotiated advance, which depended upon not merely the co-operation of the public, but was partly a result of their initiation?

II

In discussing the relationship between the asylum and the community, an obvious issue is the perception amongst the general population as to the benefits of involvement in the institutional process. The Ballinasloe asylum was broadly welcomed on its construction, despite some reservations regarding the notoriety which might attach to the town through its association with lunatic care. The employment opportunities, and more importantly, the considerable economic benefits which the asylum brought, convinced many in Ballinasloe of the wisdom of constructing it there. In 1846 for example, the asylum contributed almost six thousand pounds to the local economy in the form of wages and contracts, a considerable sum of money in a period of great scarcity.[29] However even for those individuals who were not the direct financial beneficiaries, the asylum offered other possibilities, in particular the opportunity to remove an unwanted or obstructive relative. The great expansion of the Irish asylum system is at least in part a result of the willingness of families to commit parents, siblings, and sons and daughters, who had previously been accommodated at home, but who were increasingly perceived as problematic.

The issue of family committals to pauper asylums in Ireland is muddied somewhat by the provisions of the Dangerous Lunatics Act. Strictly speaking, it was the Justices of the Peace who recommended that an alleged lunatic be removed to an asylum, thus distancing to an extent the involvement of family members. However if one examines the committal warrants themselves, and notes who made the allegation of insanity, the extent of family involvement becomes clear. To take just one year as an example: sixty two patients out of seventy two in 1879 were committed on the evidence of family members.[30] Of the ten warrants supported by statements from persons not related to the patient, there were four by masters of workhouses, one by a workhouse nurse, two by Constables of the Royal Irish Constabulary, two by the manager of Galway Gaol and one unknown. In twelve of the cases supported by relatives' statements, the warrants named relatives to whom the alleged lunatic had offered violence, but in the majority of the remainder the patients are described generally as being 'violent towards others' or 'threatened to injure self and others'. In most of these cases, particularly with female patients, members of the family were most often attacked. These figures would seem to substantiate David Wright's recent suggestion that families, rather than the asylum authorities, regulated admissions to asylums.[31] The concept of the institution being used as a means of respite for stressed carers is further supported by the significant numbers of relatives who sought the release of patients whom the physician believed to be still insane (see below). But how far did relations see in the expansion of the asylum system in Ireland an opportunity to advance themselves materially?

The question of whether the Ballinasloe asylum was routinely used as a means of disenfranchising patients is difficult to satisfactorily answer. Many patients, who laboured under genuine mental illness, alleged that they were being confined by relatives in order to secure property. The ferocious landhunger in the west of Ireland which had intensified as a result of the famine,[32] and the transfer of farms under the Land Acts,[33] had created an environment in which property became the measure both of citizenship and stability, and people would indeed go to great lengths to secure it. Under the Dangerous Lunatics Act, persons making a committal involved themselves in perjury if they deliberately provided false information to secure an admission. In theory a serious offence, in fact it appears to have been largely disregarded by the asylum administrators when detected, despite the fact that the offender should have been liable for prosecution. In September 1893, for example, a 22 year old man was admitted, accused of attacking his sister. It emerged that this was his second admission, he having been 'wrongfully sworn in ... once before in 1889.'[34] The physician could find no evidence of insanity, noting that 'The patient is quiet and rational without much intelligence.' However, the policeman who brought him to the asylum claimed that 'he [the patient] never beat the sister and she had no mark to show. She stabbed herself and accused him of it.' The man's own interpretation of events was 'the people all told his sister she would never get a husband as he had been a patient here if she did not get him in again and so get possession of the farm.' Unfortunately, he contracted dysentery shortly after his arrival at the asylum, and died on October 19th. The case is interesting for two reasons, though. Firstly, there was no immediate discharge of the man, despite the belief of both the physician and the policeman that he was sane. Secondly, the implication of the patient's remark, if his sister's intentions to secure the family farm were indeed true, is that a family history of insanity was not necessarily an impediment to marriage, if there were compensating factors such as land. The spectre of hereditary lunacy might not deter a suitor, but a resident lunatic would.[35]

The committal process, far from being a disinterested and remote undertaking on the part of official bodies, was mediated through local practice and advice. Relatives were the key source of information for the asylum administrators with regard to previous habits, medical histories, and family roles, but what is surprising is the extent to which the physician considered the broader family circumstances, and made recommendations regarding length of stay, and even treatment, on the petitions of relatives. In addition, the medical officer also consulted with other individuals, who had little to gain directly from the continued incarceration of the patient. In those cases where patients appeared to be what the physicians termed 'doubtfully insane', the testimony of unrelated parties became more important. In particular, the local knowledge of both police and nursing staff was frequently drawn upon in uncertain cases. Thus in May of 1893, when a 55 year old man was committed by his brother for an alleged attack and attempted suicide, the physician noted in the case book: 'The police say he signed away his farm to a younger brother and got sorry for it as the brother treated him badly and that the assault and threatened suicide were merely technical.'[36] The patient himself testified that: 'he had no one to care for him at home', but this apparently clear case of land grabbing went unchallenged, and he remained in the asylum until his death in July, 1898.[37] Similarly, the statement by 'Riely, attendant' that 'he knew him [a patient admitted in 1893] to be always a simpleton and rambling from home' appears to have significantly influenced the physician's decision to keep the man in the asylum.[38]

For the bulk of the men admitted in 1893, the case notes record clearly aberrant behaviour. Even allowing for a nineteenth century suspicion of irregular behaviour, it is clear that many patients were labouring under considerable mental strain; hearing voices, suffering hallucinations, and enduring great distress. This considerable group are not however the main focus of my interest here. What I wish to examine are the surprisingly large number of inmates whose condition may be said to be ambiguously described. In the opinion of the physician, they appeared to be quite sane, and yet they remained in the asylum. This applied to 15 of the 99 male patients admitted in 1893.

The practice of keeping patients in the institution, once they have been declared sane, is open to several different interpretations. The most common reason for detention, and certainly the most humane, as far as the physician was concerned, centred around an apparent reluctance to release patients whom the asylum authorities suspected would be ill-treated or neglected if they returned home. In the case mentioned above (no. 3376), it was believed that the patient would be unwelcome at home, and that the eccentricities which made his admission into the asylum possible in the first place would possibly deteriorate into rather more serious problems. In May, a 60 year old man was admitted for allegedly assaulting his wife.[39] The patient claimed that she and her family had physically abused him, and had attempted to take his farm and money from him. Almost from the start of his stay in the asylum, the physician noted that he displayed no evidence of insanity. Within one month of admission, he wrote: 'He is now clear, rational and very shrewd; takes an intelligent interest in Home Rule and other topics.' Every year between 1893 and 1903, when the man died, the case book was updated, and every year the physician recorded that he 'is in much the same state as on last note'(Nov. 1893) '... very quiet and rational' (1894) '... his condition remains quite unchanged' (1896) '... he never shows any abnormal signs and is always quiet and rational' (1899).[40]

Despite this evidence of continued sanity however, and despite frequent requests to be released, the patient remained in Ballinasloe. The main reason behind his continued detention appeared to be the physician's personal belief that the patient would fall into his former habits of authoritarianism at home, and his wife would simply have him committed again. 'He appears to have determined and arranged everything when at home and fought with his wife ... he will probably do the same again if discharged.' (1894) '... He promises if left [at] home not to try to interfere with his son and wife and give them an excuse for putting him in' (1895) '... his wife refuses to take him home as his brother committed suicide in a lake near the house, in which he also attempted to do so [this was not, incidentally, mentioned in his original warrant, but appears to have been declared by the wife some years later] and after last going home he insisted on taking up the management of everything and played havoc with their savings.' (1896). Thus in this case the issue of whether or not the patient was *insane* seemed less of a deciding factor than his reception at home, the objections of his family, and the apparent certainty of his eventual readmission.

Similarly, a fifty year old man who was admitted in September, 1893, and who was recorded as 'much improved' by December, was not discharged until October of 1901.[41] The case notes witnessed steady improvement – 'Is now much better and has lost all delusions and works steadily' (1894) '... He is clear and rational' (1895) '... Has no morbid delusions at present and is very anxious to get home' (1896) and so on, but his brother, whom he was alleged to have attacked before admission, was reluctant to take him back. After a full eight years of rational behaviour, the patient was finally discharged. It would appear that in those cases where a patient was on their second admission, relatives felt they had a stronger case for refusing responsibility, despite evidence of full recovery. A 48 year old man, who had spent four months in the asylum in 1893 for assaulting his wife, was readmitted in 1897 for the same reason. On this occasion, he made a similarly rapid recovery, and in June 1898 the physician noted that he 'is now calm, rational and coherent and anxious to get home: his wife is not.'[42] All of the subsequent notes testify to his sane state, but nobody is prepared to take responsibility for him. As the asylum were clearly not supposed to maintain sane inmates, the physician tried to have him transferred to the Ballinasloe workhouse, but the patient simply refused to go,[43] an indication perhaps that patients were not always the helpless objects of official attentions. At the asylum board meeting five months later he was officially discharged, but the physician ruefully noted that: 'Just at present he is slightly hypochondriacal but otherwise not insane and has been discharged but his friends refuse to remove him.'[44] Despite the patient's declaration a year later that 'he will not ask anyone to take him out as he is fit to go himself', the physician believed that he would once again return to the asylum.[45] He died there in May, 1906, having been declared sane since June, 1898.

Not all relatives sought self-advancement through the asylum, however. Some at least regarded the institution as a means through which relatives could be cured, not merely shut away, and they monitored the progress of patients continually. Letters querying treatment, offering advice, and sending money and food to patients inside the asylum run contrary to the notion that many relatives were unconcerned about the eventual fate of patients, although the asylum authorities frequently registered impatience at what they regarded as attempted interference in their treatment.[46] In one case, an archetypal Irish mother wrote 'within the last few days several letters teeming with emotional tenderness and asking that her son's susceptibilities to noises, crowds, strong lights and other such bugbears of neurotic individuals might be safeguarded against.'[47] Although relatives for the most part went along with the advice of the asylum staff, they were not necessarily cowed by the implicit authority of the institution, and they frequently acted against advice to, for example, remove relatives when they felt they were not benefiting from treatment. In this way, they regarded the asylum as a resource, one which could be assessed in terms of its efficacy, and used as they felt appropriate. Did this attitude also prevail, however, amongst the patients?

III

In much asylum history to date there has been an implicit presumption that such institutions operated to imprison social misfits, those individualists who refused to tailor their behaviour to societal norms, or were incapable of doing so. In the words of Yannick Ripa, 'these 'special hospitals' ... were a place for observing and silencing any behaviour which could be seen as threatening to the family or to society.'[48] However, what Ripa's analysis ignores is the fact that traffic to the asylum was two-way. Even in pauper institutions such as Ballinasloe, the most disadvantaged members of society – frequently illiterate, unenfranchised, with none of the professional status of the physician – could under certain circumstances leave the asylum against the express wishes of the staff. This applied to patients whose relatives or friends agreed to enter a bond 'for his or her peaceable Behaviour or safe Custody' before two Justices of the Peace,[49] thereby limiting the extent of control held by asylum staff. In 1893 there were 22 out of 99 male cases admitted which were discharged despite being declared still insane by the physician, and frequently against his specific advice.

It is rather difficult to determine the attitude of patients towards the asylum, and the use which they made of it. Legal confinements with the approval of the patient were rare, so that nineteenth-century admissions all involved a third party assuming responsibility for the patient in one form or another. However the patterns of admission, and particularly readmission, suggest that some individuals at least recognised the asylum as just that – a refuge from stressful, violent or otherwise uncomfortable lives. Some patients made rational, logical assessments of their lives, and decided that permanent residence within the asylum was a better option than a return to their former existences. Several of the cases mentioned above indicate that a patient could not be forced to leave the institution if they felt they were not ready. Interestingly, although many of these individuals were long-stay patients, who could arguably be described as institutionalised, several indicated their reluctance to leave the asylum within relatively short periods of time.

One such was a thirty year old admitted originally in July 1905, suffering from acute mania.[50] He recovered quickly, and was described by the physician as 'a good mechanical drudge'. From the earliest days of his admission he was reluctant to discuss his home or parents, saying that 'as he had not heard from them this long time' there was little point in contacting them about the possibility of his release from the asylum. He became a reliable farm worker, who enjoyed the responsibility he was given in the stables. When the physician broached the possibility of his discharge, he responded by feigning illness. Interestingly, this was of a physical rather than a psychological nature, so that he could continue to work but be declared unfit for release. In 1910 he 'had to be moved to hospital from the farm division as he got several

very alarming fainting fits. He has no organic disease nor enlarge-
ment of heart. He has reported attacks since he went to hospital
and says he is not fit to go home and will have to go to bed again.'
Each time his discharge was discussed, he responded with a lapse
into illness, or apparently accidental injuries such as a 'severely
sprained ankle'. He remained in the asylum until his death.
Another patient, admitted originally in December, and again five
days after being discharged cured in January, 1894, regarded the
asylum as both a safe haven from the monotony of home life, and,
more importantly, as a means of avoiding the mortal sin of suicide:
'Before his discharge he had been working regularly on the [asy-
lum] farm: He says 'he had nothing to do at home but shuffling
round the house'. He found nothing wrong with himself since he
went home but knew they did not care for him there – he does not
want to earn Hell by laying hands on his own life – He is still in
very much the same condition as on former occasion.'[51]

The physician's case notes, although most obviously useful for
gathering information on individual patients, also offer a unique
insight into staff-patient relations. The entries vary in length, and
one frequently finds that more extensive records do not necessarily
indicate a more complex case, but rather one which, for one reason
or another, the physician is especially interested in. The tone varies
from a benevolent amusement, in those cases where the patient
has a particularly good relationship with the physician, to an
intense irritation, when the requests, advice and even demands of
the staff are ignored. Despite the authority which was implicit in
the figure of the physician, it is surprising how disobedient and
disruptive patients could be. Patients refused to work when they
were asked to (a willingness to labour, and to obey orders, was
regarded as a sign of sanity), or willfully spoiled the organised
games of cricket and football. In one such case, a patient was
admitted for allegedly stabbing his brother, but he declared to the
physician that he wanted to enter the asylum as 'he needed a rest
as the life in Dublin is very fast and hard.'[52] However, the physician
could find nothing wrong with him, describing him as 'affectedly
stupid, contradictory and evasive.' Moreover, 'he is partly an
author his principal work being an autobiography' and 'he is not in
the least affected by his position but rather welcomes it as a new
experience', one which he presumably intended to put in his
autobiography. The patient simply lived in the asylum, refusing to

participate in either work or leisure, and ignoring the best efforts of the physician to turn him into an integrated member of the community. '[He] will only join in games after much pressing and then deliberately does things which he knows are against the rules (cricket football etc.), plays hockey but is useless as he is lazy and undecided . . . he slouches round the place generally evading walking exercise and will not answer my argument as to his course of conduct.' Apart from this policy of non-cooperation, the patient appeared content, declaring the year before his death in the asylum from double pneumonia that 'he does not know why he was sent here but he likes being here.' The question of whether the man was happier inside the asylum than out of it is perhaps less important than the physician's apparent helplessness to regulate his behaviour. He had in fact been discharged as 'not improved' for a short period of time, but was swiftly readmitted, to continue in precisely the same manner as before, apart from his complete refusal to tell the physician how he had spent his brief sojourn outside.

One of the most effective tools which the patients used against the physician's authority was silence. Very many refused to utter a word direct to the doctor, or replied to questions in unintelligible whispers, or spouted meaningless lines, while the physician noted that they were in fact capable of rational speech. In an obvious way, dialogue was used by the physician as a means of testing a patient's mental state, and release could be secured if patients responded verbally in what the physician regarded as the correct manner. In this context, individuals who had lost the power of speech were severely disadvantaged. A man was admitted on April 13 with a bad stammer: 'it takes him several minutes to sputter out a word in unconnected syllables: difficult words require a great effort to pronounce and cause contortion of all his facial muscles.'[53] This patient, who was incapable of describing his response to the asylum, his changing mental state, and more importantly, of asking for his release, remained in the asylum for over twenty years until his death. On admission, he had manifested no signs of insanity; however after eight years in the asylum he fulfilled the apparent expectations of the physician, and began to behave peculiarly.

Some patients however reserved for themselves the right to challenge authority through language. Apart from the several bilingual patients who continued to speak Irish in the asylum, forcing the physician to conduct his medical assessments through an interpreter,[54] there were cases in which the patient seized the verbal initiative, and went beyond the intimate physician-patient relationship to air grievances. One such individual had been noted since his admission for his prolific letter writing, and his constant haranguing of asylum staff as to the conditions under which he was kept.[55] The man's tenacity in sending letters through unofficial as well as official channels worried the physician sufficiently for him to record that he had invented 'put offs' to prevent the patient from making further contact with solicitors and relatives outside the institution in the hope of securing his release. Once the man realised that he was being deliberately thwarted, he created the following public scene:

> About 10 days ago he proceeded to act on his notions about using 'his only weapon his tongue' to procure his liberty. Accordingly in the Dining Hall, having eaten, he stands up and begins to pour forth torrents of Billings Gate[56] on each of the medical officers, assailing them with every possible epithet of offense and contumely: this also occurs in the yards and day rooms. In an exhausted moment he explained that he considers himself bound to do so to effect his discharge: he will listen to no arguments to the contrary. He has also indulged in numerous written letters of abuse.

One of the major debates of the nineteenth century in psychiatry was that of the efficacy of institutionalisation. Did asylums cure the mad, or did they merely act as a means of removing dangerous individuals from society until their maniacal delusions had passed? For many of those who supplied the testimony which committed patients, it was a moot point. Once the threat had been removed, there was little reflection. However the process of readmission raises the possibility that patients did in fact regard the asylum as a means of recovery, and recognised the benefits which a temporary respite from the outside world could bring. For some, this involved a lengthy period of trial and error. A young political activist was admitted to Ballinasloe in July, 1893, having been transferred from Mountjoy prison in Dublin. He had been serving a ten year sentence for the burning of Weston House, as part of a Land League protest. Four years into his sentence he became insane, was transferred originally to Dundrum Criminal Lunatic Asylum in Dublin, and then to Ballinasloe, as he was originally a native of

Galway. He was described as being cured, 'and appears to have been buoyed up with the hope of being discharged. His conduct is said to have been good.'[57] He had a brief maniacal episode three days after his arrival at Ballinasloe, but then became 'quiet and rational in behaviour.' He was released on August 11th, despite some misgivings on the part of the physician, but was readmitted six days later:

> On his arrival home there were illuminations and rejoycings throughout the country and a dance in his father's house. A local poet began to recite about the 'Heroes and martyrs of Weston' which threw B___ into a state of intense excitement and made him occupy all the attention of the company: He beat his father and brothers very violently and was brought back by the police handcuffed and tied down and even with that they say they never had such work.

The asylum had its calming effect, and within a few months he was deemed well enough to be discharged. Interestingly, the patient himself declared that he would come back if he felt the approach of an attack – '[he] says he would always return before he got bad as he knows when it's coming on' – and attributed his recovery to the therapeutic effect of working with the maintenance men when in the asylum. On his discharge, it was noted that he had been 'quiet, coherent and rational for almost a year.' Within just four days, he was back, 'in a state of violent maniacal excitement with various delusions.' Once again, his delusions vanished, and in a fortnight he 'is now in the same condition as before his discharge – quiet, rational, coherent and working at anything he is asked.' The patient declared that 'he will never ask to leave the asylum again', and he died there in September, 1914. In this case, the asylum seemed to offer some level of protection, not for the sane community against the insane, but vice versa.

This is not to say that traditional notions regarding the authority of the physician should be overthrown. Within the asylum hierarchy, he held the key position, and this was strengthened as the century advanced, and insanity became increasingly viewed as a medical specialisation. The physician determined ultimately how any patient should be treated, and his recommendations carried far more weight than the protests of either patients or their relatives. Moreover, it was up to the medical officer to diagnose patients, and determine their mental state, a process which could be highly subjective. When the case notes were updated, each patient was asked a series of questions relating to their length of stay in the asylum, the circumstances under which they were admitted, and their present state of mind. One apparent indication that an individual was not ready for release was a lack of expressed interest in leaving the asylum. The case notes make specific mention of those patients who do not ask to be released, and this is taken as a sign of their disturbed state, presumably on the basis that a sane individual would demand their liberation. In several cases, the failure to ask to be discharged appeared to be the sole grounds on which presumptions regarding sanity were made. One man, believed to be violent towards his sister-in-law, demonstrated complete indifference to the question of his release.[58] 'He appears to have lost all regard for his home or desire to return there and never asks for his discharge' (1895) '. . . says he does not care about getting home; they don't mind him atal [sic]' (1899) '. . . [he] does not know why he was sent but he does not fault it a bit' (1904) '. . . He would not like to go home – what good is it.' The physician concluded that the man was 'stupidly content', and he made little effort to persuade him of the benefits of leaving the asylum.

With one patient in particular however, there was a somewhat different conclusion. A 30 year old man, admitted for assaulting his sister, appeared reluctant to consider the possibility of going home. Each year, the main focus of the physician's investigation is this issue of whether the patient would go home on his own request. '. . . he is rational and coherent but thinks he is not yet well enough to 'face for home' and never broaches the subject unless it is suggested to him.' (1895) '. . . questioned about his farm and affairs he says he does not know and would rather be here than at home: I do not detect any delusions.' (1899) 'Says he felt very lonesome at home when he went there and found his father dead and his brother in America when he could not read the clock or know what day it was' (1900) '. . . says he is a bit lazy about going home and does not care to. Does not seem to have delusions now.'(1904)[59] However, in 1905, the patient became 'very excited . . . constantly demanding his discharge'. These 'demands' were now construed as indications of insanity, and the patient remained in the asylum until his death. The official attitude was rather curious. A reluctance to leave the institution was interpreted as aberrant behaviour, yet the demand for release appears to have been regarded as a challenge to the authority of the physician, and was dismissed, with the patient's excitement cited as a reason for further detention.

There was also a good deal of significance attached to a patient's willingness to acknowledge their insane state, and discuss it with the physician. One important aspect of the assessment process was the physician's use of rationality as a test for release. It was however employed in an apparently contradictory manner – patients were required to recognise and admit the 'fact' of their mental illness, before they could be released, and a reluctance to discuss the specifics of cases was taken as a sign of continuing instability, regardless of other evidence of recovery. In some senses, this strategy appeared to be an attempt to force patients to admit to the superior judgement of the physician, who was qualified to judge sanity, but it also suggests a quasi-confessional approach within the asylum, where acknowledgment of illness and a plea for assistance/forgiveness may be followed by a secular salvation and release. Thus the patient who eluded discussion of his case, despite showing little other evidence of insanity, was detained: '. . . he hears, with evident reluctance, questions on his foibles and shows a disposition to avoid them.'[60] When, however, he reached the stage some four years later where 'he talks without hesitation of the time he was sick', he is described as 'much improved mentally and anxious to get home.'

To conclude, the great expansion of the Irish asylum system in the nineteenth century was influenced by many factors, including politics, economics and the changing structure of Irish family life. Like any such development, individuals responded to asylums in a variety of ways, ranging from fear to apathy, depending on how they perceived their own position within the system. One thing is clear however. A simple interpretation of the asylum as an unproblematic means of social control is unsatisfactory. Each player in the asylum drama – patient, physician, relative, the gaol and workhouse manager – all viewed their roles quite differently, and the records they left provide us with an increasingly sophisticated understanding of not merely the history of lunacy, but the impact of the asylum system upon local and national life.

CHAPTER EIGHT

Families, communities and the legal regulation of lunacy in Victorian England: Assessments of crime, violence and welfare in admissions to the Devon Asylum, 1845–1914

Joseph Melling, Bill Forsythe
and Richard Adair

Social historians have long debated the role played by families in the committal of the insane to lunatic asylums during the nineteenth and early twentieth centuries.[1] This has formed a significant chapter in a wider debate on the changing relationship between families and formal institutions of care in what historians are increasingly likely to term the 'mixed economy of care', where the continuing significance of private provision before and during the seminal lunacy legislation of 1808–1845 is now increasingly recognised.[2] Recent essays, including some in the present volume, consider the 'community context' within which family behaviour might be understood and contribute to the history of what we might term the domestic economy of welfare in European history.[3] Such studies help to draw our gaze away from the Foucauldian concern with technologies of power within the walled institution and back towards the moral economy of compassion and sentiment which Walton found amongst working class families in industrial Lancashire.[4] Recent research also alerts us to the ability of families and others to penetrate the power structure of the asylum and to locate such welfare strategies within a longer-term perspective of institutional change.[5] Scholars in the United States as well as Britain have consistently challenged Foucauldian interpretations of the asylum as an instrument of social control and have stressed the capacity and willingness of working class families to make effective use of such facilities.[6] The essays in the present volume enable us to frame our analysis of the Victorian asylum within a longer-term perspective of social welfare provision advocated by demographic historians such as Richard Smith in studies of the relationship between ageing and the services offered by the poor law in England.[7] Smith has argued that far from viewing the advance of legislation as the elaboration of powerful systems of social control and regulation, we can more plausibly view the growth of institutional provision as responses to a 'market demand' for welfare benefits in the face of challenges to the resilience of family and community provisions for their members.[8]

If we are to follow the invitation of Smith and others to excavate the context in which welfare choices were made by calculating family units, we must uncover the roots of discrimination and compassion within the household and the community whilst recognising that specific initiatives flow from rules, values and assumptions which were common to many different areas. Whether we view such domestic economies as the locus for rational calculations about household resources, the cradle for collective sentiments which bind individuals together, or part of an ensemble of responses which made up a moral economy of class survival, there is little dispute that we can best understand the dynamics of decision-making within families and communities by detailed investigations of specific historical localities where the interplay between communal resources and institutional provision can be more precisely contextualised. Earlier research on the admissions to the Devon Pauper Lunatic Asylum in the period 1845–1914 has led us to argue elsewhere that the strategic decision to commit a family member to this lunatic asylum was influenced by a variety of social factors including period of residence within a particular parish or poor law union, membership of different types of households, gender, marital status, and 'visibility' to the authorities responsible for the administration of both the poor law and the lunacy legislation of the nineteenth century.[9] The different agents responsible for the identification and the institutionalisation of the pauper lunatic in the decades following the 1845 Lunacy Act were acting not only within the framework of rules governing the certification of an individual as insane but also according to the cultural references which informed the obligations, responsibilities and sense of place during these years.[10]

It remains indisputable that lunatic asylums provided a very particular form of 'welfare' service and that such institutions formed part of an evolving system of state provision, over the design and implementation of which their main users had very limited influence. Nor is it always clear how the rich micro-histories of the role of families and kin in the institutional provision for the insane can be integrated with the kind of broad comparative sweep of state formation which Foucault offered.[11] Foucault's work provides, therefore, a problematic legacy for historians of the lunatic asylum as well as the penal system. This is evident in recent scholarship which emphasises the interplay between the asylum and the systems of both pauper and penal regulation.[12] Comparative research on the spread of regulatory models of treatment within the modern hospital and asylum as well as the reformed prison continue to draw on the agenda set by Foucault and Norbert Elias in discussions of the European 'civilising process'.[13] This comparative research draws our attention not only to the increasing circulation and exchange of intellectual models which were available to states and professional experts of different societies in the nineteenth century, but also to the less visible and articulated world of lunacy regulation, and places the micro-politics of family and community preferences within a larger landscape of political governance. An adequate response to the challenge of reinterpreting institutional reform posed by Smith appears to require an analysis of both the demand and supply sides of the welfare equation, encompassing not merely the preferences of families but some attention to the boundaries which communities and the law set on individual behaviour. This may provide a way of avoiding a polarised view of lunacy administration as *either* an exercise of political regulation *or* as the provision of a social good for which there was legitimate demand.

The present essay attempts only a modest contribution to this task by seeking to show how prisons, lunatic asylums, workhouses and other institutions (including the local judiciary) did indeed combine to influence the provisions made for pauper lunacy in this period. We also suggest that the actions of families and communities exerted some influence on the practices of these institutions and that families were in conversation with the authorities as to the limits of what was socially tolerable.[14] These conversations were necessarily fragmented and our understanding of them is restricted by the limits of the sources which are available.[15] The admission notes of the asylum again confirm the fluidity and complexity of the process by which behaviour was deemed to be the expression of lunacy rather than the malice of the responsible criminal. As in so many other areas, including the treatment of children and young persons, the legislation of 1845 and 1890 left a large area in which local officials struggled to make sense of their legal obligations, whilst families interacted with the provision and regulation of the state authorities.[16]

Out of these engagements and conflicts between the different actors came the complicated narrative of lunacy provisions and the welfare of the insane which was recorded in the official reports of the Victorian period. As Roy Porter has noted in reflecting on his efforts to retrieve and distinguish the 'voice of the mad' during the eighteenth century, what we hear when listening for the authentic narrative of normality by which we may then distinguish the cry of the insane is not a coherent and resonant echo but rather 'dissent, discussion and dissonance, not unison'.[17] Many versions of events are available within the archival sources as well as texts which offer edited selections of these materials. We may only recreate a world of the insane by selecting partial perceptions from conflicting accounts of different agents involved in accommodating the insane. Magistrates and poor law officials were often criticised by the Lunacy Commissioners in London for their lethargy in prosecuting those responsible for the ill treatment of lunatics in private mad houses or licensed hospitals, in private dwellings and family homes, and in the premises of the poor law or county asylum itself. The Commissioners promoted a particular version of humanitarianism which equated proper care with institutional treatment though the period; the overcrowding of the workhouses and the asylums themselves raised important questions about the standards of provision which could be offered to individuals.

The point in contention during such exchanges was often the way in which the laws on the care of lunatics might be interpreted and applied. One of the more interesting but frequently neglected aspects of lunacy regulation is the distinction between violence inflicted by (or indeed upon) a raging lunatic which qualified his or her description as 'dangerous' and therefore as eligible for certification and dispatch to the asylum, and the acts of violence which were serious enough to lead to the committal of the individual for trial as a criminal lunatic. The implications of violent behaviour and the capacity of even the Lunacy Commissioners to enforce its will appear to have depended to a surprising degree on the willingness of local magistrates and even jurors to prosecute and convict, more especially where violence against the insane was graphically evident. On the other hand, the Commissioners in London were anxious to persuade the magistrates who formed the governing body of the Devon Asylum to admit a number of individuals convicted as criminal lunatics to the institution. There was considerable professional prestige to be gained by psychiatrists from contact with the legal system, whether as expert witnesses in court or as the distinguished position of Visitor in the Lord Chancellor's Department to which John Bucknill ascended on his departure from Exminster. Yet the medical staff of the Asylum appear to have been as determined as the JPs who governed the institution that Exminster should not house the criminally insane, much to the irritation of the Home Office and Lunacy Commission.

The identification of violent behaviour and the significance attached to these violent acts was therefore the subject of some negotiation between different agents rather than being a self-evident condition for the committal of the insane. If we are fully to understand the different connotations of suffering we need to keep these competing interpretations of the significance of violence in view. Our primary sources for exploring these issues are mainly those generated by the Devon County Asylum itself, located at the village of Exminster near Exeter and where around thirteen thousand people were admitted between the day of its inauguration in 1845 and the outbreak of war in 1914. The essay seeks to decode these official materials in an attempt to investigate the nature and content of the suffering which individuals and families experienced in these years and the role of sentiment in the interaction between family, individual and agents of social and asylum policy and law.

CRIMINAL LUNACY AND THE DEVON ASYLUM

Before the departure of its first medical superintendent and celebrated alienist John Charles Bucknill in 1862, Exminster Asylum was lauded by interested parties, such as the state regulator, the Lunacy Commission, as a centre of pioneering excellence.[18] The asylum was built for 400 pauper lunatics, but its population rose almost continually and by 1914 there were around 1,400 there. Indeed the buildings were constantly being extended to receive greater numbers. This particular asylum almost only received pauper lunatics and therefore almost all sent there were certified as lunatic under the 1845, 1853 and 1890 statutes.[19] Charges for their treatment and maintenance were thus met by the Poor Law Guardians established under the 1834 Poor Law Amendment Act.[20] A significant proportion of the 13,000 who arrived at Exminster had come from the workhouses of the twenty Devon County poor law unions or from the urban corporations of Exeter and Plymouth and their certification of insanity had been undertaken by the poor law medical officers prior to committal by magistrates.[21] The Relieving Officer of the Union, with assistance bought in as needed, was personally responsible for conveying the lunatic to the asylum.

A rather different route was taken by the criminal lunatic. The processing of this category of lunatic exposes many of the tensions and complexities within the classification of the insane during the nineteenth century as well as the scope for intervention by the relatives of the mad. 'Criminal lunatics' might be defendants in criminal cases found insane on arraignment or (alternatively) insane at the time of the offence. Both categories of criminal lunatic would be ordered to be held 'during Her Majesty's pleasure'. A third category of criminal lunatic was the prisoner, sentenced to a specific sentence of penal servitude or imprisonment, who became insane during that sentence. Before the opening of Broadmoor Criminal Lunatic asylum in May 1863 there were heavy concentrations of criminal lunatics at Bethlem in London (after 1814) and at Fisherton House (after 1849). Each institution can be seen as seeking a niche in a rapidly-changing market for the care of the insane, though by 1870 both Bethlem and Fisherton had ceased to receive criminal lunatics. Two-thirds of all these inmates were held at the recently-opened Broadmoor and most of the remainder were lodged in county pauper lunatic asylums.[22]

The magistrates and medical professionals of Devon were not unusual in their anxiety generally to avoid housing this class of patient. As the 1882 Commission into Criminal Lunacy observed, there was a widespread belief, that criminal lunatics constitute a specially dangerous class of persons; that they are often homicidal; that they present a form of danger which ordinary lunatics do not show, in being able to enter into combination or conspiracy; that they incite other patients to turbulence and breaches of discipline; that their presence in county and borough asylums is injurious to the other inmates ... that asylums have not the equipment or the appliances which are required for the safe keeping of such persons.[23]

The figures recorded for the Devon Asylum reflected this resistance to the accommodation of those perceived as the most dangerous and disruptive of inmates. At the beginning of 1859, for example, there were nine male and two female criminal lunatics resident at Exminster and just over three decades later this number had fallen to a total of six.[24] There was also an insignificant trickle of inmates arriving at the Asylum from a variety of prisons, numbering only seven during the whole of the 1870s. A further disincentive to housing the criminally mad could be found in the weekly charges for accepting such inmates, which was always higher than the 8–9 shillings per week paid by Devon unions for their pauper lunatics.[25]

Not only did the Home Office press for the acceptance of criminal lunatics but they also determined the date of their release. This severely reduced where it did not remove the power of discretion exercised by the Visiting Committee to release criminal patients on probation. On the other hand, it must have been apparent to Bucknill that considerable celebrity and prestige was to be derived from contact with the infamy of criminal lunacy, not only in the court room but in making special efforts to engage with this group of insane individuals.[26] The editor of the *Journal of Mental Science* displayed a keen interest in such individuals and in detecting the hidden springs of criminal lunacy and the moral insanity often associated with their case histories.[27] The antipathy to receiving criminal lunatics therefore dates from the period following his tenure at Exminster. So fascinated and confident was Bucknill of his powers of analysis that he did not feel constrained from offering his opinion by the lack of personal contact with such individuals as Nicholas Besch who was committed to a French asylum in 1854 following 'his attempt to tear out the eyes of his wife'.[28] The ambitious alienist drew a detailed and dramatic portrait of intense sexual jealousy and calculated revenge based upon the deluded belief that Madame Besch was guilty of persistent adultery with a local man.

The Exminster superintendent utilised his public voice to acquire quickly a reputation for expertise which allowed him to figure as a scientific medical witness in serious criminal cases where a defence of insanity was presented. An important opportunity arrived in 1855 when Robert Handcock of Appledore in North Devon was brought to trial for the savage murder of his wife for an imagined offence of adultery. Handcock's acquittal as a 'monomaniac' and his detention at Her Majesty's Pleasure was carefully reported by Bucknill in his influential *Journal*.[29] Other cases were often less sensational but possessed some element of literary farce or tragedy which caught the eye, as when the Exminster physician gave evidence in 1857 at a troubling case where a man had become obsessed with gazing at windmills and had maimed a child in the hope and expectation of being removed to a region where windmills might be found.[30] After Bucknill's departure in 1862 for the more elegant and prestigious surroundings of the office of the Lord Chancellor's Visitors, the Devon Asylum continued to receive criminal lunatics throughout a period when overcrowding at Broadmoor caused problems and the second criminal asylum at Rampton was not opened until 1912.[31]

Relations between the Home Office and local magistrates continued to be fraught as the London officials provided little guidance or help in the matter of criminal insanity and local magistrates themselves on occasion misused legislation to present the asylums with most contradictory situations. As Janet Saunders also found there was a tendency for some magistrates to use the occasion of a court appearance to make a penal committal order for the disposal of individuals who lacked a settled domestic residence and whose behaviour could be construed as erratic.[32] Such conduct was apparent to the Lunacy Commissioners in 1889 when their *Report* noted that at Exminster there was,

one girl here ... who was brought up before the magistrates, fined ten shillings for unlawful possession and then sent to the Asylum at once. This does not appear to us to be fair to the patient who, at the time she committed the offence, was either responsible or not, but she has been treated as if both alternatives could exist simultaneously.[33]

The majority of criminal offenders who arrived at the gates of the Asylum were far removed from the infamous celebrities who sustained the attention of contemporary newspapers and allowed psychiatrists to cut a figure within the law courts. Most were guilty of petty crimes but a very small number of murderers and other serious offenders did go to Exminster although almost all such were screened out to Broadmoor.[34] The typical Exminster criminal lunatic was a trivial offender frequently with a record of recidivist offending, who had become either physically frail or erratic beyond the reach of the punishments meted out to them in prison. The wanton violence of others made their restraint necessary but difficult. When such individuals became incapable of withstanding the penal regime, the gaols appear to have been ready to see them shunted into the asylum where they would often expire or be retained as chronic patients for lengthy periods. Edward C. was diagnosed as a 'quiet and harmless old dement' when he arrived from Devon County Prison in 1860 having served his fifteenth term for vagrancy. He had been convicted for committing the crime of being abroad without the means of self support under the 1823 *Vagrancy Act*. In fact he might just as easily have applied for relief at the union workhouse as been arrested under vagrancy legislation. Indeed he possessed no known relatives and died a month after admission. William M. came to Exminster from the same prison in that year but proved so violent that he was to be re-certified on expiration of his sentence and remained as a chronic patient twenty years later. This pattern of dispatching prisoners incapable of responding to the Benthamite and severely moralistic rationality of the Victorian gaols can also be seen in the determination of the governor in a Lincolnshire prison to secure the admission of a handcuffed Devonian to Exminster after he repeatedly tore up his penal clothing.[35] Occasionally such behaviour was resorted to by prisoners who sought better medical treatment and accommodation at the county asylum. Catherine M. was convicted of prostitution and seems to have successfully pushed for the cure of her venereal disease in Bucknill's care but miscalculated that she would be released on her expected date and 'after the monthly meeting of the magistrates she vented her disappointment at not getting her discharge by swearing at and bullying those around her'. They let her go six months later.[36]

Whilst the criminal lunatics represented only a tiny constituency, along with young children and adolescent girls, in the Devon Asylum, the administration of such groups provides some insights into the limits and capacities of different institutional regimes. The certification and retention of these minorities also casts light on the relationship between the different agents who were responsible for the certification of the insane and the degree to which families and communities could conflict or collude with the legal authorities to secure their preferred outcome. One man came to Exminster after being sentenced for only six weeks after being convicted for indecent exposure, apparently because he had acquired a reputation within the locality for 'lying about in barns and outhouses . . . frightening women'.[37] In some instances it was the family itself which initiated the legal action which led to the committal of an individual such as William F., who was sent to the Asylum after a warrant was sworn by his brother against him in 1847. He was to die there three years later.[38] The family's capacity for tolerance of this awkward individual had certainly been exhausted by the periodic violence displayed in earlier years and the asylum offered a means by which his kin could protect themselves before further violence could be inflicted on them.

Such cases of family involvement in criminal proceedings remained relatively rare in this period and in many instances it would appear that families and poor law guardians colluded to deny their knowledge of any relationship to the criminal lunatic, thereby shifting the burden of maintenance on to the County Treasurer.[39] The burden of such charges was apparent to guardians even before the passage of the 1845 Lunacy Act. When the Axminster Union transferred a criminal lunatic to the new County Asylum in 1844–45 they quickly faced a plethora of bills amounting to £42 7s 6d for Ameliora J., 'an Insane Pauper belonging to Axminster, lately tried at the Devon Assizes for a felony but acquitted on the ground of insanity'.[40] Liability of unions for prisoners with an identified settlement being certified during sentence had been confirmed by legislation in 1840.[41] Where possible, and more particularly towards the end of the period, the poor law guardians ordered their relieving officers to pursue relatives for the reimbursement of the ratepayers.[42] This provided the relatives as well as the poor law officials with a bone of contention since the release of criminal lunatics required the sanction of the Home Office and it was by no means certain that the prisoner's kin or his community (who were usually involved in the decision to release pauper lunatics to 'relatives and friends') would welcome the return of the inmate.

The consequence could be an extremely protracted and bad-tempered squabble over the settlement of the criminal lunatic, with the high maintenance costs at the county asylum as the penalty for defeat. Even Bucknill strained his usual good relations with the St. Thomas Union when he suggested in 1856 that they accept responsibility for the 'criminal lunatic', Samuel Cary R. and apply to the Secretary of State for his discharge as cured.[43] The Guardians brusquely replied denying his settlement in their union and any intention of acknowledging his claims by making such application. They relented only when a judicial order was made fixing his settlement in their union and even then refused to pay the asylum bills and fees which had mounted up in the interim. The grandees of the St. Thomas Board stubbornly contested liability until the bitter end almost a year later.[44] So acrimonious did such contests become by the 1880s that in 1884 Parliament enacted that the cost of maintenance of criminal lunatics, whether in Broadmoor or local asylums, should be defrayed by the Treasury.[45] This did not restrict the liability of poor law unions completely, as the Axminster Guardians discovered in 1900 regarding Walter T., who appears to have completed his penal servitude at the Devon Asylum between 1889 and 1900. When his sentence was spent he was promptly reclassified as a pauper lunatic and thus became a charge on the ratepayers of East Devon.

This brief survey of the passage of criminal lunatics to the Exminster Asylum in the Victorian period indicates that we can indeed see the county asylum as functioning in part to service the system of penal regulation developed within England and Wales during these decades, though this statement conceals more than it reveals since these provincial institutions were never involved with more than a tiny number of penal lunatics and were increasingly superseded by the specialist facilities at Broadmoor and Rampton before the First World War. The dominance of poor law concerns within the system of lunacy administration was apparent from a very early period in the life of Exminster, even if Bucknill saw scientific responsibilities and professional advantage in the treatment of the criminally insane. So marked were the tensions between the role of magistrates and guardians involved in pauper lunacy and the disposal of the criminal insane by the courts that the central state assumed increasing financial as well as institutional responsibility for the incarceration of this class of lunatics. In doing so Parliament confirmed the development of increasingly specialised services for those groups who were not easily managed by either the lunatic asylum or the prison. A significant contribution to this process was made by the resistance and collusive manoeuvrings of poor law officials, families, asylum medical personnel and even magistrates in a bid to avoid the financial and physical burden of criminal lunacy being levied on them. These burdens might range from the simple assumption of the maintenance of a known vagrant, to the deposit of a petty sexual offender and community nuisance in the asylum when a brief prison sentence would prove an inadequate deterrent, and the alternate identification or denial of familial relationship to a violent lunatic who placed an intolerable burden on relatives or neighbourhood. In such instances the intellectual provenance of the institutional regime was less significant than the ability of families and communities to calculate the balance of advantage between acknowledging the individual concerned and colluding with officials to deny his or her rights to belong to their settlement. Playing to maximise their benefit from the rules of the institutions they dealt with, but could not hope to control, does not demonstrate a callous disregard for sentiment. It may suggest that there was more than one solution to shared difficulties and that each group was concerned to avoid bearing the undoubted costs of criminal lunacy.

Such calculative approaches are readily comprehensible in the face of the risks which criminal lunatics could pose to the collective. The next section attempts to compare the responses outlined above with the qualitative evidence which can be derived from asylum and other sources on the part which violence played in the containment of the uncertified family member and the institutionalisation of the certified lunatic.

SUFFERING AND FAMILY CARE FOR LUNATICS IN VICTORIAN DEVON

One of the key reference points for social historians seeking to explain the significant rise in the numbers admitted to public lunatic asylums in the nineteenth century remains Andrew Scull's argument that poor families were increasingly unwilling to carry

the burden of disruptive and unproductive members as the pressures of the commercialised market economy and the availability of
places at these institutions began to be appreciated in the second
half of the century.[46] In a separate discussion of the treatment of
the elderly poor in the nineteenth century, Richard Smith has
emphasised the impact on family and community behaviour of a
tightening in poor law rules and a decline in the willingness of
family members to care for aged dependants.[47] In responding to
Scull's pioneering scholarship, researchers have usually concentrated their criticisms on the period 1800–1880 and have often
followed his lead in assuming that the later decades of the nineteenth century were overshadowed by the failure of moral treatment and the inexorable advance of hereditarian and eugenic
ideas.[48] The evidence we have gathered from the Devon experience
indicates that each perspective can be utilised in an assessment of
the changing pattern of community and institutional provision for
lunatics during our period, though each account of family calculation needs to be placed within a context where the physical and
emotional (as well as material) costs of containment and exclusion
can be registered, if not precisely measured. There are some clues
that the 1880s marked something of a watershed in the period and
that the later years can be distinguished not simply as the dark age
of eugenicist pessimism about the insane but rather as a time when
the asylums faced changing legislative and administrative reforms
as well as absorbing pressures within the poor law and medical
profession in favour of more specialist provision for different
classes of lunatics. These latter moves were reinforced by the
renewed efforts, noted by Smith and other scholars, of the Local
Government Board and local poor law authorities to limit expenditure on pauper relief and compel the relatives of the elderly and
infirm to contribute towards their upkeep.

A familiar difficulty we face in attempting to record the distress
experienced by lunatics and the changes in patterns of administration is the bewildering array of accounts and competing rhetoric
of blame and reform which marked the management of lunacy in
the middle and later decades of the nineteenth century. It was the
very dramatisation of the spectacle of the isolated lunatic kept in
barbaric conditions which served as the cue for the claims of
enlightened intervention that reformers voiced during these years.
The paradox remains that in the era of growing commercialisation

which Scull sees as the context for the weakening of family bonds, Shaftesbury and his allies made their attack on the private mad-house and the trade in lunacy the foundation for the idealisation of the public institution. This is not to deny the profound neglect and gross abuse of individuals in the years before the 1845 legislation, often uncovered and reported by the new generation of Poor Law Commissioners who investigated the conditions of the poor as well as enforced the stringent rules of less eligibility. It was Assistant Poor Law Commissioner Gilbert, who discovered in the 1830s a Tiverton woman who had been immured for some twenty-eight years in a tiny room with no fire or furniture and a Devonian man chained in the darkness of an outhouse for eight years.[49] Such scandals provided the reformers with the ammunition they needed to defeat backwoods opposition to the new asylum movement and to demand the compulsory registration of all the insane whether inside or outside the walls of an institution.

Legislative intervention implied a significant invasion in the private domain of the domestic household and the affairs of the family. The victims of hidden attics and outhouses as well as the private madhouse were portrayed as the solitary afflicted in need of comfort and treatment. The needs of the outcast lunatic were graphically illustrated in 1852 when the Lunacy Commissioners successfully prosecuted the brother of a Lewtrenchard farmer for the neglect of his nephew, Charles L., who had been chained for nine years to the floor of a wooden cell measuring only a few feet wide.[50] When Charles was liberated from his box he was 'at first so bent that he could not stand nor walk and was unaccustomed to the stimuli of light and clothing'.[51] The governors of Exminster Asylum noted that over a period of nine months in their institution 'he has been uniformly quiet and well conducted and has been regularly employed in the Blacksmith's shop'.[52] By bringing a close relative to court for the cruel neglect of a man for whom the family possibly sought to claim relief, thereby drawing the attention of senior poor law officials to his plight, the Lunacy Commissioners gave notice of a public interest in the condition of the insane and their determination to see such individuals placed in public institutions.

In his early years, when Bucknill shared the patronage and good opinion of the Lunacy Commissioners, he was anxious to use his skills as a publicist to dramatise the role of the psychiatrist as explorer of the darker recesses of mistreatment by relatives of the vulnerable lunatic. The undoubted misery of the individuals concerned cannot be ignored. He reported to his readers the case of Joseph A., who had been restrained in a tiny attic for eighteen years by his mother and brother and that of Edward L., squatting in his own waste in the total darkness of a tiny room at Bratton Fleming and where he remained for seven years so contorted by lack of space that 'his nose was almost between his knees, his legs drawn up'. On examination it was found that one of these legs was broken.[53] Such cases could only legitimate the claims of the new asylums and the Lunacy Commission to provide a therapeutic regime infinitely superior to that available in private madhouses or local communities.

Yet Bucknill was himself aware of the tensions and contradictions inherent within the legislative project undertaken in 1845. The groups who appeared to be most vulnerable to mistreatment were the very young and the elderly, since they usually depended on relatives and kin to provide basic care. It is very difficult to ascertain the extent of the physical and sexual abuse of the children and women who entered the Devon Asylum, still less of those who remained in their own communities, given the reluctance of even medical personnel to record the possibility of sexual violence.[54] Even before the eugenicists raised the spectre of idiot and imbecile children breeding a race of defectives, there was some alarm expressed when a young woman gave birth to illegitimate children after an unidentified man had 'taken advantage of her simplicity'.[55] Female children and adolescents were also at risk when they entered the service of others if they could not rely on family protection. Susan H. entered Exminster at the age of seventeen but had gone into service when only nine and was 'very ill used by her master who was punished for his conduct'.[56] In some instances the medical and clerical staff of the asylum were able to identify negligence in foreigners, as when they entered the details of twelve year old Jane R. in 1876 as 'a daughter of a French man, a Quack Doctor ... [she] has been half starved'.[57] In other instances the admission notes suggest the possibility of sexual abuse of adolescent girls rather than offering clear evidence.[58]

Even when it was clear that such children could not be easily cared for at home the magistrates who governed the asylum and Bucknill himself were reluctant to accept idiots and imbeciles for whom they could offer no specialist facilities, unless it could be shown that such young people were a serious danger to themselves or those around them. Exminster's Clerk was directed by the Visiting Justices to remind the Honiton Guardians of this point and tell them that 'James H., a patient from that Union, has shewn no disposition to be dangerous to himself or others since he has been in the asylum. That he is an idiot and about nine years of age'.[59] Even when Bucknill relaxed this rule to admit two children in 1847 (one with serious epilepsy), each died within a brief period of arrival.[60] One consequence was that children were usually admitted only when the claim of significant violence or extreme disability was confirmed by the Poor Law authorities and certifying personnel.[61] The asylum authorities realised that the risk of accepting such young people, even when in desperate need of some care, was that they were unlikely ever to leave the institution. Thus Jessie C. was accepted in 1876 aged thirteen as 'idiotic from birth and unable to speak', and was still there at the end of the century, having 'never been known to speak except on a few occasions when she has sworn'.[62]

There was less risk that the elderly would remain to clog up the arteries of the asylum over a long period of residence, but rather similar concerns were evident in the reception of such infirm individuals from their families and the Poor Law authorities. Cases of serious neglect were noted by Bucknill and he seems to have been a willing witness against the relatives who perpetrated such abuse, as when he noted on the entry of Grace W. in 1848 that she had been 'under the protection of a son and his wife who are now committed for trial for their ill usage of her and depriving her of all the necessaries of life'.[63] It was not rare to find on examination of the individuals who came to the asylum that they displayed some signs of physical abuse, as when the Visitors themselves noted that a woman arrived in 1852 'in a condition evidently showing bodily ill treatment'. She died ten days later.[64] As late as 1894 a man arrived with 'extensive bruises on chest, back, buttocks, arms and legs some of which look as if done by a stick' and rope marks revealing where he had been tied.[65] He again died shortly after entering Exminster.

Even if graphic evidence of physical abuse was absent, there were large numbers of paupers arriving in the early years in poor health and the women in particular often came (as the governors commented) in 'a state of emaciation and weakness'. This was still a problem a decade after the institution opened its doors, as the Superintendent's notes on the many consumptives amongst the admissions testify.[66] Bucknill warned his employers that the continued propensity of poor law guardians to use his establishment as 'a public infirmary' would result in abnormal death rates being recorded at Exminster.[67] Here lay a familiar conundrum for an ambitious physician who was extremely critical of workhouse medical care and reluctant to turn away elderly patients who appeared to be suffering from varying degrees of neglect. There was little prospect of cure and their presence as chronic patients not only reduced the scope for the individual treatment of others with a better prognosis but their death reflected badly on the cure rates claimed at the asylum.

A final factor which seems to have circumscribed the ability of Lunacy Commissioners, medical professionals and local magistrates to enforce the legislation of 1845 was the reluctance of local communities to comply with the spirit of the new laws where it was perceived that family rights were being infringed. The London Commission was persistently pressing asylum Visitors (themselves magistrates) to prosecute individuals under the lunacy acts where clear evidence of cruelty and neglect could be found. The local magistracy was itself chary of engaging in such actions and their scepticism was confirmed when juries at the local assizes refused to convict where family members were involved and even when those employed to care for lunatics were accused of gross neglect. As late as 1875 a prosecution was brought against a couple who had been paid by the relatives of Thomasine P. to look after her in private premises. The relieving officer of the Sidmouth Union discovered her in squalid conditions:

> she gave an unintelligibly wild and chattering answer . . . her arms which she threw about were covered with excrement . . . on the rug which she had over her being turned up the smell was so offensive that it was impossible to remain in the room . . . the bed and sacking under her were sodden with filth'.[68]

The couple were charged and acquitted at the next Devon Assizes. The evidence is impressionistic on this point but there are signs of a reduction in the reported incidents of gross abuse and neglect inflicted on lunatics arriving at Exminster from the mid-1880s onwards. This might arise from a variety of matters as the asylum medical notes shift from concerns with the social origins of the patient to concentrating much more directly on their course of treatment within the institution. It is also possible that the vigilance of the Lunacy Commission, coupled with the more detailed examination of the person prior to certification, contributed to greater standards of care being shown towards the insane in both their communities and the institutions which processed their passage to Exminster.

In many instances the responsibility for the brutal or negligent treatment of pauper lunatics lay with the local union officials and the guardians who employed them rather than the relatives of the insane. Within a few months of opening the asylum, the Exminster justices were expressing their dismay at the action of the Totnes Guardians in transporting a woman naked in a cart to their care and condemned the action which arose from 'the hardness of the Parish Officers who had refused decent clothing'.[69] It was an indication both of rising expectations and of continuing negligence that the Lunacy Commission criticised the Plympton Guardians almost fifty years later for refusing an elderly woman admission to the union workhouse and dispatching her by rail to Exminster where she was 'brought in moribund' and died within hours of her journey.[70] The anxiety of local guardians to defend the interests of the ratepayers could lead to neglect even where the families of the lunatic were striving to care for them in desperate circumstances. It required the determined intervention of a local clergyman in a village near Barnstaple to force the certification of 'a neglected idiot child'. The Lunacy Commissioners commented in their *Annual Report*, that her parents existed,

> in a state of great dilapidation and presented an aspect of extreme poverty . . . the Parents appeared to be . . . kindly disposed but obviously not in a position properly to maintain and take care of their poor idiot child, who, on account of her restlessness and violent agitation and for her own protection, had been during the past two years kept in restraint day and night . . .[71]

The Commissioners added with some acidity that the Barnstaple Guardians 'having full knowledge of the miserable state of the poor idiot . . . refused to recognise any claim to relief'. It may have been the public ignominy to which the Lunacy Commissioners exposed them on this occasion which persuaded the Barnstaple authorities to provide for their idiot children on rather more generous terms at other times.[72]

The final section of our essay pursues this theme of the responsiveness of the Poor Law to the preferences which are revealed by the records of local unions and the Devon Asylum and seeks to explore the nexus between families and communities in the representations made regarding the behaviour of an individual found to be insane.

FAMILIES, COMMUNITIES AND THE SPECTACLE OF PAUPER LUNACY

Since Walton's pioneering research on family ties and lunacy admissions in industrial Lancashire there has been considerable interest in the influence of family ties on the dispatch of pauper lunatics to and from Victorian asylums.[73] Less attention has been devoted to the communal contexts in which families and kinship networks were formed or the sources of support which were available to kin groups amongst extended kin and from membership of such institutions as church congregations and voluntary societies. The remarkable scarcity of solitary householders amongst those admitted to the Devon Asylum in this period and the disproportionate numbers of unmarried women and men coming to Exminster would suggest that household membership had some influence over the pattern of admissions. Females living in Devon at this time were not only likely to be rather more mobile than their male counterparts, but women admitted to Exminster were somewhat less mobile than the general female population but possessed a much more pronounced migration history than male lunatics.[74] Such evidence appears to point to the capacities of kin to absorb solitary individuals into their households prior to their institutionalisation as lunatics and also the greater vulnerability of the unmarried to being identified and admitted to the county asylum. Whereas men who came to the asylum were very strongly tied to the parish and union of their birth, females were less deeply enmeshed in long-standing networks of kinship and community.

Whilst these patterns of settlement provide some important clues as to the influence of household and community structures on the incidence of certification in the nineteenth-century, they offer only limited insights into the micro-politics of the events which led to the institutionalisation of individuals. Much of the admission and case note evidence gathered by the Devon Asylum suggests that many, if not most, of those coming into Exminster were in poor physical health and that the decision to certify them had been taken at a point in the family life cycle where the resources of the individual had diminished or the capacity of their kin and friends to cope with them had been depleted by some loss or change in household membership. The trigger for the formal intervention of the poor law authorities and medical opinion was often a violent act by the individual which was now presented on the certificate of insanity as intolerable. The boundaries of tolerance in such instances were not the province of the family household alone but were drawn by families in relation to the immediate neighbourhood and community. Working class and small farming families were as anxious as their wealthy counterparts to conceal the shame of insanity, lest the entire household be stigmatised as insane.[75] The fear of public shame helps to explain the barbarous isolation in which some lunatics were detained in remote attics and farm buildings. The difficulties of such concealment and the anxiety of families themselves to avoid close intermarriage made it unlikely that community knowledge of insane relatives could be easily avoided in smaller settlements.[76]

Whereas poor law authorities and the magistrates governing the Devon Asylum were reluctant to accept responsibility for convicted criminal lunatics however passive, and juries slow to return guilty verdicts on families or employees accused of brutality or neglect in handling vulnerable lunatics, there appears to have much been less reticence in dispatching an individual accused by relatives and neighbours of violent intentions. Workhouse officers were similarly anxious to transport to the asylum any inmate who displayed aggressive behaviour towards others or themselves. In many instances the testimony of relatives, police officers or workhouse masters was accepted as corroborating evidence indicating insanity. The precise nature of the violence inflicted or threatened is often difficult to fathom from the materials and this again implies that the consensus reached between family members and Poor Law officials could be at least as significant as any material facts in the committal of an individual. Richard D. was brought to Exminster in 1847 by the relieving officer and his own son after persistent violence between Richard and his wife, whose reported threat to kill him had caused 'great anxiety and seemed to prey deeply on his mind'.[77] Even young children could be dispatched once the testimony of their actual or attempted violence was agreed.[78]

The timing of the certification of the lunatic seems to have depended to a large degree on the capacity of family and kinship households to accommodate the behaviour of the individual within the cycle of life events that shaped the fortunes and resources of the household unit. The death of a key member of the household and more especially an individual who had been the primary carer of any dependent person often provided the trigger for acting in concert with the poor law officers. Parents who had cared for their children over many years were often forced by illness and old age, if not death, to relinquish their responsibilities and in the absence of other kinship or community support an institutional solution was sought. Susan K. who entered the asylum aged forty-five in 1872 was typical of many admissions recognised as having long-standing illness. She had been cared for all her life by her father, a Greenwich Pensioner, and when in extreme old age he elected to go to Greenwich Hospital she was unable to cope without family support.[79] Ann P. appears to have been cared for into advanced old age until the deterioration of her condition led to her arrival at Exminster in 1860.[80] At such points the violence of the family member often turned the scales, as when it was said that Charlotte G.'s father had become too infirm to stand up to 'violent and destructive' behaviour and became 'unable to support her', or aged householders turned to the poor law when unable to withstand their aggressive spouse.[81] The situation was particularly serious when the person certified was the head of the household or the (usually female) partner responsible for the care of the children and upkeep of the home.

It was often a crisis around family resources which compelled the family to approach the poor law and to seek assistance for their distracted relatives. The intervention of the relieving officer made a journey to the county asylum possible but by no means inevitable. Individuals might be relieved in their own homes, offered some assistance with paid carers within the community (i.e. 'boarded out'), or placed in the workhouse before they were considered for formal certification. The absence of material and human resources was the common feature of many such cases. William S.' wife had just born a 'hydrokephalic' child; his family were in destitution; his wife and children were all very sick and he himself was ill and unable to work.[82] Mary B. had just given birth when bailiffs arrived to evict her, her family having no money or resources.[83] As one plaintively explained: 'everything has gone wrong lately'.[84] After the death of her husband, Sarah S. fell behind with her rent and after the landlord seized all her goods became 'very low spirited, desponding, melancholy', it being noted on her certificate that when at home she 'would sometimes lie on a bed one or two days together'.[85] Here lay two threads that were often used to tie together the facts which indicated the insanity of a female admitted to Exminster: failure to fulfil household obligations and an aggressive or violent disregard for members of their family or community. Florence G. was admitted to Exminster aged thirty-four in 1903, having been certified (it seems) on her mother's testimony with whom she and her child lived. It was said that Florence,

> does no work of any kind, not even to attend to her child, nor housework, is dirty and neglectful of herself in every way. Sits moodily all day long. At night makes much disturbance and suffers from sleeplessness. She is violent to her mother, knocks her down . . . is uncontrollable by her mother with whom she resides.[86]

Here the documents make no reference to the father of the child, though in other instances the insanity of people admitted to Exminster was more explicitly attributed to moral weakness or to violent sexual jealousy, unrequited passion and abandonment by husbands or lovers.[87] The threat posed by women and men to the integrity of the family household or to themselves was frequently the catalyst which propelled an individual towards the asylum. The weight of grief and distress at the death of children or spouses could disable females until their 'desponding' behaviour raised fears of violence against themselves or others. Mary B. had lost two of her children in 1875 when relatives tried to relieve her melancholy by encouraging her to visit them 'for a change of air' with only slight improvement, whilst the death of three children, a son-in-law and grandchild in succession reduced Jane J. to 'melancholia'.[88] Mothers who confided to their medical personnel a deep resentment towards new born babies could find themselves certified,[89] whilst other women were stricken by the guilt at the real or imagined neglect of children in their household.[90]

The variety of sources which informed many of the certificates suggest not merely the presence of family testimonies but a wider theatre of community knowledge and involvement. Only under particular conditions would such knowledge be disclosed to the legal authorities and even the poor law authorities might collude in the restriction of information if they did not wish the full power of the criminal law to be invoked. One of the Axminster Relieving Officers confided to Bucknill in 1861, for example, that a Yarcombe woman admitted to the asylum was locally believed to have starved five of her babies to death and had been taken to the workhouse where she may have tried to strangle a sixth. Mary P. was certified in 1872 after confessing her temptation to kill her children with a razor, confirming a belief which appears to have been widespread in her village that she had drowned an illegitimate child before her marriage, thereafter 'wandering frequently by the riverside where the child was found'.[91] The status of such opinions and the media through which they were transmitted reveals something of the tension between regulation and consent that we discussed earlier. For his part, Bucknill was anxious to demonstrate a forensic ability to use such evidence whilst separating out scientific facts from community fictions. He told a Select Committee of Parliament many years after he had departed from the Devon Asylum:

> I remember a curious case of an old woman ... her house had been broken into ... I found her quite sane ... I found she was what they call a witch ... four young men of the village thought they were bewitched by her. They had broken into her home and, to take off the witchcraft, they had cut slashes in her arms and left her bleeding. They had drawn blood to remove the witchcraft. This woman was certified as having had delusions. She was quite sane and remained sane. It was a mistake.[92]

Such testimonies portrayed the psychiatrist not only as the rescuer of the vulnerable lunatic but as the arbiter of sanity within communities where traditional folk beliefs could lead to the victimisation of solitary individuals.[93] On other occasions Bucknill was keen to stress the real threat with dangerous lunatics could present to the community, recalling the case of a Devon shoemaker who was arrested 'parading the streets with a knife tied on a pole and frightening people'.[94]

The professional perspective on community sentiment given by Bucknill needs to be set against the evidence in the admission documents of community influence over the certification of individuals. Such influence was on occasion expressed through the voice of 'friends' or the reported views of neighbours, though entering the houses of 'strangers' also placed an individual on a fast track to Exminster, as when William M. came to Bucknill's care in 1847 having 'rushed into the house of strangers near Honiton by night, smashed the contents of the house and threatened to murder them all.[95] A more familiar case was that of Elias B., depicted in 1904 as 'a terror and a source of anxiety to his friends and to the neighbourhood of Tavistock'.[96] In some cases, where reports of assault or sexual violation could have provided the substance for a criminal prosecution, magistrates appear to have conferred with local medical personnel and decided on a committal order to the asylum, as when a man was found to have sexually abused village children.[97]

The decision to certify most individuals appears to have been the outcome of a dialogue between the relatives, friends and neighbours and the legal authorities responsible for administering pauper lunacy. The conduit between these two spheres of influence was provided by the relieving officer. Reports of a scandalised neighbourhood would reach him in due course and the poor law authorities could themselves form part of the imagery of insanity which figured in the lunatic's narrative. Sitwell A. was sent to Exminster in 1902, having 'talked wildly and volubly about her neighbours.'

> Said they accused her of being a prostitute and cried it in the road. Said one of the Guardians had knotted a cat and given it to one of the neighbours to whip her. She keeps her doors locked as she says she is in bodily fear of her neighbours. Shouts from her window, calling out dreadful things. Talks constantly to herself. Says her neighbours are trying to kill her.[98]

Where the violence of an individual involved relatives, community or even poor law in significant costs for supervision and maintenance then the asylum became a much more attractive solution. Before the asylum opened its doors, local workhouse masters were compelled to house violent lunatics such as the young woman at St. Thomas who was 'daily increasing in violence and requiring constant attendance and watching'.[99] Another female was brought to Okehampton Workhouse in the 1860s, 'in a most violent state, in fact dangerous to herself and others',[100] whilst the Exeter Guardians were concerned to hear that one chargeable pauper was 'exceedingly violent, smashing all the glass and everything that came in his way: persons had been employed to look after him until he could be removed to the county asylum'.[101] The costs of insanity were clearly calculated in regard to the level of violence and the expense of restraint involved.

Relatively few of those who are entered in the admission registers were found 'wandering at large' without connections in the towns and villages where they were detained. Occasionally vagrants were discovered to be lunatics and brought to the asylum, as when Charles M. appeared on the streets of Axminster in 1851 and in the absence of any settlement rights the County Treasurer funded his removal to Bucknill's care. Fifty years later the same union noted that John C. had been 'apprehended by the police as a wandering lunatic' without any knowledge of his origins.[102] It is difficult to tell if the inability of relieving officers to discover the settlement of wanderers was the result of vigorous efforts to interrogate unwell individuals or conveniently accepted where the costs fell on the county rather than their union.[103] Even some of the most exotic of wanderers returned to their native community prior to certification, as when Arthur K. came home to his mother having been absent for several years 'without fixed residence or employment'. Arthur had some brushes with the penal system, having 'tramped all over England: been to sea: been three times to Russia: twice in gaol'.[104] Poor law authorities were determined to recoup the cost of offering comfort to strangers from the responsible unions, as is evident from the bitter wrangles over settlement and removal costs throughout this period, and there must be at least a possibility that many disorderly vagrants were moved on by local officers where there seemed little prospect of ascertaining their origins.

CONCLUSIONS

The evidence presented in the admission documents used in this essay reveal some of the complexities of lunacy administration in the later nineteenth century. Recent contributions to the social history of insanity have sought to place the growth of lunatic asylums within a longer trajectory of welfare provision whilst stressing the need for a careful exploration of the micropolitics of community and institutional provision. Smith has urged us to consider the possibility of a demand-driven history of welfare services, whilst other writers have returned to Foucault's agenda in seeking to place psychiatric facilities in a long-term comparative perspective which includes the building of pauper and penal reformatories. This essay offers a contribution to these debates by considering the role not only of families but of 'friends' and communities to the application of lunacy legislation in the period 1845–1914. The particular concern here has been with the different ways in which violence was perceived and dealt with by the variety of actors who participated in the narrative of certification. In assessing the influence of 'communities' on the institutionalisation of lunatics only a few accounts of residents identified as non-relatives were selected and said little of the multiplicity of religious and voluntary societies which formed a vital part of many lunatics' lives and often featured in the accounts of their descent into insanity.[105] The loss of place or faith in such specific communities could prove as dramatic as the onset of bereavement or slippage of one's footing within a household or the respect of a neighbourhood.

The events which set a person on the road to the asylum were extremely varied but they often followed a change in household arrangements which diminished the resources available to the individual or increased the prospective costs of their maintenance. The death of carers, breadwinners or loved ones could reduce the person to a destitution for which outdoor or indoor relief was inadequate. In calculations of costs and benefits made by relatives, friends or workhouses masters, a propensity to violence was the entry on the certificate which had tilted the balance against the care of the individual outside the asylum. The meanings of violence were construed according to the needs of the moment rather than being a simple equation with the 'dangerous lunatic' identified by the lunacy legislation of the period. Despite the ambitions of Bucknill to claim a forensic expertise in cases of criminal lunacy, we have seen that neither the poor law guardians nor the magistrates who governed the Devon Asylum were keen to house violent offenders. The Exminster Visitors were as reluctant to accept criminal lunatics as workhouse masters were to accommodate violent inmates in their lunacy wards. The county asylum as well as the union workhouse remained a general rather than a specialist institution, a function confirmed by the opening of specialist facilities for criminal lunatics, idiot children and others during this period. Families and friends could often drive a bargain with the poor law authorities for the low-cost maintenance of even a violent individual before the mounting pressure of Lunacy Commissioners began to tell towards the end of the nineteenth century.

The hand of the family was strengthened by the reluctance of local juries to prosecute those responsible even for gross neglect and abuse of vulnerable lunatics. This can be read, in part, as the resistance of local communities to the invasion of traditionally private spaces by the interrogating glare of the poor law and lunacy authorities, reflected in Bucknill's concern to contrast family ignorance and distorted community beliefs with the scientific enlightenment brought by medical knowledge. More prosaically, kinship groups and the parishes or towns where they lived were the key sources of the lay knowledge of lunacy and the information laid before relieving officers and medical personnel. The violence which an individual was known or suspected to have inflicted was only formally communicated to the authorities in circumstances where the consequences could not be contained within the privacy of a household or where community values were outraged. Private violence to contain the threat of violence posed by a supposed lunatic appears to have been tolerated long after the passage of the 1845 legislation. Even criminal violence and assaults by community members appear to have been the subject of consultation between communities, medical personnel, police and magistrates and in a surprising number of cases were routed away from the criminal justice system and towards the poor law and certification.

Such a preliminary assessment of the admissions to the Devon Asylum can make only a limited contribution to the growing literature on the social relationships which made up the world of Victorian lunacy and the location of modern psychiatric institutions within the development of the penal welfare state. Much of the literature on family responses to insanity since Walton's important comment on the Lancashire experience has been implicitly addressing the influence of calculation and sentiment in caring strategies. Our reading of the Devon sources indicates that the possession of both material and emotional resources need to be seen within the life cycle of family events where the presence (and availability) of physical violence and restraint were a key consideration. Various forms of abuse by, or upon, those later certified as lunatics could be and were tolerated within limits established by families, friends and communities as well as institutions of authority and the legal system. To view such dialogues between the informal and formal regulators of behaviour as the expression of a social market 'demanding' welfare provision is no more persuasive than models which present the asylum merely as the outworks of a carceral state. As Smith and others have noted, we need detailed studies which reveal the impact of specific responses to state initiatives. The evidence from the Devon Asylum indicates that this period was one in which the legal regulation of lunacy was the subject of continued, if unequal, negotiation rather than the imposition of control or the building of consensus.

CHAPTER NINE

Community care and mental deficiency 1913 to 1945

Jan Walmsley, Dorothy Atkinson
and Sheena Rolph

INTRODUCTION

This chapter will draw together the findings from recent research into the way mental deficiency was managed in two southern English counties to show the nature of policy, provision and practice for people with learning disabilities outside the institutional context which has hitherto been the focus of most historical interest.[1] Whilst a number of commentators have placed the origins of care in the community in the post World War Two era, there is increasing evidence coming from recent scholarship to suggest that it has much longer antecedents.[2]

The contemporary rhetoric about care in the community tends to portray it as the semantic opposite to institutional care. The argument is that the institutional era, which once held sway, has been discredited, and has been replaced by care in the community. Despite findings that some care in the community can be as regimented and institutionalised as care in institutions,[3] there remains a general belief amongst social policy commentators that it is a case of institutional care versus community care.[4] Not only this, but community care is viewed as superior to institutional care. This chapter, by contrast, shows that community care is, and has long been, an adjunct both to institutional care and to family care; that the different forms of care existed on a spectrum; and that community care could be as controlling as institutional care.

The arguments in this research owe a great deal to Mathew Thomson's pioneering work on mental deficiency between the wars. In his thesis,[5] Thomson explored the implementation of the 1913 Mental Deficiency Act, particularly with reference to case files in the London Metropolitan Archives. He argued that it was too simplistic to view the 1913 Act as legislation imposed from above, and that there was considerable negotiation between the Board of Control, which had central authority over the workings of the Act; local authorities, charged with implementation in their own areas; and families, when it came to making decisions about appropriate action in individual cases. He also demonstrated that there was a range of provision far more complex than a simple dichotomy between institutional and family care, provision which warrants the name 'care in the community'. This paper builds on Thomson's work to explore the legislative foundations of care in the community, and to examine how care in the community was managed in two local authorities in the inter-war years.

THE LEGISLATIVE FRAMEWORK 1913–1945

What is distinctive about the early twentieth century response to 'mental deficiency' is the effort to extend control and care to groups which had hitherto been unlabelled, the 'feeble-minded' and 'moral imbeciles'. As will be seen below, recent research in the UK strongly suggests that, until the twentieth century, care for the mass of people now labelled as having a learning disability[6] was left to the family, supplemented by various types of outdoor relief or workhouse provision. Only the minority were housed in purpose-built institutions, mainly lunatic asylums or madhouses, and some, from the later nineteenth century, in specialist institutions such as Earlswood, the Royal Eastern and Royal Western Counties Asylums.

The first statute to be directed specifically at 'idiocy' was the 1886 Idiots Act. Hitherto 'idiots' and 'lunatics' had been managed under legislation which made institutional provision for the 'insane'. The subjects of the Idiots Act were 'idiots' and 'imbeciles', people with quite severe degrees of impairment sufficient to prevent them from being self supporting even in favourable circumstances. Around the turn of the twentieth century the gaze extended, to encompass those whose impairment was less severe, what Tredgold[7] called 'The largest and most important class of all – the adult feeble minded'.

The threat posed by the adult feeble-minded to the welfare of the nation as a whole was a preoccupation of two organisations, the National Association for the Care of the Feeble Minded (founded 1896) and the Eugenics Education Society (founded 1907). These bodies campaigned vigorously in the early years of the twentieth century for legislation to deal with the 'problem' they posed, and were successful to the extent that a Royal Commission, the Radnor Commission, was appointed in 1904 to look into the question.

Contemporary commentators employed arguments designed to appeal both to fear and to compassion in campaigning for a change in legislation. In a review of the findings of the Royal Commission and other investigators in the period immediately prior to the passing of the 1913 Act, Tredgold[8] cites research showing that mentally defective; women were abnormally fertile; that their off-spring were likely to be below average in physical and mental fitness; that illegitimacy was prevalent, with at least 40 per cent of women admitted to Rescue Homes in the period 1909–13 being mentally defective, that mentally defective women spread venereal disease; that feeble minded men were disproportionately repre-sented in the prison population; and that, in 1906, 67.8 per cent of the adult feeble-minded were paupers maintained partly or entirely at the public expense.

The Radnor Commission concluded:

> Of the gravity of the present state of things there is no doubt. The mass of facts that we have collected, the statements of our witnesses, and our own personal visits and investigations compel the conclusion that there are numbers of mental defective persons whose training is neglected, over whom no sufficient control is exercised, and whose wayward and irresponsible lives are productive of crime and misery, of much injury to themselves and to others, and of much continuous expenditure wasteful to the community and to individual families . . .[9]

There were a number of conflicting solutions proposed to the problem, but primarily the object of both the National Association and the Eugenics Society was to identify this problematic group and to inhibit its numerical growth. As Tredgold put it: 'It was high time to stem the advancing tide of degeneracy ... Their propagation must be prevented'.[10]

After some considerable lobbying and amendment the 1913 Mental Deficiency Act was passed. Its main aim was to control the feeble-minded through segregation. The Act made it the duty of Local Authorities to ascertain, certify and make provision for 'mental defectives' in their areas. There is not space to go into detail here, but it is important to recognise that in certain circumstances the Act gave extensive powers to detain people without their consent, or that of their families. Detention in institutions was high on the agenda of those campaigning for change:

> It was increasingly assumed that alcoholism, prostitution, vagrancy and to a large extent unemployment were a complex of problems with a single root – feeble-mindedness. Since this was an innate and inherited condition contemporary wisdom saw the institution as more important as a means of reproductive control than of rehabilitation.[11]

The 1913 Act is best known for its provisions to institutionalise 'mental defectives', but in fact the Act provided for three forms of 'care, supervision and control', namely institutional care, guardianship and supervision. From the start institutional care was seen, in rhetoric if not reality, as a means to an end, the provision of instruction and training, stabilising and socialising inmates, and if possible fitting them for employment outside the institution. This intention was expressed in the 1929 Interdepartmental Committee on Mental Deficiency (Wood) Report:

> The Medical Superintendent must not be content with the statutory periodical review of the patients, but should himself ensure that no case shall be retained if after a sufficient period of training there appears to be a reasonable chance of its making a satisfactory adjustment to the conditions of a simpler institution or to those of licence. Put shortly, this means that the institution should no longer be a stagnant pool, but should become a flowing lake, always taking in and always sending out.[12]

This was reiterated in a 1932 text book:

> the modern aim is gradually to restore such a person to the community provided that adequate steps can be taken to avoid his falling into misconduct or becoming a parent[13]

To this end a system of licensing was authorised which enabled an institution, with the approval of the Board of Control, to grant leave of absence to an inmate, provided the home to which they were to go was approved. The licence could be revoked at any time, and the patient returned to the institution without further formalities. Technically, for statistical and financial purposes inmates out on licence remained inmates of an institution, but licensing was a significant way in which 'defectives' could resume life outside the asylum, albeit closely regulated.

The second type of provision was guardianship, which provided for the placing of a 'defective' in the control of a suitable person as guardian whose powers were 'such as could be exercised by the parent of a child under the age of fourteen years'.[14] Guardians could be parents, relatives, employers or other adults. If a defective was placed under guardianship the local authority could provide regular financial assistance, whereas only ad hoc payments could be made, for example, for clothing, to those families which were not guardians and not in receipt of poor relief.

The third category was statutory and voluntary supervision which consisted of the visiting and overseeing of defectives in their homes by salaried officials, health visitors, school nurses, social workers or local mental welfare associations, usually affiliated in the inter-war years to the Central Association for Mental Welfare.[15] Visitors were charged with regular reporting to their local authority's Mental Deficiency Committee, and drawing its attention to cases where proper control was not being exercised so that the defective could be placed in institutional care or guardianship.

The 1927 Mental Deficiency Act, in addition, made it the duty of local authorities to ensure that any necessary training was provided for defectives in institutions, under guardianship or under supervision. through provision of Occupation and Industrial Centres. This duty was observed assiduously in some areas but was not consistently observed throughout the country.

Thus, although the primary thrust of the Mental Deficiency Acts of 1913 and 1927 was to promote the development of institutions, the machinery set in place included measures to enable the authorities to regulate and control people outside the institution – through licensing, guardianship, supervision, and occupation centres. The numerical significance of these non institutional provisions can be seen in Table 9.1.

Table 9.1 *Total numbers of people provided for under the Mental
Deficiency Acts 1926 and 1939*[16]

	1st January 1926	1st January 1939
In institutions	20,297	46,054
Under guardianship	785	no separate figures available
Under statutory supervision	15,733	43,850
Total	36,185	89,904

The figures show that large numbers of people were catered for
outside institutions throughout the inter-war period. It also demonstrates that large numbers of people who had been certified as
defective by 1939 must have been without formal certification and
provision in 1926. The Wood Committee, reporting in 1929, estimated that there were around 60,000 in need of non-institutional
care. As Table 9.1 shows, only around 16,000 individuals were
being dealt with by statutory supervision or guardianship at that
date.[17] By the Wood Committee's estimates, around 40,000
believed to be defectives in 1926 were without any state provision,
and were presumably living in 'the community'.

A consistent theme of investigators and campaigners was the
unacceptability of leaving care to families which did not have the
will, resources or know-how to control their 'defective' relatives.
Evidence supplied to the Wood Committee by its principal investi-
gator, E.O. Lewis[18] includes examples of living conditions for those
outside the system as a means of demonstrating the sort of evils
that arose when mental deficiency went unidentified and unregu-
lated. The use of such lurid case vignettes was a popular means of
stirring up interest in the problem of mental deficiency in
publications by members of the Eugenics Society.[19] Lewis also used
them as warnings that poor families were not in a position to
supply the control deemed necessary to prevent procreation by
defectives and social problem families.[20]

COMMUNITY CARE

This chapter aims to look 'beyond the walls of the asylum' to build
a picture of policy, practice and individual experience of mental

deficiency in the past. There was very little research interest in provision outside of hospitals for those with learning disabilities until the 1990s. Thomson explains this by the inclusion of mental deficiency in the study of psychiatry, which inevitably brought with it a focus on medical intervention and treatment. Just as mental handicap was the Cinderella of the National Health Service, so its history has also been the Cinderella of the study of medicine, social policy and sociology. A number of eminent scholars of twentieth century social policy, for example, make no reference to it.[21] Others have misplaced the origins of community care, seeing it as the product of the 1954 Royal Commission[22] or as 'a reaction to criticisms of institutional forms of care . . . confirmed in the field of mental health in the late 1950s . . . firmly established by the planned contraction of hospital provision'.[23] Means and Smith[24] characterise history of community care before the late twentieth century as one of neglect. There were instances of neglect, but this is by no means the whole story because the Mental Deficiency Acts actually did extend regulation to those living outside the walls of the asylum.

Modern definitions of community care embrace both *formal* provision – statutory, voluntary or private services based outside of institutions to support care for adults who require assistance in the tasks of daily living – and *informal* provision – the material and emotional assistance supplied by family and friends. If community care is thus seen as care *in* the community and care *by* the community interwoven in various ways, then it is futile to search for the origins of community care in recent times. Changing definitions of community care in legislation and policy documents in the late twentieth century, away from a fairly limited definition associated with deinstitutionalisation to a more all embracing notion of networks of care, have opened the way for historians to begin to re-examine care outside of institutions, and to discover the often complex interweaving of familial and other sources of support.

Recent historical scholarship has revealed that in early modern times 'idiots' and 'fools' were largely, in Rushton's memorable phrase, 'buried in the family'[25] their very existence hard to perceive. Jonathan Andrews' work on providing for the 'mentally disabled' in early modern London[26] has shown the significance of families. He writes: 'In the majority of cases, and in a notably larger proportion than others identified as 'lunatic', the family was relied upon to provide'.[27] Nevertheless, Andrews identifies rudimentary parish support to some 'idiots and fools', for example the financing of nursing or lodgings, and the giving of small sums of money. Whether one can go so far as to term this 'community care' is debatable, but one feature has resonance with a modern criticism of community care – the over reliance on families until they break under the strain. Research by Oonagh Walsh, Lorraine Walsh, David Wright and Janet Saunders[28] on care for 'mental defectives' in various parts of Britain and Ireland during the nineteenth century also points to a striking continuity in the primacy of solutions which rely on the family with inputs from other sources when it was unable to fulfil the role adequately or at all.

Thomson's work on the problem of mental deficiency between the wars[29] strongly suggests a change of direction in terms of community care in the 1920s as a result of the 1913 Act, and the eugenics agenda. As noted above, the Mental Deficiency Acts contained provisions which enabled care and control to be provided for those outside institutions. Thomson views developments in the 1920s as the state appropriating community care with the specific aim of more effectively controlling defectives. The ideal of some contemporaries is well illustrated by Evelyn Fox, Secretary to the Central Association for Mental Welfare who described community care thus in 1930:

> Community care should vary from the giving of purely friendly advice and help to the various forms of state guardianship with compulsory powers ... It should include the power of affording every kind of assistance to the defective – boarding out, maintenance grants, the provision of tools, travelling expenses to and from work, of temporary care, of change of air, – in a word all those things which will enable a defective to remain safely in his family ... If the state has undertaken the duty and responsibility of active interference in the life of an individual by supervision, compulsory attention and so forth, it must undertake the corresponding duty of making his life as happy as possible.
>
> The effective control of a defective at home does inevitably mean a restriction in his complete freedom to go in and out as he pleases, to make what friends he chooses, to select what type of employment he likes out of those that are open to him. To impose these limitations ... without at the same time giving compensating interests and amusements is to court disaster.[30]

Fox's vision well illustrates the complementarity of care and control in policy relating to mental deficiency. Indeed, her humanitarian arguments for compensation for loss of freedom are couched in such a way as to appeal to the desire to more effectively curb the threats they pose, and are consonant with the eugenically inspired alarms about the rising tide of deficiency which threatened to overwhelm the nation. However, Thomson's research also shows that a simple view of community care as the development of facilities outside of institutions is an oversimplification.

Although the 1913 and 1929 Acts set up mechanisms for local authorities to develop supervisory systems outside of institutions, the development of formal provision for people certified as defective and not sent to institutions between 1913 and 1945 was patchy. While Thomson's research into the archives of the LMB reveal a fairly extensive structure of professional and voluntary effort, the latter co-ordinated by the London Association for Mental Welfare, the situation in the provinces was often less sophisticated.[31] In order to illuminate the reality of care (and control) in the community two local authorities with a relatively sophisticated structure are examined.[32] In terms of the Board of Control, Somerset and Buckinghamshire were 'good' local authorities in that they emerged in annually published tables as having high levels of ascertainment, certification, supervision and institutionalisation. From the point of view of the people subject to the different regimes such qualitative judgements are less easy to make.

SOMERSET: AN INTERVENTIONIST LOCAL AUTHORITY

Somerset was one of 17 local authorities singled out for praise by the Board of Control in 1925 for having set up institutional provision under the Act.[33] Dorothy Atkinson's work suggests that Somerset's interventionist stance was determined by events prior to the passage of the 1913 Act,[34] and, by 1900, there was a good deal of activity to extend and improve provision for the estimated 420 'idiots' in the county, excluding those resident in lunatic asylums.[35] A report prepared by the Boards of Guardians in 1900 claimed that of these 420 idiots, 217 were living in workhouses, and 203 living with friends or relatives. Disquiet about idiots in workhouses apparently had two causes. The first, expressed by a JP in 1900, was that it was unproductive:

many adults of this class now in our workhouses may possibly never have been there at all had they early in life received some specific training in developing their mental capacities[36]

The other was that it was detrimental to other workhouse residents:

others are to be found in workhouses where they are unfit and undesirable companions for other inmates[37]

Disquiet about those living with families and friends echoes the concerns identified by the Radnor Commission in 1904 – fears of crime, venereal disease, illegitimacy and profligate breeding.[38]

There was already at least one poor law institution in the county which specialised in 'idiots and imbeciles'. This was in Frome. It catered in 1891 for 17 males and 19 females, and by 1911 had expanded its accommodation to 41 beds. There is evidence that other Boards of Guardians looked to Frome to take their idiots and imbeciles.[39] Specialist attendants ideally 'with experience of the care of the insane' were recruited.[40]

Once the 1913 Act was passed the infrastructure was there for rapid expansion, both on the institutional and on the community front, to the extent that by 1927 the numbers of people under the Act totalled 1,667, well over three times the number estimated to be in existence in the county in 1900. Despite the early development of specialist institutions in Somerset, the vast majority of people under the jurisdiction of the Act (1,134) in that year were living with their families under statutory supervision. The evidence from the county records suggests that the existence of specialist institutions gave impetus to the expansion of provision at all levels, not just institutional placements.

As well as its network of institutional settings Somerset had in place, by the late 1920s, a sophisticated array of provisions for ascertained 'mental defectives'. These included local authority day and residential special schools, Occupation Centres, run by the Voluntary Association for Mental Welfare, arrangements for the statutory and voluntary supervision of large numbers of mental defectives living with their families, and local authority supervised licensing and guardianship schemes for people who would otherwise be in institutional care.

The Somerset Mental Deficiency Act Committee was chaired throughout the period of study by Miss Norah Fry (later Mrs

Cooke-Hurle). She was also a vice-president of the Central Association for Mental Welfare. Many of the ideas and good practices
introduced and debated at the major annual national conferences
of the Central Association were incorporated into policy and
practice in the local context. In 1920, for example, the Central
Association, with the backing and assistance of the Board of
Control, had embarked on 'active propaganda to get Occupation
Centres started by Local Mental Welfare Associations'.[41] The
following quotation highlights how this idea had taken root in
Somerset:

> The Somerset Association for the Care of the Mentally Defective have
> under consideration a scheme for the establishment of Occupation
> Centres for Mental Defectives, under which it will be necessary for them
> to appoint a full-time experienced Instructor, who can organise the
> training of defectives on simple lines.[42]

In March 1929, the Mental Deficiency Committee minutes noted
that the Somerset Association was already running Occupation
Centres in Bridgwater, Frome, Street, Taunton and Weston-Super-
Mare, and would increase their provision of places if additional
financial assistance were to be given. The Committee recommended an increase in financial support, and an Occupation Centre
was subsequently opened in Yeovil. The Occupation Centre had a
pivotal role in the provision of community care in Somerset in the
inter-war years. It enabled many people otherwise at risk of
institutional care to live at home with their families, and was part
of the support and supervising arrangements which kept people
with learning disabilities under surveillance. As a contemporary
commentator noted, the Occupation Centre was 'one of the most
satisfactory means of keeping in touch with defectives living in
their own homes or under guardianship'.[43]

There was a growing realisation in the county during the 1920s
that institutional care could not be provided for everyone. It was
too expensive an option and, in many instances, was unnecessary.
Occupation Centres, Voluntary and Statutory Supervision, licensing and guardianship schemes, together formed a cheaper, community-based alternative system of surveillance. This system
existed not only to offer advice and support to mental defectives,
and their families, but to prevent the former from marrying and
having children.

In 1926, the Board of Control argued against mental defectives being able to marry:

> The procreation of children by unmarried defectives, deplorable as it is, has not, as a rule, the same evil consequences to the children as the marriage of defectives. In the former case, children brought up apart from their parents . . . can attain full development . . . morally, physically and mentally. On the other hand, those who are the offspring of married defectives remain under the control of persons who are incapable of taking care of them, and they are consequently exposed to the hardships, neglect and ill treatment that the mental condition of their parents renders inevitable.[44]

This argument found a resonance within Somerset, and a Special Sub-Committee of the Mental Deficiency Committee was set up to look at the interconnected issues of marriage, sterilisation and segregation. The Sub-Committee recommended in its 1927 report that legislation be introduced to prevent 'the marriage of the unfit'. This recommendation was based on its argument that 'an unmarried mentally defective girl admitted to a Poor Law Infirmary for confinement can be dealt with drastically under the Mental Deficiency Act and segregated for life. A known mentally defective girl though can get married, and have large numbers of defective children, each of them being maintainable'. The Sub-Committee's report argued therefore for legislation to outlaw such marriages:

> Legislation should be promoted in order to make illegal the marriage of any mentally defective person under care or treatment in an Institution or Certified House or Approved Home, or whilst placed out on licence therefrom, or under Guardianship under the Mental Deficiency Act, 1915.[45]

The question of sterilisation was also debated in the 1920s. The Central Association for Mental Welfare considered the arguments for and against sterilisation, concluding in 1926 that sterilisation would have little impact on the problems associated with mental deficiency, especially on the 'social evils' of theft, arson, assault, murder, vagrancy and destitution. In fact the Central Association's main concern was that sterilisation would in itself lead to the additional problems of immorality, promiscuity, prostitution and the spread of venereal disease.

The debate for and against sterilisation was also taken up in Somerset by the Special Sub-Committee. The debate, in the local context, took into account the relative costs of care and, in particular, the burgeoning costs of institutional care. Would sterilisation help reduce those costs? In its 1927 report, the Sub-Committee rejected compulsory sterilisation on the grounds that it would not lead to a reduction in institutional care and, therefore, would not be justified in terms of reducing public expenditure. Instead, the Sub-Committee opted for a 'voluntary sterilisation' scheme, whereby mental defectives would be able to choose 'voluntary sterilisation' as a means of avoiding compulsory segregation for life in an institution, or as a condition for discharge from such an institution, for both men and women.

The policy of segregation continued throughout the inter-war years, as it was still thought to be the most appropriate provision for many. The Central Association for Mental Welfare had argued against sterilisation in 1926, but had argued instead for more institutional care of mental defectives in segregated institutions alongside their 'mental equals' and away from the 'positive cruelty' of the outside world.

In Somerset, the Special Sub-Committee argued in favour of outlawing the marriage of defectives, and the voluntary sterilisation of defectives, partly because of the escalating costs of providing segregation in suitable institutions. The Sub-Committee's report stated: 'All forms of institutional treatment are costly. At least half the cases sent to Institutions are sent there solely to prevent propagation'.[46] The Sub-Committee argued that it was, indeed, 'very desirable' to reduce the number of mental defectives in the next generation, but that to do so by the removal and isolation of mental defectives to achieve this end would required 'the segregation of an immense number of mentally defective persons'. It concluded that: 'Segregation alone, in order to be effective, would have to be undertaken on so vast a scale that it would be likely to prove beyond the financial capacity of the public.'[47] The Special Sub-Committee was also convinced that special care and training in segregated institutions would not enable mental defectives to 'return home and earn their own living as ordinary members of the community'. In 1927, it was widely assumed that institutional care meant permanent segregation, and this was a costly, and in some ways ineffective, means of catering for mental defectives. There was a clear impetus in Somerset to develop cheaper community-based options which would prevent or delay admission to institutions, and others which would facilitate the possibility of some mental defectives being able to leave institutions for supervised positions in the community.

These community-based options were much in evidence during the 1920s, and many mental defectives were being dealt with in the community as the Mental Deficiency Act had intended. The Thirteenth Annual Report of the Somerset Association for Mental Welfare, published in 1927, listed 212 cases that it was dealing with under statutory supervision and 917 cases under voluntary supervision. The report stated:

> It is clearly impossible, even if it were desirable, to provide institutional care for all our defectives, so that there must necessarily be a considerable proportion left in the care of their relatives for whom the Association are required to provide supervision. All Mental Defectives need care and control for their own protection, or for the protection of others, and for the majority this can only be provided satisfactorily in an Institution, but supervision, if properly carried out, may postpone the necessity for removal to an Institution. Supervision is simply a means of preventive care for the less urgent cases.[48]

As well as preventative work, the Somerset Association was interested in following up mental defectives who had received some institutional training, suggesting that such training was beneficial to the defectives concerned. This point was also made in the Association's 1927 Annual Report:

> Experience has proved that Defectives are much more likely to succeed under Guardianship or Supervision after they have received a period of training at a Residential Special School, or an Institution, in good habits, self control, obedience and in some trade or occupation. The County Mental Deficiency Act Committee have placed 45 Mental Defectives out on licence from Institutions, and only 11 have been recalled.[49]

Institutional care continued to grow during the 1920s in Somerset but so did community care, and at a faster rate. Table 9.2 illustrates the growth in community placements in this period, including the number of people allowed out of institutions on licence, people living with their families under statutory and voluntary supervision; and those on Guardianship orders. The growth in the number of mental defectives allowed to live in the community in Somerset is in line with the recommendations of the Wood Committee Report,

Table 9.2 *The range of provision for mental defectives in Somerset, 1924–1929*

	Institutions	Guardianship	Supervision by Somerset Association for MW	Licence
1924	294	15	930	
1925	316	23	972	
1926	399	22	1,131	
1927	458	30	1,134	45
1928	457	37	1,128	39
1929	475	41	1,109	48

1929, which recommended the greater use of community-based alternatives.

In an unpublished study of people discharged from three long-stay institutions in Somerset in the years 1971–81, Dorothy Atkinson traced the use of licence and guardianship in the earlier institutional careers of the 126 people involved. In all, eight men had spent varying amounts of time out of the institutions 'on licence' doing farm and factory work; working in a residential school and a hospital; and working as a gardener. Fourteen women had spent some time away from the institution on licence, predominantly as domestic workers in private households, but also working in a hospital, a laundry and a residential school.

Some people did sufficiently well on licence to have this revoked and be placed instead on a Guardianship order. This meant discharge from the institution to the care of a named Guardian, either an agent of the local authority or a named private person, usually a close relative. This was the situation for three of the male licensees and three of the female. Other people on licence fared less well, being returned to the institution for a number of reasons, for example: 'because of homosexual practices'; 'for associating with the opposite sex'; 'he was seen talking to a schoolgirl'; 'pregnancy'; 'an incestuous relationship with her father'.

In the same study, a further 14 people spent some time away from the institution on guardianship orders, but all were subsequently returned to institutional care when the community placement failed. The reasons given were similar to the ones cited for revoking licences, for example: 'interfering with little girls'; 'pregnancy'; 'associating with undesirable men'. Some of the concerns of the 1920s about sexuality and pregnancy were still evident in the casenotes of people on licence, and on guardianship orders, through the 1930s and 1940s. Those concerns had been expressed early in Somerset.

> Frequent visits should be paid by an experienced visitor, and any tendency to form friendships likely to lead to marriage or immorality should be reported at once, in order that recall to the Institution or a change of Guardianship can be effected in time.[50]

The evidence from Somerset, in the inter-war years, shows how community care existed alongside institutional care, not in opposition to it. The reality was that many people lived at times in the community, and at other times in the institution, passing to and from depending on personal and social circumstances. The two case studies below from Dorothy Atkinson's research, illustrate the interconnectedness of the community with its institution(s). The careers of the two people concerned range across the spectrum of family home, care in the community and institutional care. The details, comments and quotations are taken from contemporary records.

'William Carter' was born in 1917. His father was a farm labourer, and his mother a charwoman, 'of poor mentality'. He was the eldest of five children; two younger sisters also later went into institutional care. It was stated that this was 'a poor family, with poor home conditions'. William attended the village school until in 1927, aged 10, he was examined by the Assistant School Medical Inspector, and found to be 'a high grade feeble-minded child'. He was excluded from school with the recommendation that he attend a special residential school.

William was admitted to the Somerset Special School in Street in 1928, and spent two years there. He was later admitted to a special residential school in 1930, and in 1933, aged 16, was admitted to an institution. William later spent several years outside the institution on licence, with a number of employers, mostly farmers. Extracts from some of his early licence reports suggest that his experiences were mixed, and that some placements were more congenial than others:

1939: 'He appears happy . . . his work is satisfactory'.

1942: This is a very simple youth, who is very slow . . . He appears quite happy . . .'

1945: 'He looks defective. He is slow and unreliable at his work. He is occasionally sulky and insolent . . .'

In later years, William left the institution completely to live in the community – but that is outside the period of this chapter. His career until that point shows the spectrum of family, community and residential care which operated in Somerset in the inter-war years.

'Winifred Bolton' was born in 1918. Contemporary records describe her father as 'an unsatisfactory alcoholic labourer', and her mother as 'weak mentally; an unsatisfactory housewife'. Winifred's older sister was also later admitted to an institution. Winifred herself attended the local school for two and a half years, until she was certified as 'feeble-minded'. She was excluded from school in 1925 and later that year started attending the Bridgwater Occupation Centre. She was there for eight years, attending daily, and continuing to live with her family. She was described as 'sullen and obstinate at times . . . she is simple, slow and easily led'.

In 1934, Winifred's parents withdrew her from the Occupation Centre. She was re-examined and said by the medical officer to be 'in need of institutional care and training' on the grounds that she was 'exposed to grave moral dangers'. In 1934, aged 16, Winifred was admitted to an institution. The doctor responsible for the admission stated: 'She is dull and apathetic. She lacks planning, foresight and reasoning powers'. In 1943, Winifred went out on licence as a live-in domestic worker for 'Miss Young' in Keynsham. This placement lasted three years, and was ended for health reasons. Winifred returned to the institution. Years later, she left the institution completely to live in the community.

Winifred and William were born just as the 1913 Mental Deficiency Act was becoming operational. Their careers demonstrate the two-way interaction between community and institution, where whole lives were – like theirs – lived alongside, inside and outside the walls of the asylum.

BUCKINGHAMSHIRE: THE ROLE OF VOLUNTARY ORGANISATIONS

The voluntary sector, whose contribution to the working of the Mental Deficiency Act was co-ordinated by the Central Association for Mental Welfare (CAMW), had an important role in some local authorities, particularly in ascertaining defectives, but also in fulfilling Evelyn Fox's vision of community care as both aiding and controlling defectives.

The role played by local branches of the CAMW is well illustrated by the case of Buckinghamshire, one of the first counties to form a Voluntary Association. The formation of a Buckinghamshire branch of the Association for the Care of the Mentally Defective began as early as 26 March 1914, at a Conference of Authorities and Persons Concerned with the Administration of the Mental Deficiency Act 1913, held in Aylesbury County Hall. Conference delegates included all members of the County's Mental Deficiency Committee, representatives of Poor Law Unions, Education Committees and Evelyn Fox, Secretary of the National Association. It was moved at that Conference that a branch be set up, to include representatives of all Boards of Guardians, Medical Officers of Health (ex officio), the County Education Committee, School Medical Officers, 'experts in social work', all members of the County Blind Association, the County Nursing Association, Deaf and Dumb Association, National Society for Epileptics, and the Central Aid Society of High Wycombe. Later, the Discharged Prisoners Aid Society was also invited to join.[51]

At the first meeting of the Association, held less than a month later, on 17th April 1914, it was agreed to divide the county into four divisions, each with a Divisional Council to be made up of a visitor from each parish, members of the County Association resident in the Division, and poor law medical officers. Each Division had its own secretary. A list inside the front cover of the Minute Book (undated) shows that very few parishes had a vacancy for a visitor. Other than some (male) vicars parish visitors were invariably women – vicars' wives, or members of the local aristocracy, such as Lady Leon at Bletchley Park who was both visitor for Fenny Stratford parish, and secretary of the North Bucks division. Once such an extensive network of people was in place, it was relatively straightforward for the Association to begin its work. The aims of the Association were:

(a) to promote co-operation in the care of the mentally defective between statutory authorities, Education Committees and Voluntary Societies working for their welfare

(b) visit and befriend every mentally defective person in need of advice and assistance
(c) promote the training of visitors
(d) educate public opinion as to the need for more institutions and other means of safeguarding and training mental defectives.[52]

The Association obtained a paid secretary, Mr H. Fisher, in 1919, but its work began much earlier. Mrs James, Honorary Sec., alluded to this in her address to the 1935 Annual General Meeting:

> We may feel proud that the Buckinghamshire County Council was one of the first to form a Mental Deficiency Committee and to start the work energetically before the war and its complications delayed all fresh developments.[53]

There was no hesitation in getting started. In response to an enquiry as to how many defectives had been dealt with by the Voluntary Association for Mental Welfare (VAMD) in November 1914, only seven months after it was constituted, the Secretary replied that they had dealt with 200. The visitors apparently set about the task of ascertaining defectives with some zeal. Once a visitor had identified a possible defective, s/he referred the case on to the Divisional Secretary who was empowered to employ a medical practitioner to give an opinion, at a maximum cost of 2s 6d per case. If the Divisional Secretary thought it worth pursuing, she would refer the case on to the statutory Mental Deficiency Committee for a decision on formal certification. Ascertainment by visitors considerably overestimated the incidence of mental defect. For example, in 1923–24, 74 new cases were reported to the Association, of whom 42 were formally certified; in 1924–25, 71 new cases were reported and 41 were certified.[54] Certification required the agreement of two doctors that mental defect was present. However, the Committee instituted supervision for those reported as defectives prior to obtaining a medical report. This was formalised as friendly or voluntary supervision by the 1930s, a practice encouraged by the CAMW as preventive. There were 85 such people in 1935, compared with 146 people under statutory supervision in that year.[55]

Lord Onslow, Chair of the VAMD made particular reference to the work of the Association's members in 'the preliminary investigation of cases':

The members who lived in the vicinity of mental defectives were able to exercise tact and diplomacy and it was far better that neighbours, who were well known to be philanthropically disposed, should make the preliminary investigations.[56]

Unfortunately, no records of the responses of the suspected defectives or their families have come to light. It seems likely, however, that in some cases being a VAMD visitor was a busybody's charter. A Mrs B was reported as a suspected defective by Mrs Dallow, a visitor in 1917. It was stated that she was neglecting her three children while her husband was at the front line in the First World War. She was not certified, but was placed in the workhouse, and her three children boarded out.

Once cases had been referred to the VAMD regular reports were made on their progress. Considerable persistence was shown. For example, the parents of Charles H of Aston Clinton initially requested an institutional place for him in 1916, but subsequently withdrew consent. The visitor was advised by the Executive Committee secretary to try again after harvest when he might be out of work.[57] The Association busied itself in seeking out suitable institutional places for certified defectives.[58] The Secretary reported to the Executive Committee in October 1916 that dealing with one new case had entailed writing 110 letters. Members of the Association also spent time chasing parental contributions to the care of their offspring in institutions, occasionally interceding with the Mental Deficiency Committee on behalf of parents whom visitors considered were genuinely unable to pay.

There is evidence of a constructive approach to care on the part of the Association. The case of Hilda Mary H, aged 9, came before the Committee in 1919. The visitor requested money to obtain hospital treatment for her, reporting that 'she seems quite intelligent only unable to express herself owing to paralysis'. This is an instance where the Act had been misused to certify a child with a physical impairment, but she benefitted to the extent of obtaining treatment her family could not otherwise afford.[59] The Association also made grants of clothing, and arranged for home tuition – though in the case of Edward M, this had been put in place before he had been seen by doctors who judged that he was not certifiable.[60]

The VAMD was active in promoting the use of guardianship.

The first person was placed in guardianship in 1919. However, the use of this option was limited due to a shortage of suitable applicants. In 1926, the Executive Committee agreed to advertise for guardians in Women's Institute Parish magazines, offering 20s per week for cases requiring constant care and supervision, plus clothing. (By way of comparison, an institutional place cost between 17s and 23s per week). There are instances of a constructive and flexible use of guardianship. Violet P., for example, was not certifiable, but had expressed herself fearful of going home after leaving Newport Pagnell workhouse. The Executive Committee arranged for her to go on trial as a domestic servant to Mrs. Bull, a member of the Association.[61] Annie R had been granted leave of absence from Newport Pagnell Poor Law Institution. Miss Gardiner, rescue worker at Bletchley Rescue Home, took her in pending a situation for her, and the Committee agreed to pay 10s per week to Miss Gardiner for her care. By 1936 there were 49 people under guardianship in Bucks.

The Committee was active in overseeing the work of the county's poor law institutions (PLIs) which were certified by the Board of Control for housing mental defectives – Winslow, Aylesbury and Newport Pagnell. On the whole, the use of poor law institutions was deplored, but in counties where no colony existed it was a necessity. The VAMD concerned itself with standards in these institutions. During 1917, Winslow Poor Law Institution was visited five times. The Report to the 1917 General Committee meeting stated that the patients were well looked after, but there was not enough to do: 'due to shortage of staff the patients could not be trained as the visitors would like'.[62] By 1919, lady visitors had organised classes in Winslow Poor Law Institution – raffia-binding, weaving, jam pot covers, sewing and knitting for the 'girls', whilst 'boys' did weaving, mat-making and work on canvas,[63]and by 1924 visitors were receiving inmates of PLIs out on leave. The Association continued to lobby energetically for more facilities – a colony, occupation centres, special school classes for children. In their absence, it appears there were great efforts made to make up the shortfall by the voluntary organisation.

The picture painted in the records of the Bucks VAMD is one of intense county-wide activity, locating defectives, and pressing for their care, supervision and control. Overall, the tone is benign, presenting the interventions of the Association's members as in the interests of those people who became the subjects of its attention. However, it is important to recall Evelyn Fox's words: these were compensations for loss of liberty. As Lord Onslow reminded those present at the 1925 AGM, it was

> a very great blot on the name of the English people that they had so many defectives in their midst ... somewhat of a national peril ... an increasing number of mental defectives every year ... far too much ignored by all the people who lived around them and who lived in the very midst of mental deficiency[64]

The numbers in the county apparently bore out his fears, with an average increase of 60 per annum certified over the period 1920–36. However, it is probable that this increase was as much due to the work of activists as it was to a genuine proliferation of defectives in England's green and pleasant land.

CONCLUSION

The focus in this chapter has been on the role of local authorities and voluntary organisations in providing community care for people with learning disabilities in the inter-war years. However, it is important to note that families were the very bedrock of the system. They were often poor families, and were vilified in the public writing of the eugenicists – yet they were needed and relied on to be the primary providers of care in the community. Even Somerset, one of the Board of Control's star performers, never had enough institutional places to house all identified defectives, and there was early recognition that – even if it had been desirable – the sheer cost of providing institutional care for all made it an impossible ambition. This left families in the invidious position of being essential to the grand scheme of things but, at the same time, as the objects of suspicion and surveillance.

The detailed accounts from two local authorities have shown the variation in provision for mental deficiency during the period under scrutiny. Certainly, Thomson's view that the Mental Deficiency Acts laid the framework for an annexing of community care by local authorities appears to be borne out. The picture is of necessity only partial, and additional locality studies of the type attempted here are the best means of fleshing out the picture. However, it seems possible, from our studies of Somerset and Bucks (and from comparable work in Norwich and Norfolk[65]), to concur with Thomson that community care from 1913 to 1946 was not a distinct solution to the 'problem' of mental deficiency, nor was it a separate entity from institutional care. Instead, our evidence, like his, suggests that 'the two forms of care developed in an interactive process'.[66]

The case studies presented in this chapter are from Local Authorities which were active in various ways in implementing the Act. There were many where the level of activity was far lower, especially in the 1920s. In such Local Authorities ascertainment and certification rates were low, and institutional provision for a few 'urgent' cases the only option. It is in those areas where 'neglect' was the hallmark. Whether it was preferable from the point of view of those individuals and their families to be left undetected and unprovided for is a moot point and one which cannot be explored here for reasons of space. Suffice it to say that any neat equation between 'good' Local Authorities in Board of Control terms and the experience of 'defectives' cannot be assumed. There is some way to go before a satisfactory picture of 'community care for mental defectives' can be painted.

CHAPTER TEN

Rhetoric and reality: community care in England and Wales, 1948–74

John Welshman

INTRODUCTION

The concept of community care has come to have an increasingly prominent role in contemporary health policy. As is well-known, the 1989 White Paper, *Caring for People*, defined community care as 'providing the services and support which people affected by problems of ageing, mental illness, mental handicap or disability need to live independently in their own homes or in 'homely' settings in the community'. It stated that the Government was 'firmly committed' to community care, but noted that friends, family, and neighbours shouldered the heaviest burden, and argued that voluntary organisations should contribute more to the 'mixed provision of care'.[1] Academics working in social policy and sociology have attempted to assess the effects of these policy changes on health provision, particularly for the elderly.[2] Janet Finch and Dulcie Groves, for example, have produced an important feminist critique of the gender bias inherent in the role of women as carers, while Roy Parker has suggested that the very ambiguity of community care has been a factor in its appeal.[3] And there have also been attempts to assess the way that the 'new' community care has been implemented, including through local case-studies.[4]

If those working in sociology and social policy have explored the contemporary meaning and role of community care, historians have also begun to examine the history of mental health outside the walls of the Victorian asylum. In many respects, interpretations of

the history of community care have reflected contemporary concerns, with the key question being why community care became
such an important element in policy rhetoric from the mid-1950s.
The early accounts argued that while there were problems in
introducing community care, it was primarily a progressive movement associated with increasing criticisms of institutional care and
with a pharmacological revolution.[5] Later Andrew Scull and others
emphasised the attractiveness of community care to policy-makers
concerned about ever-rising costs of health care within a capitalist
welfare system.[6] But more recently historians have argued that the
stress on community care preceded the fiscal crisis of the 1970s,
and the tendency has been towards more balanced accounts of the
reasons why community care came into prominence.[7]

There are other sources on which the historian of community
care is able to draw. The official history of the National Health
Service, for example, has provided a more sophisticated analysis
than was available previously of policy formation and implementation in this field, and detailed accounts of the history of mental
health legislation are now available.[8] At present, local studies of
the development of mental health services remain in their infancy,
though there have been some important exceptions. Hugh Freeman
has suggested that Salford managed to provide effective community
care services, in part because of the attitude of the local Medical
Officer of Health (MOH).[9] On the other hand, Chris Ham has
been more critical of mental health policy in the area administered
by the Leeds Regional Hospital Board, claiming that central
government showed greater commitment to community care than
local authorities.[10] And more recently Mathew Thomson has
claimed that in the interwar period the London County Council
created an integrated network of institutional and community
services that was arguably more efficient than the system introduced by the National Health Service.[11]

There is no shortage then, of work on community care in
twentieth-century Britain. However surprisingly little is known
about the ways that policy evolved and was implemented, particularly at the local level, and several questions deserve further
consideration. Why did the Ministry of Health and Department of
Health and Social Security (DHSS) promote community care? Was
the policy linked to the pharmacological revolution of the 1950s, or
was it simply a response to the rising costs of hospital treatment?

How effectively did local authorities implement a policy of community care and how far was provision subject to regional variations? And finally, what were the motivations of those organisations and individuals who were critical of community care? Although community care also embraced domiciliary services for the elderly, this chapter concentrates on the services for the mentally ill and 'handicapped' that have been the concern of the book as a whole. It examines the evolution of policy in England and Wales between 1948 and 1974, explores its implementation through a case study based on the Midlands city of Leicester, and looks at the way that community care became a forum for other concerns about public health, social work, and general practice.

THE EVOLUTION OF POLICY ON COMMUNITY CARE

Although the evolution of policy has received some attention from historians, many gaps remain in our understanding of why community care has proved so attractive at different times. Certainly it is clearly the case that in the medieval and early modern periods, much of the responsibility of caring for the insane was shouldered by the family and community rather than by specialist institutions.[12] In this sense the rise of the Victorian asylum, and the move towards institutional care, may be something of an anomaly when seen in a longer time-span. This suggestion is supported by the tentative moves towards community care for both the mentally defective and the mentally ill evident in the early twentieth century. Since the 1890s, Local Education Authorities had been empowered to make provision for mentally defective children. Moreover under the 1913 Mental Deficiency Act, local authorities were given responsibility for mental defectives under guardianship orders, and the 'supervision' of cases when neither institutional care nor guardianship was deemed to be necessary. The new Mental Deficiency Committees often worked in conjunction with voluntary organisations affiliated to the Central Association for Mental Welfare. In some respects, these moves towards care in the community, and the trend towards widening definitions, a loosening of statutory restraints, and a more flexible response were reflected in the 1927 Mental Deficiency Act and in the Wood Report (1929).[13]

Changes in provision for the mentally ill have always occurred at a slower rate than for the mentally defective, perhaps because there has been greater fear of the former and more public sympathy for the latter. However here too, the 1890 Lunacy Act was followed by some 'progressive' developments. These included the opening in 1923 of the Maudsley Hospital to voluntary patients, the work of the Mental After-Care Association (though its efforts were confined to London), and the Royal Commission on Lunacy and Mental Disorder (1924–26). Also significant were changes within mental hospitals themselves. Here there were innovations in design and planning, and an emphasis on new forms of treatment such as insulin coma therapy, chemical and electrical convulsion therapy, and psychosurgery, including lobotomy or leucotomy. Outside institutions, the period saw a gradual growth in after-care and psychiatric social work, particularly following the 1929 Local Government Act. Changes in perceptions of hospital care were reflected in the 1930 Mental Treatment Act: it made additional provision for voluntary treatment, and encouraged psychiatric outpatient clinics and observation wards.[14]

The significance that historians have attached to these developments has changed over time. It was inevitable that Kathleen Jones for instance, writing shortly after the 1959 Mental Health Act, would highlight any tentative moves towards community care. However as doubts have surfaced about the wisdom of releasing some patients into the community, historians have become more sceptical. Mathew Thomson for example, has argued that community care was an ambiguous concept that was linked to wider ideas about care, community and citizenship in early twentieth-century Britain.[15] This analysis is borne out by a closer reading of the Wood Report on mental deficiency, published in 1929. Its authors used the expression 'community care', and promoted measures that included day schools, occupation centres and industrial centres. Yet while they were keen on care in the community, and recommended that colonies and hostels should replace the larger institutions, they also promoted sterilisation and segregation alongside a policy of 'socialisation'.[16] Thus Thomson is correct in arguing that community care, segregation and sterilisation are all open to both reactionary and progressive interpretations.

Although it is important not to exaggerate the extent of these developments, it is clear that there had been some experiments in community care in the period before 1939. Moreover the Second World War itself served to focus attention on the mental health needs of both children and adults. Henceforth provision was affected by the administrative restructuring that accompanied the establishment of the National Health Service. Under its tripartite system, the hospitals were administered by Regional Hospital Boards, general practitioner services by Executive Councils, and public health by local authorities. Section 28 of the Act stated that local authorities might 'make arrangements for the purpose of the prevention of illness, the care of persons suffering from illness or mental defectiveness, or the after-care of such persons', and Section 51 that they were responsible for provision under the Lunacy and Mental Treatment Acts, 1890–1930, and the Mental Deficiency Acts, 1913–38.[17] It is arguable that Section 28's permissive powers gave local authorities a framework for developing a system of community care. On the other hand, responsibility for mental health services was now divided between the local authorities and the new Regional Hospital Boards, and it is possible that a more integrated system for mental health care existed before rather than after 1948.

At the local level, local authorities transferred responsibility for patients from Mental Deficiency Committees to Health Committees, and appointed former public assistance personnel as mental welfare officers. However, while there were some signs of change, the Ministry of Health also adopted a cautious approach to the development of services. A 1949 circular on occupation centres, for example, noted that progress would be 'conditioned by local circumstances including resources available and the financial considerations involved in each case'.[18] Although some local authorities provided after-care and social clubs, few employed psychiatric social workers and other specialist staff, and the severe restrictions on capital expenditure meant they were unable to build occupation centres or short-stay hostels. In 1951–52 for instance, local authorities in England and Wales spent only £1.3m on mental health, and although hospital waiting lists grew longer, only 211 occupation and training centres had been established.[19] The Ministry of Health sought to use voluntary organisations to plug these deficiencies, but even it concluded that mental health was a new departure for most local authorities, trained staff were scarce, and progress slow and uneven.[20] Thus mental health suffered from the decrease in spending on local authority health services that characterised the 1950s, and little was achieved before the publication of the Royal Commission on Mental Health's report in 1957.

Even though progress was uneven at this time, a number of wider factors generated support for a policy of community care. As we have seen, the main treatments for mental patients before 1950 had been insulin coma therapy, electroconvulsive therapy, and leucotomy, but the discovery of neuroleptic or anti-psychotic drugs such as Chlorpromazine, marketed as 'Largactil', represented an important breakthrough.[21] Secondly there were signs of changing attitudes towards mental health with the World Health Organisation report of 1953, and trends within mental hospitals themselves, including the 'open door' movement. The more sceptical approach to institutional care that was later to be propagated by Erving Goffman's *Asylums*, and by Thomas Szasz and Michel Foucault, was already apparent.[22] Thirdly there was growing anxiety about demographic changes, including the rapidly increasing numbers of elderly people, and the 1959 general election campaign reflected concern over the costs of hospital care.[23] Finally the reports of the Jameson and Younghusband Committees had raised questions concerning the roles of health visitors and social workers. While historians disagree over whether the pharmacological revolution was more important than concern about rising costs, together these factors help to explain the re-emergence of community care in policy rhetoric.

Many of these issues were reflected in the 1954 Parliamentary debate on mental health, and in the report of the Royal Commission on Mental Health published in 1957. The Royal Commission stated that hospitals should provide for patients who required specialist medical treatment, but that local authorities should be responsible for preventive services, social work, and community care. It was particularly enthusiastic about community care, stating that services should be available to all who could benefit from them, and that there should be no need for formal 'ascertainment'; the approach should be 'a positive one offering help and obtaining the co-operation of the patient and his family'. The Royal Commission noted that medicine increasingly emphasised 'forms of treatment and training and social services which can be given without bringing patients into hospital as in-patients, or which make it possible to discharge them into hospital sooner than was usual in the past'. Its most significant recommendation was that there should be a shift in emphasis from hospitals to community care, and it argued that restrictions on expenditure should not be allowed to delay the development of this policy.[24] Implementation of many of its recommendations would be delayed, but the Royal Commission was nonetheless an important milestone.

The Ministry's circular of May 1959 encouraged local authorities to implement the proposals of the Royal Commission, and many of its recommendations were reflected in the 1959 Mental Health Act. As Clive Unsworth has shown, the Act repealed previous legislation and introduced a single code for all types of mental disorder; in this sense it overturned the 1890 Lunacy Act and advanced many of the principles of the 1930 Mental Treatment Act. In addition, it seemed to create a legal basis for local authorities to provide preventive services, establish residential alternatives to hospitals such as occupation and training centres, and appoint mental welfare officers. The powers were permissive but indicated that the Minister could force local authorities to take action. The Act dismantled formal procedural safeguards, and also had a broader strategy of reintegrating the mentally disordered into the community.[25] The Ministry now claimed that the 1959 Mental Health Act had laid the basis for community care, and that local authorities were providing more residential accommodation, adult and junior training centres, and other services. In his reports for 1957 and 1958, for example, the Chief Medical Officer (CMO) wrote that 'the future of the mental health service depends on the community services', and that 'long hospitalisation is out of fashion in mental medicine as it is in general medicine and surgery'.[26]

Although the 1959 Mental Health Act set important legal precedents, it failed to ensure adequate financial backing for the development of mental health services. In fact the new block grants, which gave local authorities greater freedom in allocating resources, actually increased regional variations in provision. Internal files reveal that although the Ministry of Health stressed community care in its published documents, it realised provision in most areas was poor and slow to improve. In August 1959 for instance, the Ministry's inspectors found that some local authorities feared a flood of discharged hospital patients and thought that the introduction of the block grant would impede the development of services. Others were concerned about training, and about the way that the care of mental patients was sometimes delegated to health visitors.[27] Many of the proposals that local authorities offered in response to the 1959 circular were regarded even by the Ministry as unsatisfactory. A list compiled in June 1960 noted that 29 local authorities were not planning to extend their services, had inadequate staff, were making slow progress, or were too small to make effective provision. The list included Middlesborough, Bootle, Leicester, Suffolk West, and Bath, and arguably indicated that mental health services were poor in most parts of England and Wales. Even in the case of those authorities whose proposals had been approved, the Ministry doubted how quickly and how successfully the proposals could be translated into practice.[28]

The policy of community care was revived by the Minister of Health, Enoch Powell, in the early 1960s in the context of the planning of hospital services. In March 1961, at the annual conference of the National Association for Mental Health (NAMH), he announced a reduction in hospital beds for mental illness, a policy change that was amplified in a circular issued three weeks later. The Hospital Plan unveiled in 1962 confirmed that the Ministry of Health's plans for community care were directly related to a proposed reduction in the number of hospital beds for the mentally ill and 'subnormal'. These plans showed that the number of hospital beds would be reduced over the following ten years so that by 1975 there would be 1.8 beds for the mentally ill and 1.3 beds for the mentally 'subnormal' per 1,000 population. The Ministry stated that these aims were 'complementary to the expected development of the services for prevention and for care in the community', and argued that local authorities should provide more residential hostels and training centres, and employ more social workers. It observed that significant variations remained between local authority services, but also concluded that voluntary effort had not yet reached its full potential.[29]

The policy of community care was given additional impetus as a result of the Hospital Plan, but it embraced both domiciliary services for groups such as the elderly, and other alternatives to hospital care, and it was still not clearly defined. These problems became apparent when the Ministry asked local authorities to draw up plans for health and welfare services for the next ten years, and published them in the *Health and Welfare* White Paper of April 1963. The report recommended that local authorities should employ more social workers, provide training centres for mentally subnormal children and adults, and centres and hostels for the mentally ill. The summary revealed that over the following ten years, local authorities planned to increase the number of junior training centres from 345 to 424, adult training centres from 281 to 483, and hostels for the mentally subnormal from 47 to 464. They intended to expand centres for the mentally ill from 23 to 103, and hostels from 18 to 211, and anticipated a capital building programme of £35.8m for the mentally subnormal and £9.8m for the mentally ill.[30]

In part the purpose of the White Paper was to provide the Ministry with information about the existing level of services. One of its civil servants admitted in August 1962 that the statistical evidence of need was 'flimsy in the extreme', and that inconsistencies in the returns had made it difficult to reach accurate conclusions. He admitted that 'the plain fact is that we expect ourselves to learn a great deal from study of the ten year plans as a whole'.[31] One of the most useful features of the White Paper was that it did reveal the poor state of existing mental health services. In 1961, for example, local authorities employed only 1,128 social workers, or 0.024 per 1,000 population. Yet *Health and Welfare* admitted that 'no attempt was made either to indicate common standards to which the plans should conform or to suggest modifications before publication'.[32] Perhaps in part as an acknowledgement of the weaknesses of *Health and Welfare*, revised ten-year plans were published in 1964 and 1966. The Ministry seemed more concerned than previously about regional variations in services, and now stated that its aim was to work towards a situation where 'an acceptable standard of services' was provided throughout England and Wales. The published plans showed that local authorities planned to increase the number of adult hostels from 72 to 387, expand the number of junior hostels from 50 to 158, and spend around £345m on a capital building programme. As well as moving towards smaller institutions, the local authorities anticipated that they would appoint additional staff, with the number of mental health social workers increasing from 2,398 to 3,778 by 1975.[33] As was later remarked, *Health and Welfare* was not a plan. Rather it simply amalgamated the stated intentions of local authorities, did not provide adequate costings, and therefore failed to provide a credible framework for community care.

Even so, it is important to try to establish whether the publication of the *Health and Welfare* plans did actually signal a greater commitment to community care on the part of the Ministry of Health and the new DHSS. They certainly continued to promote community care, both in the field of mental health, and for the elderly. In 1962, the CMO noted that without more trained social workers, local authorities would be 'seriously handicapped in carrying out to the full their growing responsibilities for community care'.[34] Two years later, the Ministry suggested that hostels should be an integral part of mental health services, and that the selection of residents and adoption of policies on care and rehabilitation demanded a 'team' approach. In 1965, the CMO argued that 'if the community mental health services are well developed, the hospital component, though it must be active, need not be large'.[35] There were some signs that this was not simply rhetoric. The amount that local authorities spent on mental health services, for example, did increase in the late 1960s, from £21.9m in 1967–68, to £26.9m in 1970–71. Yet at the end of 1964, local authorities in England and Wales still only provided 31 hostels for the mentally ill, and in 1968 the DHSS admitted that waiting lists had increased and that 'a further considerable expansion of the mental health services will be required before the needs of the mentally disordered in the community can be met in full'.[36]

In part the DHSS was responding to the Seebohm report (1968) which represented the first serious examination of health and welfare services since the legislation of the late 1940s. Although the committee had been set up to consider services for the family, it ranged beyond its remit and was critical of much of the provision by local authority health departments. On the specific question of community care, it noted that psychiatrists were increasingly interested in the social context of mental health and supportive of community care, and local authority spending on mental health had increased, from £4m in 1959–60, to £17m in 1966–67. However the report thought that the term 'community care' had been used in unfortunate ways, and pointed out that this area still represented a tiny fraction of health service expenditure as a whole. While some areas had developed efficient services, in others progress had been hampered by serious shortages of staff, buildings, money, and by a lack of interest on the part of the general public. Overall it concluded that 'the widespread belief that we have 'community care' of the mentally disordered is, for many parts of the country, still a sad illusion and judging by the published plans will remain so for years ahead'.[37]

The Seebohm committee used the alleged failure of local health departments on community care to bolster its recommendation that responsibility for mental health should be transferred to Local Education Authorities and the new Social Services Departments. These recommendations were implemented in the 1970 Local Authority (Social Services) and Education (Handicapped Children) Acts after which mental health was no longer a primary responsibility of the local Health Committees. The personal mental health services along with adult training centres became the responsibility of local Social Services Departments, while junior training centres for the mentally 'handicapped' were transferred to Local Education Authorities. Interestingly, some of the recent changes in the meaning of community care date back to this period. The Seebohm Committee had stressed that there should be more community participation in social services, while the Aves Report had drawn attention to the importance of voluntary services. It was in the context of these changes that a Sheffield survey concluded in 1973 that 'care in, by, as part of, and in co-operation with the community can develop most fruitfully if it is linked with the insights of community development'.[38]

Some of the Secretaries of State for Social Services, such as Sir Keith Joseph, did appear to have a genuine commitment to community care. Perhaps as a result, reports that tried to chart the direction of future policies were more honest than previously about the existing level of services. The White Paper *Better Services for the Mentally Handicapped*, for example, published in 1971, revealed that community care was not yet a reality. It suggested that the new training centres and residential homes were of high quality, but that little had been done to provide training centres for mentally handicapped adults, residential care for adults and children, or help for families. Overall it concluded that 'the developments recommended by the Royal Commission 14 years ago are far from being accomplished', and suggested that 'what is needed is faster progress to overcome the present deficiencies'.[39] These findings seemed borne out by the statistics. By 1973, local authorities in England provided 97 day centres and 167 homes and hostels for the mentally ill, and 367 adult training centres and 302 homes and hostels for the mentally handicapped.[40] While progress had been made, it was clear that in most areas provision was not adequate to implement community care.

An important question is whether services for the mentally handicapped had developed more quickly than those for the mentally ill, and some answers were provided by the White Paper *Better Services for the Mentally Ill*, published in 1975. In the foreword, Barbara Castle admitted that despite the 1959 Mental Health Act, 'supportive facilities in a non-medical, non-hospital setting are still a comparative rarity', and spending on local authority provision was dwarfed by expenditure on hospital services. In general the paper was cautious, noting that little could be done in an era of financial restraint, and admitting that 'the scope for making progress during the next few years will be very limited'. It conceded that community services were still minimal, and that the failure to develop adequate social services was perhaps the greatest disappointment of the previous fifteen years. The document claimed that community care was still a valid concept, but concluded that while some local authorities had developed day and residential services for the mentally ill, others provided no facilities, and nationally the total level of provision fell short of the guideline figures.[41] It is not possible here to assess how far the creation of Social Services Departments, and the 1974 health service reorganisation, helped or hindered the implementation of community care. However it seems clear that in 1975 even the Government accepted that the ideal of community care had not become a reality.

COMMUNITY CARE AND ITS IMPLEMENTATION:
A LOCAL CASE-STUDY

While the reports and internal files of the Ministry of Health and DHSS indicate the development of policy, the implementation of community care can best be examined through a case-study of an individual local authority. Located in the East Midlands, Leicester was a major provincial urban centre with a population of around 285,000 at the 1951 census, and an affluent city with prosperous hosiery, boot and shoe, and light engineering industries. By the early 1900s, it had gained a reputation as a 'progressive' local authority. Arguably, annual MOH reports and other documents reveal little about the relationships between the mental hospitals and local authority services that hold the key to community care.

Yet used with care, it is possible to assess how quickly national developments filtered down to the local authority level, to see if there was any 'bottom-up' policy-making, and to chart continuities and changes in provision in our period. Leicester was a 'progressive' local authority within the deprived Sheffield region, and provides an unusual case-study in the implementation of community care.

As in other areas, the emergence of community care in the 1950s was only one stage in the longer-term history of mental health provision. There is evidence that private madhouses had existed at Wigston Magna in the county and at Belgrave Gate in the city, and other new institutions for the insane had been established in the late eighteenth and early nineteenth centuries, including the Leicester Infirmary Asylum (1794) and the Union Workhouse (1839). But by far the most important of these was the Leicestershire and Rutland Lunatic Asylum (1837), later replaced by a new mental hospital at Narborough (1907). With regard to the mentally defective, the local authority had begun to make provision for children in the 1890s, and a voluntary after-care committee had also run a home for 'feeble-minded' girls. Following the 1913 Mental Deficiency Act, the local authority opened three small hostels, and in 1923 purchased a large house and estate named Leicester Frith; provision was subsequently supervised through a Mental Deficiency Committee.[42] In general it seems likely that Leicester's provision for mentally defective children and adults compared favourably with other cities, not least because of the influence of local eugenists such as C. J. Bond and R. B. Cattell.

This history forms the backdrop for later developments. With the National Health Service Act, local hospitals were taken over by the Sheffield Regional Hospital Board, including the asylum at Narborough, now called the Carlton Hayes Hospital, and various units and hostels at Leicester Frith, now named the Glenfrith Hospital. At the local authority level, Leicester's Health Committee took steps to comply with the legislation by appointing a mental welfare sub-committee, and approving its proposals under Section 51.[43] In April 1949, the Health Committee agreed to appoint a psychiatric social worker and other staff, and to employ one of the Regional Hospital Board's psychiatrists on a part-time basis. At this time, mental health was supervised by two people; a 'worker' who was responsible for administration and an occupation centre for children, and a health visitor who visited homes and prepared reports on the 500 cases covered by the Mental Deficiency Acts. But there were some improvements in provision. From the interwar years, the local authority had run an occupation centre for children in a church hall. They learnt sewing, handicrafts, and cooking, and in general the centre was ill-equipped and overcrowded; its supervisor admitted that the main aims of the training were for the children to be 'obedient and happy'.[44] A new school named after Emily Fortey, a prominent Labour councillor who had previously campaigned for better health services for children, was opened by the Minister of Health in September 1956.

The opening of a large new school was an impressive achievement at a time when shortages of materials and restrictions on capital expenditure made it difficult for local authorities to replace obsolete institutions. Moreover thinking on mental health policy at the local level can be seen to have been affected by Ministry circulars and by the recommendations of the Royal Commission. A circular issued in 1952 for instance, had encouraged local authorities to provide temporary respites for relatives by admitting mental defectives for up to two months to local mental hospitals. The recommendations of the Royal Commission further blurred the boundaries between the hospital and the community. In March 1958, Leicester's MOH concluded that in future, patients would be admitted to hospitals more informally, they would stay for shorter periods, and the dividing line between homes and hospitals would be less clearly defined.[45] Later in the year, he again reviewed policy on hospital admissions, noted that many pupils at the Emily Fortey school were over 16, and argued that crèches, sheltered workshops, and training centres were needed for children and adults.[46] The MOH reports indicate that there was an increasing awareness of the potential of workshops and hostels, of the importance of integrated services, and of the need for psychiatric expertise. In this respect the Leicester case-study suggests that in some local authorities more 'progressive' ideas did quickly filter down to the local level.

However while the MOH was in tune with contemporary thinking on mental health, services on the ground improved more slowly. The emphasis of the Emily Fortey school on furniture repair, woodwork, and cookery suggested that there were important continuities with the regime of the old occupation centre. Moreover in

general, during this first decade, the needs of children were priori-
tised over the claims of adults. The local authority continued to
classify mental defectives as 'idiots', 'imbeciles', the 'feeble-minded'
and 'moral defectives', and followed a policy of supervision,
licence, and guardianship. It had not yet opened an occupation
centre for adults, or other institutions such as day centres or
hostels. Although the Health Committee appeared to have
ambitious plans, its members were aware that improved provision
for community care would require extra money.[47] It agreed with
many of the MOH's proposals, but it was wary about incurring
additional expenditure, asked the Association of Municipal Corporations to lobby for additional grants, and pointed out to the
Ministry that it did not benefit from increases in the block grant
for mental health services.[48] In revealing the results of the administrative separation of the Regional Hospital Board and local
authority services, the slow pace of the development of junior and
adult training centres, and the effects of curbs on capital spending,
Leicester was probably typical of most local authorities.

Although the local authority achieved little in the field of mental
health in the first decade of the National Health Service, the *Health
and Welfare* White Paper did force it to consider its existing
provision and future plans. After discussions between the Health
and Welfare Committees and the Sheffield Regional Hospital
Board about anticipated needs, the proposals were approved by
the City Council in October 1962.[49] According to the White Paper,
Leicester planned to expand the number of places in junior and
adult training centres for the mentally 'subnormal', increase the
number of social workers from 15 to 23, and embark on a capital
expenditure programme of £58,800, but did not plan to provide
more centres and homes.[50] The revised plans for the period
1965–76 revealed that Leicester planned to further increase places
in training centres for mentally subnormal adults, and to follow a
capital building programme of £2.5m. Compared to the earlier
plans, it anticipated employing more district nurses and social
workers, but fewer health visitors, home helps, and midwives.[51]

As at the national level, it is important to find out how Leicester's *Health and Welfare* plans fared in practice and whether the
local authority was able to implement community care before 1974.
In some respects, practice at the local level simply reflected
national legislation; following the Mental Health Act for example,

local doctors no longer used the terms 'mental defectiveness' and 'mental deficiency'. But there was also evidence of local initiative that contradicts the image of stagnation in mental health at the local level. The local authority monitored practice elsewhere; in 1960 for instance, the mental health sub-committee visited adult training centres in Holland.[52] New services included a health visitor who had special responsibility for mental health, a scheme for following up 'handicapped' children, and a new mental health social club set up in 1962.[53] More importantly, new centres, hostels and training centres were opened in both adapted and purpose-built premises as restrictions on capital expenditure eased in the late 1960s. The question of what actually went on in these new institutions requires additional research. But on the ground the new facilities included a short-stay hostel for adults opened in December 1965, a hostel for mentally 'subnormal' adults, and the junior training centre that was opened in 1970. Thus in its creation of new institutions, and provision of other community services, Leicester to a certain extent took up the opportunities offered by the Royal Commission and 1959 Mental Health Act. Perhaps most interestingly, it seems to be the case that at the end of the day the children and adults who attended occupation centres returned to live with their families, thus raising the question of how far a 'mixed economy' of care was implicit in policy at this time.

In other respects, provision remained unimpressive through the 1960s. The plans for an adult training centre were delayed by the Ministry's restrictions on capital expenditure, and it was housed temporarily in a working men's club and a disused warehouse before it finally opened in 1965.[54] Despite the new institutions, other services still relied heavily on the resources of voluntary organisations such as the Red Cross, in part because staffing continued to pose problems. The evidence of waiting lists, and of hospital admissions and discharges, provides a means of assessing the success or failure of community care policies. Some of the new institutions did have long waiting lists, such as the Emily Fortey school, suggesting the existence of a reservoir of unmet need. Similarly the MOH argued that the high re-referral rate indicated that patients who required longer support were leaving hospital prematurely. In 1969 for example, he wrote that 'costly hospital admission and treatment is being undermined by the inability of the local authority services to maintain adequate support for the patient on his return to the community'.[55] As we have noted, this system was fractured further after April 1971 when responsibility for mental health services was divided between the Local Education Authority and the new Social Services Department.[56] Thus while some new institutions had been opened, the number of places in junior and adult training centres remained inadequate, and problems of resources and finance still hampered the development of community care.

Although the criteria used to assess the success or failure of community care policies require further discussion, it would appear that up to 1974, Leicester was able to implement its plans for community care with only limited success. In the field of mental health it established a mental health services sub-committee, replaced the occupation centre with the Emily Fortey school, and showed much interest in the recommendations of the Royal Commission and in the 1959 Mental Health Act. It submitted modest but realistic plans for *Health and Welfare*, and the pace of development accelerated in the 1960s, with the opening of the adult training centre, short-stay hostels, and other institutions, the provision of social clubs, and the appointment of additional staff. Yet hospital and community services remained split between the Regional Hospital Board and the local authority, and progress was hampered by shortages of trained staff, and by the restrictions on capital expenditure. Despite the implicit assumption that the family would act as a locus of care, the emphasis was on new institutions rather than on support services in the home. Overall, while the local authority showed much interest in the potential of community care, it had only partly realised its ambitious plans by 1974. Clearly it is very difficult to generalise from the experience of a single local authority. But since Leicester was generally regarded as being a 'progressive' County Borough, its experience in the area of community care hints at a gloomy conclusion for other local authorities in England and Wales.

COMMUNITY CARE AND ITS CRITICS

It was ironic that responsibility for community care was foisted onto the local authorities, the most demoralised branch of the National Health Service, and this was one of the points frequently made by those who were critical of policy. Who were these individuals and groups, what were their motives, and what interest groups did they represent? Does their work help to provide a more objective history of community care?

Some, such as the young Kathleen Jones, were researchers based in university social administration departments. In 1954, for example, she provided a case-study of mental health in Lancashire in one of her first published articles, and in 1960 a general history of mental health services. Before 1948 services had been provided through the Lancashire Asylums Board with after-care being the responsibility of Mental Welfare Associations, but responsibility was then split between the Regional Hospital Board and numerous local authorities. Many of the mental health workers employed by the local authorities had previously been Poor Law relieving officers, and there were few psychiatric social workers. Some cities such as Oldham had tried to integrate hospital and community services, but in other areas there was no system for referring cases to social workers. Jones argued that improvements in the efficiency of the after-care service could prevent relapses on the part of the patients, but also pointed to a range of problems.[57] The book published in 1960 has been castigated for being overly progressive in tone. But she also drew attention to variations in provision, was critical of co-ordination, and again noted that most mental welfare officers were former public assistance relieving officers. She concluded that although services had expanded rapidly in some areas, others 'have been slow to develop their mental health services beyond the minimum statutory requirements'.[58]

Psychiatrists also had much to lose and gain from the introduction of community care. Some of Jones's findings were supported by Jack Tizard who was based at the Medical Research Council's Social Psychiatry Research Unit at the Maudsley Hospital in London. In 1956 he argued that 'the gross overcrowding and barrack-like austerity of most mental-deficiency hospitals' kept down waiting lists, and he concluded that a more radical approach, that used clinics, hostels and sheltered workshops and was more in line with contemporary thinking on mental health, was required. Yet Tizard pointed out that few local authorities had made adequate provision, and that 29 had no occupation centres.[59] A second survey by Tizard found that provision in London for mentally 'subnormal' children was satisfactory, but that occupation centres were still based in church halls, and only 19 per cent of adults had attended them in 1955. He argued that the pay and conditions of staff were poor, parents were critical, and social workers overworked, and he recommended smaller institutions and better support for families.[60]

Some of the contributors to Freeman and Farndale's 1963 collection on mental health used local case-studies in an attempt to evaluate services, while others were sceptical about the degree to which community care had become a reality. The authors of a research project on mental health services conducted by Political and Economic Planning argued that the move to community care was taking place against a background of 'permissive legislation, vague policy, unsettled opinion and some controversy'. In particular, local authorities had little guidance and few standards, and there was no method for assessing need.[61] Hugh Freeman, then a consultant psychiatrist at the Salford Royal Infirmary, noted that local authorities employed few psychiatric social workers, mental welfare officers were poorly trained, and health visitors knew little about mental illness. He advocated junior and adult training centres, hostels, and mental health centres, and emphasised that mental health services should be integrated.[62] Catherine Colwell and Felix Post found from a follow-up survey of patients discharged from the geriatric unit of the Bethlem Royal and Maudsley hospitals that although 39 per cent of these patients had symptoms that required support from community services, they received little after-care because services were limited and there was a shortage of trained social workers.[63]

But the most famous and influential attack on community care in this period was that mounted by Richard Titmuss. As is well-known, Titmuss had been the author of a magisterial history of wartime social services, and from 1950 had been Professor of Social Administration at the London School of Economics. Titmuss had wide-ranging interests and was arguably the most perceptive thinker about community care in this period. In the case of the mentally ill, he suggested that the main factors in the emphasis on community care had been the National Health Service, the reaction against institutional care, John Bowlby's stress on the family as a therapeutic agent, Treasury policy on capital expenditure, and local research and initiatives in places like Worthing and Nottingham. At the same time, it was not clear who was responsible at the local level, and resources were inadequate. In particular, discharge rates from hospital had greatly increased, mental hospitals were doing more work than ever before, hospital discharge rates were being seen as misleading indices of efficiency and productivity, and the family was being romanticised.[64] Titmuss pointed out that a key problem was the shortage of social workers, and that community care was not necessarily any cheaper. In May 1959, for instance, he wrote that 'if community care is not to spell community irresponsibility, what is first needed is a definitive policy and legislation, then leadership, then a willingness to spend the money required'.[65]

Titmuss had been in close contact with the NAMH from the late 1950s, and he repeated many of the same points in a famous address to its annual conference in March 1961, on the same occasion when Enoch Powell outlined government plans to eradicate the Victorian asylums. Titmuss noted that community care evoked 'a sense of warmth and human kindness, essentially personal and comforting', but he argued it was misleading and misunderstood in local government circles. He pointed out that in 1959–60, local authorities employed only 26 full-time psychiatric social workers, and claimed that allowing for price changes, demographic movements, and the increase in mentally ill people, local authorities were spending less on community care than ten years earlier. He commented that 'to transform the bad old mental hospital into the therapeutic institution will be an expensive business', and recommended increased grants to local authorities, better funding for social work courses, and a Royal Commission on the training and recruitment of doctors. Titmuss concluded that by shifting the emphasis from the institution to the community, a situation was being created in which 'we are transferring the care of the mentally ill from trained staff to untrained or ill-equipped staff or no staff at all'.[66] Titmuss's speech was immediately reprinted in the *Spectator* which noted in a leader article that community care was a 'fine concept', but that 'at present there is only a skeleton army, heavily overworked and wretchedly paid'.[67] It subsequently received much press coverage.

These observations on the direction of community care reflected wider issues that included Titmuss's belief that the numbers of social workers had to be increased, preventive medicine should be built around GPs rather than MOsH (Medical Officers of Health), and social workers should be amalgamated in new departments in local government. In a speech given at Torquay in April 1964, for example, Titmuss noted the 'little empires of power' that existed in local and central government, and in voluntary organisations, and he argued that questions about the role of GPs and MOsH in community care for the elderly should lead to a wider enquiry about the deployment of health and welfare services.[68] Similarly, in a speech at Eastbourne in April 1965, Titmuss noted that in local government there was 'too much 'balkanised' rivalry in the field of welfare'. He rejected the idea of family service departments, and again argued in favour of social service departments, claiming that 'if that overworked term 'community care' has any meaning then it must have something to do with the provision of services which are essentially social, essentially personal and primarily local'.[69]

These suggestions were received enthusiastically by social workers, but critically by MOsH and some GPs. General practitioners had themselves been in a poor position in the 1950s, as several surveys had demonstrated, and they were only beginning to regroup in the early 1960s. The Gillie Report on the future of the family doctor (1963) had argued that community care demanded closer communication between psychiatrists, GPs and the staff of local authorities, and it envisaged the GP as the co-ordinator of hospital and community care services.[70] Titmuss countered that there was no evidence that doctors were establishing contacts with social workers independently of MOsH, or that they were assuming a leadership role with respect to community care.[71] At the same time Titmuss looked more favourably upon GPs than local MOsH, and this was reflected in his influence on the Seebohm Committee and its subsequent endorsement of Social Services Departments. Given the failure of community care in this period, it is arguable that Titmuss's ideas had relatively little impact on policy formation and implementation. However his comments on community care both illustrate wider rivalries between public health, general practice, and social work in the 1960s, and provide a striking resonance with many current-day concerns.

CONCLUSION

While the antecedents of community mental health services can be located in earlier documents including the Wood Report on mental deficiency, it was from the mid-1950s that the Ministry of Health and DHSS actively promoted a policy of community care. The timing reflected the pharmacological revolution, increasing criticisms of asylums, concern about the costs of hospital care, and the growing professionalism of groups like social workers. The new emphasis was in line with the recommendations of the Royal Commission on Mental Health and other policies including a planned reduction in the number of hospital beds whose natural corollary was an expansion of smaller institutions and domiciliary services. Indeed the emphasis on community care was inextricably bound up with wider questions about the future of hospital medicine. The Ministry of Health promoted this policy through its circulars and annual reports, and in 1963 it also got local authorities to plan their health and welfare services over the following ten years. In the late 1960s, the restrictions on capital expenditure were relaxed and the new DHSS placed more emphasis on research and on more standardised services. In some local authorities, including Leicester, there were some important achievements: they built junior and adult training centres and short-stay hostels, employed more psychiatric social workers, and pioneered admission policies that blurred the distinction between the hospital and the community. Significantly more progress was made in the period after 1960 than in the previous decade.

Nevertheless the central government departments and local authorities only partly realised their ambitious plans in the period up to 1974, and the meaning of community care remained elusive. Although the National Health Service Act provided local authorities with the basic framework for a policy of community care, the Regional Hospital Boards that ran hospitals were remote from the local authorities that administered community services, and public health in general became a backwater after 1948. Mental health services that were dependant on new buildings were severely hampered by the restrictions on capital expenditure in the 1950s, while the shortage of psychiatric social workers meant that many local authorities still relied on public assistance personnel. The *Health and Welfare* plans indicated that many local authorities lacked ambition and the Ministry did not seem willing to coerce those whose services were of poor standard. Moreover the comments of observers such as Titmuss, the report of the Seebohm Committee, and the White Papers on the mentally ill and handicapped revealed that in most local authorities community care was more apparent in rhetoric than in reality.

It is important to note that significant changes in community care have occurred since the mid-1970s. Of these arguably the most important has been the shift from the idea of care in the community to care by the community. It has been claimed that in the earlier period community care was an elusive concept, but whether it was defined as domiciliary services or alternative institutions, the implication was that these would be provided by local authorities. In the 1990s on the other hand, White Papers and other policy documents now talk about care within and by the family, and by the private sector rather than public agencies.[72] This seems correct in relation to the role of the private sector. However there was also an implicit assumption by policymakers in the earlier period that families would play a role as carers, and this is confirmed by the Leicester case-study where it seems that the children and adults who attended training centres and occupation centres returned home each evening. Thus it is arguable that although national and local sources are silent about the role of the family, the continuities in the 'mixed economy' of community care may be as striking as any changes. Certainly while the consequences of new policies for community care can only be guessed at, its history in England and Wales since the Second World War does not inspire optimism in the future.

CHAPTER ELEVEN

Mental health policy, care in the community and political conflict: the case of the integrated service in Northern Ireland

Jim Campbell

INTRODUCTION

In the last thirty years there has been a sustained debate about the complex processes which inform our understanding of mental health policy in Britain and Ireland. From Goffman's interactionalist analysis of the asylum, to liberal, Marxist and post-structuralist perspectives on deinstitutionalisation, a range of contrasting arguments have been used to explain post-war mental health policy. Explanations for the accelerated discharge of psychiatric patients during this period include the influence of academic and social critiques of institutional living, changes in social attitudes, the discovery and use of psychotropic drugs and shifts in professional discourses.[1] Although there are some causal factors which seem to be more determinant than others – for example Jones'[2] attribution of humanist motives to nineteenth century philanthropists or Scull's[3] critique of capitalist political economy – there also needs to be some recognition of the specificities of nation, region and locality. Finnane's[4] analysis of the growth of the asylum in post-famine Ireland illustrates this point. In his account he unravels a number of processes, working at different levels within the Irish social and legal system, which can account for rising admissions during the period. Of particular importance was the different tax base which funded the asylum system in Ireland, the use of judicial committal and the much more influential engagement of relatives in the negotiation of admissions and discharges than was the case in Britain. Underlying the State's unwillingness to challenge a system of care which seemed to rapidly outpace available expenditure was the unpalatable fact that the administration was unable, politically, to change a tax base which was dependent on landlord rather than ratepayers' contributions. Prior's[5] account of the history of mental health policy in Northern Ireland after partition in 1921 also offers an picture of a system influenced by particular forms of social and political change. From 1921 onwards psychiatric care in Northern Ireland was gradually transformed from an approach closely attached to the nineteenth century Irish universe of asylum provision towards gradual convergence with a British system of health and social welfare. This convergence, however, was uneven and subject to sudden shifts in the political relationships between London and Belfast.

In this chapter mental health policy and practice in Northern Ireland will be discussed in the context of one such moment – the introduction of 'Direct Rule' in 1972, and the 'integrated service' as a mechanism for delivering mental health care. Although there are a number of parallels which can be drawn between Northern Irish and British systems during the last twenty five years, this chapter will focus on the sense of difference and uniqueness of politics and social policy in Northern Ireland. Shaped by historical contingency, social change and a set of diverse legal and organisational structures, the 'integrated service' in Northern Ireland delivered a system of institutional and community care which was centrally organised and very often well-funded. These agencies were, however, less able to develop mental health services which involved patients and communities in the planning and delivery of services. It was also notable that those working in the integrated service were not encouraged to find ways of resolving the underlying conflict about the State, nor were they fully equipped to deal with the psychological traumas caused by 'The Troubles'.

THE INTEGRATED SERVICE

Although Northern Ireland is constitutionally part of the UK, since its inception in 1921 it has experienced long periods of social and political conflict, culminating in the present Troubles. The State's attempts to establish a sense of 'normal' social and political life in the last 75 years have largely failed because the core concepts of nationhood and citizenship have been contested both within and outside Northern Ireland. Since the establishment of Northern Ireland there has existed a tension between the perceived rights and responsibilities of a large Catholic, nationalist minority and a Protestant, unionist majority which, until the introduction of Direct Rule by Westminster in 1972, had almost total control of political and social power. The conflict in Northern Ireland, is however, the result of more than just ethnic or religious conflict, what is often ignored in historical and political accounts are aspects of class and gender. For example the Poor Law Relief riots of the early 1930s brought impoverished Catholic and Protestant workers to the streets in defiance of the State. It was largely women who led the 'Peace Movement' of the 1970s and the progress of current political discussions has been influenced by women's groups and political parties representing working class paramilitaries. It is also a mistake to assume that the conflict is one of just two 'warring communities' because the British, and to a lesser extent, the Irish political establishment have been involved in the management and at times, exacerbation of the conflict during this period (Whyte,[6] Gaffikin and Morrissey[7]).

The rationale for the creation of the integrated service can be best explained by central government's attempt to resolve political and social conflict in Northern Ireland through Direct Rule from Westminster. There is substantial evidence to confirm that the local Northern Irish administration prior to 1972 had colluded in sectarian discrimination, particularly through the emasculation of electoral rights, repressive policing and lack of access to housing for Catholics. The introduction of Direct Rule can be viewed as a benign attempt to apply liberal democratic principles to a corrupt region within the UK. There is, on the other hand, some debate about how successful this political strategy has been. An alternative interpretation of these events focuses more closely on the central State as an actor with responsibility for the events which led to, and reproduced, conflict. Aspects of these forms of discrimination still exist today. For example Catholic unemployment has remained consistently higher that Protestant unemployment and security forces have been implicated in human rights abuses throughout the period of Direct Rule. These problems, however, must be judged against the backdrop of intense violence carried out by republican and loyalist paramilitary groups. In hindsight it now appears naive to have assumed that Direct Rule would have automatically resolved the causes of conflict in Northern Ireland (Birrell and Murie[8]).

The integrated service was established in Northern Ireland in 1973 in the midst of this crisis of State. The term integrated service is described in this way because, uniquely within the islands of Britain and Ireland, health and personal social services are brought together under one administrative structure. This replaces the split in responsibilities between local and health authorities which occurred in Northern Ireland prior to 1972, and which currently exists in the rest of the United Kingdom. McCoy[9] has traced the history of the integrated service and describes three broad phases in its development. The first decade was characterised by professional expansion within a system which was corporatist and centralised. Each professional group had a clear structure of line-management within four health and social services boards. Thus, each board contained a mental health programme of care in which psychiatrists, clinical psychologists, social workers, nurses and professionals allied to medicine practiced together. In this period boards had primary responsibility for the planning, monitoring and delivery of care. A second phase can be identified, lasting roughly from the mid 1980s to the early 1990s, during which policy focused on the need to decentralise services and introduce techniques of general management into the organisations. It was then that the first discernible attempts were made to develop coherent services in the community for people with mental health problems. Arguably the most far-reaching changes have occurred since the early nineties when the integrated service was transformed to accommodate the community care reforms recommended by the Griffiths Report. In the last decade community care policy in Northern Ireland, informed by the white paper *People First*,[10] has prepared the way for health and social services boards to separate the functions of purchasing and providing services, and to generate the conditions for an internal market in health and social care. These changes created new partnerships between the statutory, voluntary and private sectors, the establishment of independent residential unit inspectorates and the devolution of income support budgets to teams of care managers in newly created community health and social services trusts. Subsequent Orders in Council redirected boards' powers to these self-managed trusts.

Throughout this history, structures of health and social welfare in Northern Ireland have tended to be hierarchical, bureaucratic and staffed by cadres of professions whose agencies were generally detached from the influence of local communities and their politicians. This is hardly surprising because the prevailing organisational and professional discourses of the service emphasised the importance of being objective and detached from the conflict. Interestingly this overarching sense of detachment allowed professionals from both sides of the community, Protestant and Catholic, to work alongside each other in a relatively peaceful working environment. This can be contrasted with the violence and sectarianism experienced in other forms of employment in Northern Ireland. It should not be assumed, however, that prejudice, fear and discrimination do not exist in health and personal social services, rather such feelings tend to be hidden within professional discourses and rarely acknowledged in organisational policy. The service is designed to deal with social and health problems technocratically, through the application of law and bureaucratic regulation. This leads to a general avoidance of issues about the State's role in managing the conflict. In particular these services have failed to address the ubiquitous presence of sectarianism which runs through all aspects of Northern Irish life,[11] and have largely failed to build partnerships with the working class communities who have suffered most from the conflict.[12]

The integrated service is also characterised by a paradox in how power is accessed and used. At one level professionals have been largely ineffectual in changing the course of violent conflict in Northern Ireland because the service was designed to remain aloof from this conflict. At the same time policy-makers and professionals have been allowed substantial powers in making decisions about the service on behalf of patients and clients. For example, at a time when mental health service users have made some advances in redressing the imbalances in professional power within psychiatric systems throughout Europe and North America, this process has been slow to take place in Northern Ireland. In a study of 92 mental health service users, Campbell and Donnelly[13] found that users were generally unaware of the roles of professionals who dealt with them and were ignorant of ways in which complaints could be made about the service. Although there were relatively high levels of satisfaction with services received, it was clear that service users were only minimally involved in the planning and delivery of services. It appears that the excessive powers of boards and trusts in Northern Ireland in some ways reflects the centralising nature of a political system which is rarely accountable to local politicians, communities and citizens

DELIVERING COMMUNITY CARE

The range of mental health services which developed within this unique structure has had to face considerable organisational change in the last decade. The processes which led to the rapid decrease in psychiatric bed numbers and development of services in the community in Britain can be identified in the Northern Ireland context, but with some local variation. It can be argued, for instance, that The Mental Health (NI) Order, 1986 offers more protection for patients' rights and community-based alternatives to psychiatric hospitals than equivalent British legislation. This is achieved through a number of mechanisms:

- The Order is designed to encourage assessment of mental ill-health and risk in the community rather than the hospital setting – for example it is the General Practitioner (GP) rather than psychiatrist who makes the medical recommendation during compulsory admissions to hospital.
- The Approved Social Worker is given additional powers to override the nearest relative in some circumstances. This is a possible safeguard against collusion between nearest relatives and medics.
- The assessment period in hospital allows possible 'regrading' and is a protective factor in terms of the patient's civil rights
- The Mental Health Commission has powers to investigate community-based facilities and can inquire about the treatment and care of voluntary as well as detained patients

The way the legislation is operationalised by professionals has been strongly influenced by a rapid fall in available psychiatric hospital beds, documented by Prior.[14] In the early 1960s over 6,000 beds existed in Northern Irish psychiatric hospitals. Two five year strategic plans drawn up by the Department of Health and Social Services in 1986 and 1991 directed boards to reduce substantially hospital bed numbers. In the first of these plans the target of a 20 per cent reduction was exceeded well within the required period. The second five year strategic plan targetted a baseline of 1500 beds by 1997. In the year 1995/6 only 1521 psychiatric beds remained in Northern Ireland. The current five year plan proposes that, '. . . long-term, institutional care should no longer be provided in traditional psychiatric hospital environments.'[15] Although the psychiatric system in Northern Ireland has operated with a gradually reducing complement of hospital beds, this does not mean that admission rates have dropped. Rafferty[16] argues that the deinstitutionalisation which has taken place in England and Wales in the post war period should be understood in terms of the relationship between 'stock' and 'flow'; hospital bed numbers have been reduced at the same time as admission rates have risen. One side-effect of a similar process which has occurred in Northern Ireland is the difficulty which practitioners increasingly experience in trying to find places in hospital, not only for voluntary patients, but also those of need of compulsory admission. Limited numbers of beds and the paucity of community resources may be subtly changing the way the Order is being used by professionals. Byrne[17] has described how a growing number of applications for assessment by ASWs are taking place in the setting of the psychiatric hospital rather than the community. Even though the Order requires that exactly the same legal process takes place in hospital as it would be in the community – with GP and nearest relative or ASW involvement – this makes objective decision-making and the protection of patients' rights more problematic.

Outside the hospital the debate about the control of people with mental health problems living in the community has intensified, particularly after a public inquiry[18] which criticised the events surrounding the murder of a young person by a patient, discharged from a psychiatric hospital in Northern Ireland. The Report not only highlighted gaps in systems of care and protection, but also reopened the earlier debate about the reasons for the exclusion of personality disorder from compulsory admission, during the review of the previous legislation.[19] In this case the patient had a long history of involvement with child care services and, later, psychiatric and learning disability programmes. After a limited period in the psychiatric hospital, the patient left against medical advice and almost immediately killed the young person. Psychiatrists and other mental health staff informed the committee that he could not be held in hospital against his wishes because he had been diagnosed as having a personality disorder and was thus not mentally disordered, in the terms of the legislation.

The debate which followed the Fenton Report in fact intensified the controversy about the validity of excluding people with personality disorders from compulsory admission to hospital. The argument for the exclusion was that problems which people with personality disorders face are generally best dealt with in the community because such conditions are associated with problems of living, not mental illness. The alternative position is that psychiatric professionals should not be allowed to neglect their responsibilities to a group of vulnerable, often very disturbed people, left to exist on the margins of Northern Irish society with little access to appropriate care and treatment. What this debate has revealed about the integrated service is a lacuna in the planning of services for adults whose problems do not fit within traditional programmes of care – family and child care, elders, learning disability, criminal justice, health and disability. Often people with personality disorders eventually find themselves in contact with forensic psychiatry teams who operate at the interface between the criminal justice and mental health systems. In partial recognition of this gap in service the establishment of a medium secure psychiatric unit has been identified in the Department of Health and Social Services' most recent five year strategic plan.[20]

It might be assumed that the integrated service was in an advantageous position to manage the general problems associated with psychiatric deinsitutionalisation, given the way decisions were made centrally and because mental health professionals tended to work within one organisational structure. This situation can be contrasted with the British system of mental health care in which the absence of a unitary authority, in which psychiatrists, psychologists and community psychiatric nurses are employed alongside social services staff, has prevented good practice in the community mental health field.[21]

In the first decade of the integrated service multidisciplinary teams were usually located in large psychiatric institutions but since the mid 1980s there has been gradual relocation of resources and professionals into the community. This movement of personnel has coincided with the gradual reduction of acute and continuing care beds in hospitals. Although the organisational rhetoric of the integrated service implies consistency and continuity in service delivery, a degree of variation exists. Some mental health programmes have been organised in large geographical units whilst others are located in smaller patch-based units and at primary health care level. The mixture of professionals within these teams also tended to vary, according to the discretion of managers and professional groups within hospital and community trusts. At times teams have pursued an integrated, democratic style of work whilst others have adhered to the more traditional approach in which the consultant psychiatrist retains considerable professional influence in decision-making processes. Community mental health teams usually deal with generic mental health problems and refer more complex problems to specialist services which may be organised at board, trust or provincial levels. These include services for people with addictions, eating disorders and psychosexual problems. There are also psychotherapeutic services and teams for psychiatry for older people and children and young people.

Despite the promises inherent in a policy-making process which was centrally directed and closely managed by groups of established mental health professionals, there is some debate about how well community care services were funded during this period of rapid deinstitutionalisation. The new purchasing/providing split which followed the health services reforms in the early 1990s has introduced new types of services, particularly within the voluntary sector, but the provision of day care, residential care and care management programmes still remains patchy and uneven in some areas.[22] Prior[23] argues that community care policy has only been partially successful in Northern Ireland because resources still remained locked in large institutions. Although bed numbers have been substantially reduced, psychiatric hospitals continue to use a disproportionate amount of the mental health budget. The cost of running outdated establishments helps explain some of this expenditure. In Northern Ireland the six psychiatric hospitals established during the high point of asylum building in Ireland in the last century remain standing and in use. Organisational resistance to change has been, to some extent, reinforced by the continuing existence of a powerful medical discourse which strongly influences strategic decisions.

It is perhaps surprising that the public and professional representations of the integrated service as an efficient and responsive service have not been fully tested by through research. The Clinical Standards Advisory Group (CSAG), in a national review of standards of care for people with schizophrenia, acknowledged the benefit of the integrated service in the one district in Northern Ireland which was included in the study.[24] A particularly strong argument about the failure of mental health policy in Britain has focused on the inadequacy of viable financing initiatives and the associated problems of planning caused by the organisational split between health and local authorities. Evidence suggests that these difficulties may not be as great in Northern Ireland perhaps because of the centralised nature of the policy process. For example the Department of Health and Social Services used bridging finance of £34m during the initial years of accelerated deinstitutionalisation to assist in the transition towards community-based services.

Following this period, the Department commissioned research to evaluate the process and outcomes of this policy. Included in the study were all former long-stay patients discharged from the six psychiatric hospitals in Northern Ireland, between 1987–92.[25] The researchers found that former patients did not experience dramatic changes in functioning and quality of life as a result of the move from hospital to community, but that there were variations in the quality of services offered. For instance those placed in voluntary and statutory residential units were more likely to receive more comprehensive social and therapeutic services than others living in the private sector. In some respects the results were less encouraging than similar, although not equivalent, English studies. For example, the community care provided in Northern Ireland was on average cheaper than in England and the study found no direct evidence that the integrated service had provided a more comprehensive or efficient service to these patients, although this was a relatively minor research question within the overall context of the survey. Similarly there has been considerable public and professional attention paid to the issue of people who are both mentally ill and homeless in Britain. Donnelly and McGilloway,[26] in their study of homeless people residing in hostels in Belfast, found high levels of psychiatric morbidity and unmet need. Service users reported that they found the community psychiatric nursing and social work services accessible, but contact with GPs and the Northern Ireland Housing Executive less satisfactory. They also reported that, despite the fact that many of the clients surveyed had been in contact with the criminal justice, psychiatric and child care systems, there was a lack of a co-ordinated approach in dealing with their needs and an unevenness of access to social and health services.

In conclusion, it can be argued that agencies which deliver health and social care in Northern have had moderate success in managing deinstitutionalisation. This task has been made easier by the use of centralised planning and funding mechanism. Nonetheless there is some evidence to suggest remaining high levels of social and health need and gaps in service delivery in the community.

RESPONDING TO CONFLICT

The conflict in Northern Ireland has had a profound impact on the social and economic life and mental well-being of its citizens. In the years since 1969 over three thousand five hundred people have died as a direct result of 'The Troubles' and tens of thousands have been traumatised, physically, psychologically and emotionally. Research carried periodically during 'The Troubles' has revealed various aspects of psychological and psychiatric morbidity, as well as some unexpected research conundrums. What emerges is an image of a society which at times seems quite resilient in the face of violent events, but also one which contains substantial numbers of people who have been psychologically and emotionally traumatised. Lyon's study during the early phase of 'The Troubles' found evidence of psychiatric morbidity amongst patients who had first hand experience of being caught up in bomb explosions, but also an apparent capacity on the part of most of these patients to make a good recovery.[27] In a more rigorous survey involving larger populations later on in the conflict, Loughry et al[28] identified substantial levels of Post Traumatic Stress Disorder (PTSD) in patients affected by 'The Troubles'. Community-based studies carried out by Cairns and Wilson[29] reported that many respondents who had experienced violent events used psychological coping mechanisms, for example denial and distancing, to survive emotionally. The use of psychoanalytical ideas to understand the nature of social conflict has been rarely used in the Northern Irish context. However, in the course of psychoanalytical groupwork with Catholics and Protestants, Benson[30] has reported the range of intense thoughts and feelings expressed by participants. Group discourses were often modified to enable a therapeutic milieu to exist, but the implicit references to fear and hatred were often attributable individual experiences and perceptions of contemporary, violent events.

Although it is at times difficult to describe and quantify the multifaceted nature of this violence, there seems little doubt that it has had a considerable impact on all aspects of life, in Northern Ireland. What is notable about how mental health services have responded to the conflict is the way in which policy appears to treat and care for some individuals and groups rather than others. In examining the history of the State's response to the conflict, it can be argued process of selection is, understandably, shaped by broad political agendas. When social conflict erupted in Northern Ireland in 1969 attempts to provide health and social care for those suffering from the intercommunal violence was hampered by the absence of viable administrative and political structures. The local devolved government had neither the capacity nor strategic understanding to deliver comprehensive services in the midst of such a breakdown of civil society. Darby and Williamson[31] have discuss how, in the early period of 'The Troubles', services were strained to breaking point in trying to deal with massive shifts in population, and the paralysing effects of sectarian threat and violence. Health and social care professionals were left somewhat isolated from core organisational direction, but nonetheless managed to provide essential services to those most in need. This made for some unusual partnerships between statutory services and local communities. For example, professionals working in areas where the most intense conflict was taking place, often had to establish their role and function in negotiation with emerging paramilitary groups. This adjustment was necessary if they were to have any chance of gaining entry to communities which were suffering most from 'The Troubles'. Once the conflict became 'more manageable', the immediacy of contact with community groups was replaced by a more bureaucratic approach typified in the working practices of the integrated service.

Perhaps because of organisational rigidity of the integrated service, and its proximity to the State, some traumatic events were not adequately addressed by statutory services. One example of this was the lack of an organisational response to the event known as 'Bloody Sunday', when marchers who had been involved with or near a civil rights march in Derry in 1971 were shot dead by the British army. The trauma for survivors and family members has been exacerbated because of an alleged failure in the legal process in ascertaining responsibility and guilt for these events. This problem has only recently been recognised by the UK government through the establishment of a second judicial inquiry into the events. The example of Bloody Sunday helps to illustrate the restrictive compass of the integrated service because comprehensive State services were neither offered to, nor perhaps expect by, this community, despite apparently high levels of psychological need.

Such events illustrate the complex interrelationship between health care delivery and the contested nature of the State in Northern Ireland. Where death and injury was caused by 'terrorist' rather than State activity, then services were more likely to be provided by the State. Thus traumas inflicted on security forces personnel and their families tended to receive some help from dedicated psychiatric and social services within their respective organisations. In other cases, for instance when civilians were traumatised by violence carried out by paramilitary groups, few services, until recently, have been organised to meet their specific needs. Paramilitary groups, as a result of the construction of these victimologies, have tended to meet the needs of their members and families on a self-help basis, partly because of an inherent distrust of the State, but more obviously because the State will not provide and fund specialist services for these organisations. Even with the growing professionalisation and expansion of the integrated service from the 1970s onwards, mental health professionals were slow to address the needs for victims suffering as a result of political violence. When services were provided they tended to be piecemeal and conventional, rather than comprehensive, innovative and flexible. The first point of contact for someone who has suffered from the traumas of violence in Northern Ireland tends to be the GP who then makes a choice to treat or refer to generic psychiatric services. Although discrete forensic psychiatric teams service courts and prisons there is little recognition of the impact of the peculiar social and political circumstances factors on the criminal justice system in Northern Ireland. This is despite the fact that the care and treatment of paramilitaries and security forces personnel is carried out by professionals in the mental health and criminal justice sectors in Northern Ireland.

Many psychiatrists, mental health social workers, probation officers, psychiatric nurses and psychologists have had contact with people traumatised by 'The Troubles', but here remains a institutionalised and professional resistance to consider the deep seated problems in operationalising mental health policy in a society which has experienced so much conflict. It should be no surprise, therefore, that many ethical and professional dilemmas for exist for practitioners. Smyth and Campbell,[32] for example, describe how Approved Social Workers often have to work alongside the security forces when carrying out their legal functions. Some compulsory admissions to psychiatric hospital require the attendance, not just of armour-plated Land Rovers and armed police, but an equivalent British Army presence, simply because the police need protection in some areas where there is a strong paramilitary threat. Healy[33] describes how she and her colleagues have struggled to find ways of working with young people and their families who have experienced traumatic events. She recognises the need to acknowledge the painful experiences of the conflict which are internalised by professionals. These intense feelings and thoughts should be dealt with before attempting to work with people who are psychologically traumatised. Healy argues that the use of 'reflective teams' can help support individual therapists to understand the relationship between personal identities, professional roles and social circumstances of clients. The existence of such dilemmas confirm the impression that the integrated service has operated within a well-resourced, highly skilled organisation, but that no serious attempt has been made to acknowledge the impact of civil conflict on professional judgement-making. It is almost as if agencies have not given staff the permission to recognise that bridges can be made between professional and citizenship roles. Without this support these transitions are, understandably, difficult to make.

As 'The Troubles' moved through different stages, the statutory and voluntary sectors have gradually developed strategies in response to major traumatic events, especially bombings and shootings in which deaths have occurred. The voluntary and community sectors in particular have recently adopted a key role in working with individuals, families and communities who have been traumatised by violence. These sectors tend to have developed closer relationships with 'victims' and are often viewed as more trustworthy than the statutory sector; this is especially the case where groups identify themselves, or are identified by others, to be in opposition to the State. Statutory bodies have modified services in an attempt to respond to traumatic incidents in recent years, but always within the parameters laid down by the State and the existing ethos' of statutory boards and trusts. A good illustration of this adaptive process is the way in which crisis teams developed in Northern Ireland, particularly after the Kegworth disaster. This disaster happened when an aircraft crashed in England on a flight from London to Belfast, killing and injuring many people. Following this event, four crisis teams were set up in the Eastern Health and Social Services Board to deal with traumatic incidents in Northern Ireland. Since then these teams have responded to violent events, using the therapeutic and organisational lessons learned from Kegworth.[34] When a bomb was planted by the IRA, killing people on Shankill Road in Belfast in 1993, these multidisciplinary teams provided a range of services to survivors, their families and the local community. Another example of a statutory response to the conflict was the involvement of crisis teams following the Remembrance Day bombing in Enniskillen, when mourners died following an explosion in 1987. What was notable about the subsequent development of services in this case was the more purposeful attempt to resolve collective grief through cross-community meetings and groupwork.[35]

It is only in the context of the current political process, thirty years since the start of the present 'Troubles' in Northern Ireland, that the broad range of problems faced by people traumatised by 'The Troubles' is finally being acknowledged. The fact that statutory services may now be more responsive as a consequence of these political change only serves to highlight their close alignment with the State in the past. In the opening page of the Agreement document there is an acknowledgement of the position of those who had suffered:

> The tragedies of the past have left a deep and profoundly regrettable legacy of suffering. We must never forget those who have died or been

injured, and their families. But we can best honour them through a fresh start, in which we firmly dedicate ourselves to the achievement of reconciliation, tolerance, and mutual trust, and to the protection and vindication of the human rights of all.[36]

In a recent Department of Health and Social Service Report[37] on existing services designed to meet the social and psychological needs for people traumatised by the violence of the last thirty years, the failure of the past is acknowledged. There is a recognition that statutory services have generally not been successful in addressing many of the needs of people who have suffered from violence. The Report describes the lack of awareness of, and publicity about existing services, including the growing range of community and voluntary sector activity. There is some concern that the work of these services has been hampered because of inadequate funding. Although there are examples of good practice, for instance in the work of some crisis teams, there remains a degree of mistrust of the State sector by some groups. More specifically waiting lists for psychology services were found to be excessively long and there is a concern that counselling services were in need of regulation and monitoring. A continual theme which runs through the Report is the failure to acknowledge fully the depth and breadth of pain which many people in Northern Irish society have experienced.

If the recommendations contained in this Report were to be carried out in full, it would mark a new departure in the way mental health services respond to effects of the conflict. It implies that the people who have been traumatised will be more visible and their needs recognised in the planning process. In engaging with this process mental health professionals working in the integrated service will have the opportunity to work more closely with individuals and communities they treat and care for.

CONCLUSION

The way in which community care policy for people with mental health problems developed in Northern Ireland since 1972 can be explained by a number of regional and national factors. By the time 'The Troubles' started a process of convergence with British mental health policy had already taken place in previous 50 years.

Even at the height of the political conflict the perennial themes of deinstitutionalisation, legislative reform and the construction of new forms of services in the community preoccupied the minds of policy-makers in Northern Ireland. In this respect, mental health professionals and administrators shared the same concerns as their British counterparts. Nevertheless, the contested nature of the State inevitably produced local variations in Northern Irish mental health policy. However unusual it may seem, it was somehow understandable that mental health services were unable to provide innovative and flexible responses to the conflict because professionals were employed by agencies which were organisationally detached from local communities. The integrated service on the other hand was moderately successful in translating policy into provision which enabled people with mental health problems to live outside the hospital. It could be argued that organisational consistency and rational planning are the hallmarks of mental health policy in Northern Ireland during this period. How the integrated service will develop depends on whether the series of cease-fires and the tentative political processes will resolve the conflict in Northern Ireland. There is some indication that political change is already altering the way in which mental health policy will be delivered. In its recent strategy document the local administration has recommended approaches which encourage community development and social inclusion in the delivery of health and social welfare.[38] These developments will challenge the rationale which underpinned the establishment of the integrated service in 1973 determine the shape future of Northern Irish mental health policy.

CHAPTER TWELVE

Outside the walls of the asylum? Psychiatric treatment in the 1980s and 1990s

Sarah Payne

INTRODUCTION

Care in the community for people suffering from psychiatric illness has been central to mental health policy in Britain for a number of years. Community mental health services have developed alongside the running down of institutional psychiatric care and a shift in the location of in-patient treatment from the large scale hospital to the smaller unit.[1] The principle of caring for people with mental health problems outside of the hospital has been welcomed, particularly by user groups and survivor networks[2] and despite some dissenting voices, there has been for some years an apparent consensus over the objective of providing most of the care needed beyond the walls of the asylum.

As we move into the next century, however, this agreement concerning the ideal of community care has been challenged by the apparent failure of these policies for some groups within the mentally ill population.[3] A series of high-profile acts of violence carried out by people in psychiatric treatment in the community has brought a reassessment of the objectives of this policy. Similarly, reports of self-harm and suicide amongst those discharged from hospital suggested that community care was failing.[4] In addition, in a period of increasing levels of homelessness in Britain, there has been growing concern that people discharged from the psychiatric hospital form a significant proportion of the homeless.[5] Studies which have attempted to assess the extent to which those who have left institutional psychiatric care are surviving on the streets, rather than having found safe alternatives in the community, are often inconclusive due to difficulties in assessing the causal direction of any association.[6] However, there is little doubt that a large number of those without permanent homes are also suffering from severe mental illness and that they are also unlikely to improve in such conditions.

Thus the debates in the 1970s and the early 1980s over how best to deliver care in the community for those diagnosed as mentally ill – debates which focused on the overlapping nature of the services, on issues of funding, and on overcoming the opposition of local communities, for example – have begun to be replaced by other debates. The focus now is on risk management, the need to identify patients representing a risk – to others and to themselves – and the need to design services to manage such a group.[7] Thus there has been a growing divide, in media representations of the mentally ill and in policy responses, between patients who are seen as appropriate cases for community care, and those who are not. The apogee of this comes with the Labour Government's planned White Paper on mental health policy, which aims to develop a range of solutions to meet the needs of what are being seen as different categories of patients. The debate leading up to White Paper is framed around concepts of risk and danger, as was evident from an early leaking of the Paper's contents, when the *Daily Telegraph* revealed: 'Care in the community is scrapped – more secure units for mentally-ill patients who pose danger.'[8]

This chapter discusses community mental health care policy in the 1980s and early 1990s prior to the White Paper on mental health services. In exploring these issues the focus is on the changes in service delivery brought by the shift to community care and the failures which were being increasingly highlighted during this period. During the run up to the new White Paper particular groups of patients were being identified in terms of the risk they posed to the community and the failure of community care to adequately respond to the needs of these patients. Mental health policy by the mid-1990s had begun to construct the notion of the dangerous mental health patient as different to the less troublesome, less ill patients.

This is associated with an increasing use during the 1980s and 1990s of the term 'worried well', to refer to the less problematic patients. However, whilst this term had been used dismissively in North America since the early 1980s to refer to relatively affluent patients – often women – who paid for private psychiatry and psychotherapy, in Britain the worried well were constructed as those treated within the state funded system for minor, insignificant illness. Whilst this group were not synonymous with the worried well patients in the US, they were also more likely to be women, and this contrasts sharply with the fact that those represented as dangerously mad were more likely to be men.

Thus these developments were not 'gender neutral', and this needs further exploration. The ways in which services changed during this period helped to construct a particular gendered notion of mental illness – in which women were seen as the majority of the worried well whilst men made up the majority of the threateningly mad. This is associated with changing patterns of treatment, and also with media representations of the mentally ill through the reporting of particular acts of violence. The gendered impact of changes in mental health policy in the 1980s and 1990s is, therefore, also critical to an understanding of changes in the services and their implications both for individual men and women within the mental health system and for the ways in which mental health issues came to be viewed, in the run up to the 1998 White Paper.

PSYCHIATRIC CARE IN THE 1980S AND 1990S

Most people suffering from mental health problems are treated in the community, in the primary health care system,[9] and this has been the case since the development of the state funded primary health care system. Approximately four times as many people are seen each year by a GP for mental health problems compared with the number seen by psychiatrists.[10] People with what are primarily described as more minor mental illness are likely to remain in the care of their General Practitioner throughout their illness.

Changes in the delivery of mental health services in the past twenty or thirty years have had a greater effect on those who have been diagnosed as suffering more severe and enduring mental health problems, and in particular those diagnosed with psychotic conditions, who in the past were most likely to have been hospitalised for long periods of time. For this group there have been far reaching developments in mental health policy, with an increasing emphasis on services in the community. People diagnosed as suffering from senile and pre-senile dementia, for example, from which recovery is unlikely, are also less likely to be hospitalised in the early stages of their illness than before.[11] People with severe depressive illnesses may still receive in-patient treatment – but much less often than in the past. These shifts in the kinds of illness that are treated inside the hospital are directly associated with the reduction in the availability of in-patient treatment. However, different groups of patients have been affected in different ways.

CLOSING THE PSYCHIATRIC HOSPITAL?

The mental health system of most developed countries turned increasingly towards non-institutional care during the latter half of this century.[12] In England the number of psychiatric beds fell between 1954 and 1982 by 55 per cent, from 152,000 to 72,000. This fall continued into the 1990s, so that by 1993–94 there were only 43,000 beds available,[13] a reduction of 72 per cent over this period in total. If this trend continues, there will be less than 20,000 beds left by the year 2000.[14] Many of the bed losses were in the large scale hospitals, which were replaced by smaller units attached to general hospitals.[15] The ten years between 1972 and 1982 saw the closure of over 40 of the larger psychiatric hospitals in England – those with more than 1000 beds.[16] Another 45 psychiatric hospitals, of all sizes, are due to close by the year 2000.[17]

This dramatic reduction in the provision of facilities for in-patient psychiatric treatment did not mean that psychiatric admissions decreased. On the contrary, the total number of psychiatric admissions actually increased, so that whilst in 1964 there were 155,000 admissions to psychiatric hospital, a rate of 347 per 100,000 population, by 1984 there were 192,000 admissions, a rate of 409 per 100,000 population. By 1993–94, this had increased further to 224,000 admissions, a rate per 100,000 population of 462.[18] Between 1964 and 1993–94, then, total psychiatric admissions increased by nearly 50 per cent. Thus the reduction in in-patient psychiatric facilities in Britain in the last forty years was accompanied by an increase in the number of cases treated. This did not indicate a growing epidemic of psychiatric illness, but changing patterns of admission and discharge, and in particular a faster turnover of in-patients. In 1993–94 figures from the Department of Health on the hospital psychiatric services describe a 'throughput' in psychiatric bed use over the year of 5.5 compared with 2.5 in 1983.[19]

The pattern for many patients, however, is one of admission to psychiatric hospital and discharge which is then followed by subsequent readmission at a later date. If one compares figures for first admissions, which include only those who have not previously experienced in-patient psychiatric treatment (available until 1986) with figures for total admissions it is clear that the vast majority of the increase in psychiatric admissions over this period is accounted for by the readmission of those who have already been treated as in-patients and discharged from hospital – the phenomenon of the so-called 'revolving door'.[20]

If we break these admission statistics down by age and sex, however, an interesting picture emerges, for not all patients are equally prone to this pattern of admission, discharge and readmission. The most notable feature of age and sex-specific patterns of in-patient psychiatric treatment is that whilst women continue to dominate the statistics for in-patient treatment – as has been the case for a long time – in some age groups men have overtaken women. Amongst younger age groups there are now more admissions of male patients than of female.[21] For example, figures for psychiatric in-patient treatment from one health authority show more episodes of hospital treatment for younger men than for women in the same age group. In 1993–94 the treatment rate for men aged 20–24 was 348 per 100,000 population compared with 291 for women; between the ages of 25–34, the male treatment rate was 435 per 100,000 compared with a population rate of 418 for women.[22]

In addition, amongst the older population, men have overtaken women as the major recipients of in-patient psychiatric treatment. Thus over the age of 75, there were more first admissions and total admissions per head of population for men than for women by the mid-1980s.[23] However, admissions for women for diagnoses of senile and presenile dementia have remained higher than those for men. Instead, admissions to psychiatric hospital amongst older men for other conditions have increased – the over-representation of men amongst the over 75s is not explained by an increase for one sex in admissions for dementia, but relates to an increase in other kinds of illness, depression in particular.

These gendered differences in patterns of in-patient treatment at the same time as the number of available beds has decreased are important, although difficult to interpret. It may be that scarce resources are being 'rationed' in favour of men by the psychiatric profession; and it may be that men – particularly in the younger age groups – are seen as presenting as more of a threat or a risk to the community and are therefore more likely to be removed from the community than women. Certainly studies suggest that those who are admitted are more highly disturbed in comparison with earlier years,[24] and mental health professionals are more likely to view male patients as in need of in-patient treatment as a form of control.[25]

It may also be that the provision of psychiatric services in the community benefits women more than men – for example, with more self-help and support groups aimed at women than men.[26] Amongst the older population, higher admission rates amongst men may reflect a greater difficulty in finding other residential accommodation for men who are suffering from mental difficulties; or a greater reluctance on the part of families to provide care for men with some forms of illness, whereas women are more often cared for in such circumstances.

PSYCHIATRIC CARE IN THE COMMUNITY

At the same time as hospital provision has decreased, there has been an increase in services in the community for those diagnosed as suffering from psychiatric disorders. The terms used to describe this care are open to a number of definitions. Just as 'community care' has a wide range of meanings, many of them bearing little relation to the kinds of help or care actually received by vulnerable people living on the outside, so community mental health care covers a wide range of mental health services outside the institution.

The debate over community care issues in general in the 1980s and 1990s was informed by a feminist critique which highlighted the way in which care in the community largely meant care by the family and, in most cases, this meant care by women.[27] This critique has become more complex with the increasing recognition of the part played by male carers[28] and the intricacy of caring relationships. However, it is important to recognise, in relation to community psychiatric care, that the majority of those diagnosed as suffering mental health difficulties are caring for themselves, rather than being cared for – particularly amongst younger age groups.[29] This raises a different set of questions in terms of the formal provision of care in the community. In discussions within the mental health system the term community care is largely taken to mean the provision of medical treatment and social service support rather than the (often or largely fictitious) notion of the wider community providing 'care'.

Much of the early debate over community mental health services focused on the discharge of long-stay patients from the psychiatric institution, and the closure of long-stay hospitals.[30] The focus in these accounts was the issue of rehabilitation and how the transfer to the community could be managed, and also how best to provide support. 'Decarceration' was seen as a solution to the problems experienced by long-stay patients[31] – the poor quality of life experienced by those in a total institution, the appalling conditions of most psychiatric hospitals, and the ways in which the asylum system itself created illnesses such as 'institutional neurosis'.[32] Studies showed that patients experienced an improvement in their quality of life outside the hospital.[33]

Despite the importance of these issues, community care for people with mental health problems in the 1980s and 1990s has had to face particular challenges. In recent years the majority of those receiving psychiatric care from services outside the psychiatric hospital have never been long-term in-patients. Instead, those with severe and enduring mental illness are likely to have had numerous hospital admissions, each lasting a relatively short length of time. Thus in discussions about care in the community there are a number of distinct issues which relate to different groups in receipt of this care. Former long-stay patients have a separate set of needs on discharge compared with new patients suffering from serious mental illness. Reintegration into a community left twenty years ago is a different matter to the attempt to construct alternatives which enable someone in an acutely ill episode to remain supported outside of hospital treatment.

What then do we mean by care in the community in the last decade of the twentieth century? Psychiatric care in the community encompasses care delivered by a range of professionals and funded from a range of sources. It includes treatment from a general practitioner and the primary health care team, incorporating, for example, psychotherapy and counselling, relaxation clinics, addiction counselling and stress management support.

More specialist psychiatric community services are often provided within a medical framework, sometimes in a hospital setting. For example, when the psychiatric hospitals were being run down and beds lost, there was an increase in the provision of psychiatric treatment in the hospital on an out-patient or day patient basis. Day cases initially increased but have in the last twenty years decreased again, whilst out-patient attendances have continued to increase, from 192,000 new cases in 1983, for example, to 248,000 in 1993–94.[34] A recent study of treatment by day hospital compared with in-patient treatment found few differences in terms of outcome, but those treated in a day hospital had the advantage of being able to maintain their contacts in the community.[35] The initial recovery was quicker amongst in-patients but the rate of relapse was higher.

Recently there has been an increasing emphasis on mental health treatment further out in the community, beyond the asylum, delivered via community mental health teams (CMHTs). CMHTs vary in style and practice from area to area but largely are sector-based and include mental health professionals employed by the health authority (psychiatrist and psychiatric nurses) and staff employed by the social services (in particular, psychiatric social workers or approved social workers).

However, there has been a growing concern over the amount of care provided in the community, and whether it is enough to meet the needs of those who require services.[36] In the first years of the shift towards non-institutional care, the reduction in psychiatric beds was achieved more rapidly than the creation of places in day hospitals and day centres.[37] Estimates of the number of cases treated nationally in the community suggest that more than 100,000 long-term mentally ill people are now living in the community.[38] Of these, more than a quarter have no contact with specialist psychiatric services and depend on their GP for all care.

PSYCHIATRY AND COMMUNITY CARE

Whilst the move towards community treatment has continued, the psychiatric profession's reactions to this trend have been varied. Some have resisted the idea.[39] Others have argued the need to move with the patients into the community – if only because this is the way to retain professional control. Tyrer for example, sees community care as: 'both an opportunity and a threat. The opportunity offers psychiatrists greater responsibility for planning and directing services; but the threat is loss of influence if we delegate this task to others'.[40]

Psychiatrists are clear that their role in mental health teams should be as a leader, or at least as the 'major player' if these initiatives are to succeed.[41] Thus the shift towards community care has been accompanied by a particular concern amongst psychiatrists over a dilution of their central role in determining the shape of mental health services: as Pilgrim warns it is important to recognise that 'conservative psychiatrists [are] fearful of losing their territorial power base'[42] and that this fear affects the intervention of psychiatry in policy debates.

Prior[43] explains psychiatry's willingness to move into the community as in part the result of a shift in psychiatry's focus. The increasing use of a behavioural model of therapy has, he argued, destroyed the old asylums from within as psychiatry lost the rationale for institutional care. Others, however, have argued that psychiatry was seeking to lose a role that it had grown into, that of warehousing the chronically ill inside the asylum, in order to realign the profession more closely with medicine.[44]

In practical terms, solutions to psychiatry's dilemma over their location in the emerging community-based system have ranged from an increasing involvement of the profession in services based in primary health care, to a system of home-based treatment which takes the asylum into the home. The location of psychiatry in mental health services in the primary sector has been unevenly spread, with psychiatrists tending to be based in fundholding practices, larger practices and in areas where one or more GPs has a specialist interest in mental health problems.[45] This increase in the number of psychiatrists working in community settings appears to have been associated with reduced hospital admissions,[46] – however, this is affected by the model used. Where psychiatrists operate what has been termed a 'shifted outpatient model' the patients seen are largely those who were seen before as outpatients in the hospital – thus the location of treatment has changed but not the patient profile. In other situations where psychiatrists operate a system of shared care with the GP retaining overall responsibility, patients include people with conditions which would have been treated in the community in any case.[47]

Many of the studies of referrals by GPs to community mental health services have found that GPs refer patients to specialist mental health services at a lower level of disorder when those services are based in the community, compared with referrals to hospital based services.[48] On the one hand this would appear to reflect success, as patients are diverted from hospital treatment with earlier intervention. However, there have also been criticisms that community care, through a shortage of places, is failing those who need it most, the seriously mentally ill.[49]

A number of psychiatrists have set up 'home-based' treatment services, which provide intensive care in an acute phase of illness for those who would otherwise be admitted. Reports of the success of such schemes, which have been started in various locations during the 1980s and 1990s, have suggested that this approach to the severely mentally ill results in fewer hospital admissions, and more satisfaction for both carers and users, whilst outcomes are similar to in-patient treatment.[50] Not surprisingly, perhaps, the lower costs of such programmes compared with in-patient treatment have also been emphasised.[51] However, a review of home-based services in the US suggests that for many patients, problems of employment, domestic circumstances and coping mechanisms continue to present difficulties.[52] In addition, for some patients, particularly women, the home itself is an insecure or dangerous place – for example, in circumstances of severe poverty or violence – and in these surroundings people require a safe place to recover outside the home.

POLICY DEVELOPMENTS IN COMMUNITY PSYCHIATRIC CARE IN THE 1980S

Community psychiatric services grew during the 1970s and early 1980s in Britain, developing in a fragmented way which varied from area to area, following the policy recommendations of the 1975 White Paper, 'Better Services for the Mentally Ill'. The 1983 Mental Health Act increased the support for care outside the institution for people with mental health problems. As we have seen, there was slow progress towards the targets contained in the 1975 White Paper.

One significant factor in the debate over community care policy was the 1986 report on community care by the Audit Commission, which was highly critical both of what had been achieved in terms of community mental health provision and also the inherent weaknesses and problems in the services, which were seen as fragmented, poorly co-ordinated and with unclear lines of control and responsibility.[53]

Major changes in the organisation of community care were heralded by the White Paper on the future of community care, *Caring for People*,[54] which followed the 1988 Griffiths report.[55] The 1989 White Paper introduced the idea of 'case management' for all vulnerable groups, including those who were receiving psychiatric care. 'Care management', as it become known, followed the use of 'Case management' in the US as a way providing services for patients suffering from severe psychiatric illness through the appointment of a manager who determines the needs of the individual and constructs a package of services to meet those needs.[56] The system was not evaluated prior to being introduced in Britain nor was it piloted here. Studies of the efficacy of case management in the US have suggested that there is no significant difference between patients receiving case management and those in the ordinary system in terms of the patient's quality of life, need for medication and relapse rates.[57]

'Care management', in common with other British policy provisions,[58] did not create a right to receive services. Although care managers are required to consider what is needed without reference to what is available, government guidelines have encouraged local authorities not to inform individuals of the outcome of their care assessment so as to avoid legal action they might take.[59]

The introduction of care management has also slowed down the process of discharge for many in-patients, due to the unavailability either of a care manager to arrange for a care package or the unavailability of services in the community for the patient after discharge[60] – although studies prior to the introduction of care management also show slower discharge due to the lack of after-care services.[61] Thus whilst in 1994 the Audit Commission gave cautious support to the new community care, arguing that there were signs of initiative and imagination in the use of devolved budgets, it remained critical of delays in discharging patients due to problems in arranging the necessary assessment by a care manager prior to discharge.[62] Furthermore, the introduction of care management without additional resources may have led to an increase in psychiatric admissions, as a result of closer monitoring of patients in a system in which alternatives to in-patient treatment are scarce.[63]

In the same period, another policy change in the 1990 NHS and Community Care Act introduced an internal market to both health care and the social services, with the creation of purchasers or commissioners, as they later became known, who were given responsibility for purchasing appropriate services, and providers who were given responsibility for the actual provision of services. In health services this produced two sets of purchasers: the Health Authorities, purchasing for their area and their population, and the newly created fund-holding GPs, purchasing services needed by patients on their practice list. Hospital Trusts acted as the main providers, offering services on a contract basis, although other providers – in the private and voluntary sector – could also sell service provision. The internal market was also introduced in the local authority social services where the local authority would act as the broker responsible for finding services from a range of providers.

This new system, with both sets of changes being introduced in the same few years and with little or no piloting beforehand, gave rise to particular difficulties for the mental health system. For one thing, the changes left responsibility for medical treatment with health authorities and responsibility for social care with the social services. In the past, this split between a nationally funded health care system and a locally funded social care system had been seen by many as a major source of the difficulties experienced both by those receiving care and those trying to deliver care. Now, after the 1990 Act, both of the key agencies involved in the care of those diagnosed as suffering from severe mental illness were involved in an internal market. Fragmentation was an inevitable product of the market system introduced as a result of the 1990 Act – with implications for mental health patients and their access to services. What resulted was a patchwork of service providers in both health and social services,[64] which created further problems in ensuring that patients' needs were being met. Furthermore, as Paton[65] argues, the internal market introduced 'perverse incentives' for both purchasers and providers in the mental health system, particularly when purchasers commission services but, if the services fail, the public complain to the hospital which is seen to be at fault.

Funding for community care services has also been the focus of debate as emphasis on these services has grown. Community psychiatric care is very much the poor relation in terms of expenditure by the NHS on mental health services. Whilst the proportion of NHS expenditure going to the mental health services has fallen slightly in recent years, to just over ten percent of the total, the division between services has remained fairly constant. Over three quarters of NHS funding for mental illness goes on the provision of in-patient and hospital treatment (some estimates put the proportion even higher, at ninety percent), less than a quarter goes towards funding the services provided in the community.[66] Thus the proportion of total NHS expenditure going to support community mental services is failing to match the increasing demand for such services. It is perhaps unsurprising that the perception of community psychiatric services as being in crisis has simultaneously grown. In the words of Lord Acton, in the House of Lords debate on the Mental Health Amendment Bill in 1998, there is a vicious circle:

> most resources are tied up in providing hospital beds; thus there is no spare capacity to develop community services; thus people are unsupported in the community and so are admitted to hospital; thus hospital beds are full, so most resources are tied up in providing hospital beds, and round and round and round the circle goes.[67]

GENDER AND COMMUNITY CARE

Community care services were not only suffering from problems in funding and the new organisation of the services, as a result of policy changes. There were also increasingly clear gender differences in who the services were reaching, and these differences were also significant in the growing crisis by the end of the 1980s and the beginning of the 1990s.

Women are over-represented in figures for treatment for mental health problems at all levels of the service, whilst community surveys also report more women than men suffering from symptoms of psychiatric illness.[68] The last few decades of this century have seen an increasing awareness, prompted particularly by feminist analysis in this field, of the gendered dimensions of mental health and treatment for psychiatric services. Much of the literature has focused on explaining women's apparently greater vulnerability to mental illness – asking whether women are more prone to mental distress than men as a result of their biological difference, their help-seeking behaviour, or economic and social factors such as the stress associated with poverty, domestic work, and childcare. Feminist writers in particular have argued that a medical stereotype in which women are seen as inherently closer to mental illness has resulted in a mis-treatment of women as psychiatric patients when their problems are structurally caused.[69]

The extent of women's over-representation in figures for psychiatric treatment varies in different service sectors, and has varied across time, and this may relate to this medical stereotype. Men are more frequently referred to specialist psychiatric care than are women at the same level of illness.[70] Thus it seems likely that judgments regarding the need for treatment and the nature of that treatment are being made not only on the basis of diagnosis and severity of illness, but other factors. A recent study of GPs' referral patterns suggested an important gender difference in the use made of psychiatrists once in the community. Whilst GPs refer more men, and more young men, to hospital based psychiatric services, GPs are more likely to refer women to specialist care when the psychiatric service is based in the community.[71] There may be a range of reasons for this, including the GP's perception of domestic and childcare responsibilities as an impediment to hospital attendance. However, studies also suggest that GPs refer less severely ill patients to the community based psychiatrist than to the hospital practitioner.[72] This in turn may impact on admission rates and may help to explain the changing patterns in psychiatric admissions in recent years. Thus an unanticipated outcome of the shift of psychiatrists into the community may be an increase in the hospitalisation of men, and young men in particular, as they are seen more often by hospital based psychiatrists and pass more easily through the final filter to in-patient treatment.

Whilst GPs refer women more often to psychiatrists in the community, a study by Sheppard[73] found that GPs were also considerably more likely to refer women than men for assessment for formal or involuntary admission to in-patient treatment under the 1983 Mental Health Act. The same study also found that more of the women referred by GPs had social problems which underlay their mental health difficulties: 'GPs seemed to be seeking a medical solution to these women's problems'.[74]

As noted above, one critique of community mental health services in the medical literature focused on a shift of specialist psychiatric care from those suffering from severe and enduring illness – such as schizophrenia – to a patient group described as 'the worried well'.[75] However, an underlying and unexplored aspect of this criticism that services for depressed patients are increasing inappropriately is that most of these worried well are women, whereas in the past men were the more likely 'beneficiaries' of specialist services.

An additional factor in the shifting pattern of psychiatric treatment for each sex is the extent to which the voluntary sector has developed to provide alternatives to treatment for mental health service users. Whilst pressure groups have been critical of the mainstream mental health services, highlighting the patient's loss of self-determination and autonomy within the system and the dangers of many treatments, women's health groups have also drawn attention to the specific threats for women. In particular, research carried out by MIND showed that mixed-sex wards in psychiatric hospitals left women vulnerable to assault and fearful whilst remaining as in-patients.[76] Although the mixed-sex open plan wards are to be phased out, shared day-time accommodation remains problematic for many women. A number of self-help and voluntary groups for women have been created in the last couple of decades, often by women who are 'survivors' of the state funded health care system and by women health workers.[77] Thus one reason for the different trends in psychiatric admission patterns for women and men may be that there are more services available to support women in crisis in the community, and that alongside the formal health care system there is an increasing number of services which are designed specifically to meet the needs of this particular group of people, and which women can turn to in times of need. Many of these operate on a self-referral basis, and this may also act to reduce women's rates of admission where women are able to receive support earlier on in an illness and avoid becoming more seriously ill. Whilst many services in the voluntary sector are also over-stretched and may only take a limited number of new patients, other services – such as drop-in sessions, coffee mornings and discussion groups – may still be able to provide much needed support sooner rather than later for women in need of help.

THE FINAL STRAW: THE CRISIS IN COMMUNITY PSYCHIATRIC CARE

We turn now to look at the final phase in the run up to the White Paper on mental health services to be published by the Labour Government. By the late 1980s and early 1990s there was an increasing debate within the medical literature over the provision of community care, and who was being served by new developments. There was increasing debate over alternatives to in-patient treatment and the treatment of the severely mentally ill. However, there was also increasing public as well as professional concern over the failure of funding to match needs, and the perceived shortfall both in in-patient provision and in places in community services.

Thus the last decades of the century see a growing and highly public debate – in the national media and with widely publicised contributions from the medical profession and mental health workers – in which the notion of the risk posed by the mentally ill is re-stated many times. At no point in the debate does the question of gender become explicit – but in the reporting of high profile incidents of violence the dangerous patient is identified as male. And during this debate the issue of power – to detain a patient, to retain a patient in hospital, to enforce medication – is also central.

The increasing sense of crisis in the psychiatric services in the 1990s was linked to a number of different factors. There was seen to be a crisis in hospital provision, resulting from the decreasing number of psychiatric beds. A survey of in-patient psychiatric facilities in London, for example, in 1990, revealed that more than a third of the districts in Greater London were operating with a bed-occupancy rate over 100 per cent – one had a bed-occupancy rate of 117 per cent, considerably higher than the 85 percent recommended rate for 'optimal efficiency'.[78] Official reports such as the Biennial Report of the Mental Health Act Commission and the House of Commons Health Committee were identifying this crisis in provision.[79]

In the in-patient sector psychiatrists were warning of two problems stemming from the bed shortage. Firstly there was the concern that an increasing proportion of in-patients in the wards were acutely disturbed and as such presented a risk to themselves and to others. Thus an item in the news pages of the *British Medical Journal* in 1994 stated, 'Psychiatric services are dangerous, warn doctors',[80] quoting psychiatrists in both London and Bristol as claiming that patients' safety was being jeopardised by the lack of secure beds for these severely disturbed people.

The second problem identified during the early 1990s by the psychiatric profession was that the bed shortage prevented the early admission of some patients who needed in-patient treatment whilst forcing the premature discharge of others who needed to remain. The 1994 House of Commons Health Committee report also highlighted this concern, citing one psychiatrist's evidence: 'those who can be best managed in the community, although it may not be ideal at that point, are discharged . . . I think that if you had the space clinical wisdom would say that one would wait another week, another ten days'.[81]

Not only were there problems with finding in-patient beds, many of the beds found were inappropriate – in acute wards in the general hospital, for example, rather than longer stay provision. One estimate suggested that there were up to 3000 new long-stay patients, over a third of whom were being treated in acute wards rather than more suitable conditions.[82] Alternatives to in-patient admission during times of crisis were also too rarely available to those suffering severe mental health problems, despite recommendations by the Mental Health Act Commission[83] that such services needed to expand rapidly.

A study of these new 'short stay' patients caught up in the revolving door of admission and readmission found that despite the fact that the majority were living in independent accommodation, the majority were living alone, without paid work and in a poor condition.[84] Most were in contact with mental health professionals but the study found they received little day to day support.

The concern voiced over the shortage of appropriate in-patient accommodation came from both the profession itself[85] and also from pressure groups such as the National Schizophrenia Fellowship[86] and Schizophrenia, A National Emergency (SANE). SANE was founded by Sunday Times journalist Marjorie Wallace and was particularly well placed in the late 1980s and early 1990s to use national media to get across the message that community care was failing to meet the needs of this group of the population.

Whilst the psychiatric profession might be seen to have a vested interest in retaining a central role for in-patient treatment, where their own control is clear and unchallenged, the involvement of other groups who claimed to be representing patients and their carers was significant in the public debates over the need to retain or increase the provision of institutional care.

Meanwhile, the community care system was also in crisis. The Fifth Biennial Report of the Mental Health Act Commission[87] highlighted a number of areas in which there were 'worrying gaps' in the provision of community care services for the mentally ill. Some CMHTs, particularly those in the inner cities of Britain, were particularly stretched[88] and were increasingly forced to operate a form of triage which ensured that community support and treatment went to those who were seen as in most need rather than all of those in need.[89]

At the same time as demand on the CMHT was becoming impossible, studies suggested that the work of the community psychiatric nurse had changed, as a result of their move from an institutional base to a base in the primary health care setting, and that there had been a decrease in the proportion of 'schizophrenics' who were being treated by a CPN.[90] The combination of these factors produced a growing shortage of care for one group in particular – those with severe and enduring mental health problems.

A study of routes to in-patient admission in Inner City London found that more had been admitted via the police than through their GP, and a high proportion were self-referred on a walk-in basis. Only 15 per cent were in touch with community mental health services.[91] Community mental health services increasingly were seen, particularly in high stress areas, as serving a completely different population to those they theoretically had been set up to serve.

Whilst concern and publicity about problems with the mental health services was growing in the 1980s, a more severe crisis was precipitated in the early 1990s by a series of incidents involving patients who had been recently been discharged from in-patient psychiatric treatment. These incidents received considerable publicity not only around the time they occurred but also over years to come with the ensuing public inquiries and court cases. In December 1992 Jonathon Zito was killed by Christopher Clunis, a 'known schizophrenic', three months after he had been 'released into the community with little medical supervision'.[92] This was quickly followed by an incident in which Ben Silcock, also being treated in the community for psychiatric illness, was badly mauled after climbing into the lions' enclosure in Regent's Park. There were a number of other cases, all highly publicised, in which people diagnosed with severe mental health problems and in particular with psychotic illnesses were found to have committed acts of violence against the public or, in some cases, against care workers.[93]

The policy response to the case of Ben Silcock was prompt, with the Conservative Health Minister, Virginia Bottomley announcing a review of the workings of the 1983 Mental Health Act and the possibility of community treatment orders (CTOs) to enforce treatment for patients outside the hospital. CTOs had been proposed by the Royal College of Psychiatrists in the 1980s as a solution to the problem of patients who failed to take medication whilst in the community.[94] Under the 1983 Act there was no legal power for the medical profession to force patients to medicate. The only solution was formal admission to hospital under the 1983 Act – clearly problematic where there were too few beds. In the following months the RCP moved away from CTOs[95] and the eventual legislation, the 1995 Mental Health (Patients in the Community) Act introduced a system of supervised discharge for in-patients who had been detained under the 1983 Act. The objective of supervised discharge was to increase the planning and co-ordination of services for people under supervision and as such the new arrangements were seen as supporting the existing care management approach.

Before the 1995 Act patients were often discharged from hospital on the condition that they continue to take their medication. The use of this extended leave to create a system of control over patients in the community – by admitting a patient overnight, for example – had been challenged in court.[96] However, such a solution was difficult not only legally, but also where beds were in such short supply. The need was for a policy which avoided admission altogether, whilst retaining the power of supervision. The language of both the legislation and policy guidelines reinforced the idea of dangerous patients and the risk they posed to others as well as to themselves. The new process gave a responsible medical officer the power to institute a review of the patient's treatment, where the patient was seen as constituting a risk either to themselves or to others.

In the same period, an associated policy development created through Department of Health guidelines rather than legislative change introduced 'at risk' or supervision registers, of those who were seen as being at risk of suicide, self-neglect or likely to commit a serious crime.[97] These developments were given additional weight by the inquiry into the care and treatment of Christopher Clunis, which reported in 1994. The report highlighted the shortage of funds for community mental health services, and recommended an increase in the number of community workers, but the report also supported the use of both at-risk registers and supervised discharge.[98]

Both the new registers and supervised discharge were criticised by civil liberty groups, mental health pressure groups and workers in the services who argued that such new powers represented an unacceptable degree of control over those diagnosed as mentally ill.[99] With supervision registers, it was argued that not only would an individual not necessarily know if they were on such a list (although guidelines held that patients should be told, there would be exceptions to this) but also that being registered on such a list was not linked with additional resources to help the individual.[100] Similarly, supervised discharge was criticised for failing to tackle the fundamental problem of inadequate resources in the community, whilst removing individual's rights.[101] In addition, the new powers were criticised for the way in which they reinforced an emerging notion of the dangerous mad, from whom the public needed protecting. Whilst there were high-profile cases such as that of Clunis featuring random acts of violence against the public, the vast majority of acts of violence are committed by those who are not diagnosed as mentally ill. The most significant risk for those suffering from mental illness is the risk of suicide and self-harm, and risks of violence against them by members of the public.[102]

In addition to the new regulations, there was also a range of different funding initiatives to meet the criticisms of underfunding in this sector. In 1995 funding of £10 million – to match £10 million found by the NHS – was announced to create a Mental Health Challenge Fund. The Mental Illness Specific Grant (MISG) which followed this development aims to provide funds for projects devised specifically to meet the needs of the severely mentally ill. The MISG aims to create an improvement in joint planning between health and social services. The amount available increased each year with a 23 per cent increase in 1996–97, an additional £11 million on the previous year.[103] Problems over the geographical distribution of mental health community services – with specific problems in high use areas, and the inner cities in particular – are to be tackled by a 'Target Fund' which will be directed to parts of the country where there is greater need.[104] Further funds, an additional £10 million for community based mental health services in London, were promised by the Health Secretary at the time of the Clunis inquiry report,[105] to meet the criticisms of underfunding in the capital. In addition, the Conservative government announced funding to help meet the needs of homeless people for psychiatric care, thorough the Homeless Mentally Ill Initiative (HMII) which would be targeted particular on problems in London.

Despite this additional funding, criticisms remained. The difficulties in community care have affected in particular those with severe and enduring mental health problems who are finding the services in the community inadequate for their needs. In particular groups such as MIND, the mental health pressure group, have highlighted the fact that there are still few alternatives to in-patient treatment for people in times of mental health crisis. Such services as are available may not be appropriate where they are heavily medicalised, or where there is little understanding of the needs of particular groups – of women users, or people from minority ethnic groups, for example.[106] Services for people in a period of mental health crisis need to be safe, easily accessible, and provide secure support during such a period. Thus additional funding alone is not a solution, where the mental health treatment remains within a system which views risk in terms of the risk patients are seen to present to others rather than the risks patients present to themselves. Within this risk-based approach, psychiatrists are identified as the profession who can judge such risks and who should make decisions about treatment,[107] yet as pressure groups like MIND argue, the risks to the patient of the treatment should also be considered.

CONCLUSION: COMMUNITY CARE INTO THE NEXT CENTURY?

Thus despite the growing use of community care for people with mental health problems, by the end of the twentieth century we have begun to see a tentative backlash in which the need for institutional care for a particular group of these patients – those seen as dangerous as well as mad – is being resurrected. The latest developments in mental health services seem to identify two groups – those who are identified as suitable for community based services and those who need increased surveillance to ensure the safety of the public is not compromised. Within such a framework, the emphasis is on risk – the risk posed to the patient herself or himself, through actions ranging from neglect to suicidal behaviour, and more obviously the risk posed to others through the violent actions of the patient. At the same time, this particular sub-group is becoming more clearly identified as the male, often young, schizophrenic. And the power of the psychiatrist remains unchallenged – as the primary assessor of this risk and as supervisor of the supervision process. Psychiatry's fears about the threat posed by move to community care have largely been removed by the construction of another 'threat' and the location of the psychiatric profession at the centre of the shifts in policy. It seems certain that community psychiatric care will continue to dominate mental health services, if not expenditure on mental health treatment. However, the role of the hospital – and hospital based psychiatry – continues to occupy a central role and for some groups at least, will continue to represent a significant feature of their lives.

Notes

CHAPTER ONE

1. Andrew Scull, *Museums of Madness: The Social Organization of Insanity in Nineteenth-century England* (London, 1977), 13–14.
2. Michel Foucault, *Madness and Civilisation: A History of Madness in the Age of Reason* (New York, 1972).
3. David Rothman, *The Discovery of the Asylum* (Boston, 1971).
4. For a revision and extension of this thesis, see Scull, *The Most Solitary of Afflictions: Madness and Society in Britain, 1700–1900* (London, 1993).
5. Kathleen Jones, *Lunacy, Law and Conscience, 1774–1845* (London, 1959); Jones, *Mental Health and Social Policy 1845–1959* (London, 1959) reprinted as *A History of the Mental Health Services* (London, 1972); *Asylums and After: A Revised History of the Mental Health Services from the 18th Century to the 1990's* (London, 1993).
6. Mark Finnane, *Insanity and the Insane in Post-Famine Ireland* (London, 1981).
7. Jones, *Asylums and After*, 92; Andrew Scull, 'From Madness to Mental Illness: Medical Men as Moral Entrepreneurs', *European Journal of Sociology*, 6 (1975), 219–61; Finanne, *Insanity and the Insane*, chapter 1.
8. Richard Hunter, *Psychiatry for the Poor. 1851 Colney Hatch Asylum. Friern Hospital 1973: A Medical and Social History* (London, 1974); William Llewellyn Parry-Jones, *The Trade in Lunacy: A Study of Private Madhouses in England in the Eighteenth and Nineteenth Centuries* (London,1972); John Crammer, *Asylum History: Buckinghamshire County Pauper Lunatic Asylum-St. John's* (London, 1990).

9. Russell Barton, *Institutional Neurosis* (London, 1959); Erving Goffman, *Asylums: Essays on the Social Situation of Mental Patients and Other Inmates* (New York, 1961).

10. Michel Foucault, *Madness and Civilisation, passim*; Thomas Szasz. *Age of Madness: the History of Involuntary Mental Hospitalization* (New York, 1973).

11. Some notable doctoral theses which focus on specific institutions in Britain and Ireland include: Janet Saunders, 'Institutionalized Offenders – A Study of the Victorian Institution and its Inmates, with special reference to late-nineteenth century Warwickshire', Unpublished PhD thesis, University of Warwick, 1983; Michael A. Barrett, 'From Education to Segregation: an inquiry into the changing character of special provision for the retarded in England, c.1846–1918', Unpublished PhD thesis, University of Lancaster, 1987; Richard Russell, 'Mental Physicians and their Patients: Psychological Medicine in the English Pauper Lunatic Asylums of the Later Nineteenth Century', Unpublished PhD thesis, University of Sheffield, 1984; Jonathan Andrews, 'Bedlam Revisted: A History of Bethlem Hospital, c1634–1770', Unpublished PhD thesis , University of London, 1991; Peter Bartlett, 'The Poor Law of Lunacy: the administration of pauper lunatics in mid-nineteenth century England with special reference to Leicestershire and Rutland', unpublished PhD thesis, University of London, 1993 ; David Wright, 'The National Asylum for Idiots, Earlswood, 1847–86' unpublished D.Phil. thesis, University of Oxford, 1993; Andrew Saris, 'The Proper Place for Lunatics: Asylum, Person, and History in a Rural Irish Community', Unpublished PhD thesis, University of Chicago, 1994.

12. Arthur Foss and Kerith Trick, *St Andrew's Hospital Northampton: The First 150 Years (1838–1988)* (Cambridge, 1988); Jonathan Andrews et al., *The History of Bethlem* (London, 1997).

13. Jones, *Asylums & After, passim*. For a similar reliance on parliamentary papers, see also Phil Fennell, *Treatment with Consent: Law, Psychiatry, and the Treatment of Mentally Disordered People since 1845* (London, 1996).

14. Phil Fennell, *Treatment Without Consent*.

15. For edited volumes on the history of psychiatry in Britain and Ireland see Andrew Scull (ed.) *Mad-Houses, Mad-Doctors and Madmen: the Social History of Psychiatry in the Victorian Era* (London, 1981); Scull, *Social Order/Mental Disorder: Anglo-American Psychiatry in Historical Perspective* (London, 1989); W. F. Bynum, Roy Porter and Michael Shepherd (eds) *The Anatomy of Madness: Essays in the History of Psychiatry* (3 vols.) (London, 1985–7); German Berrios and Hugh Freeman (eds) *150 Years of British Psychiatry, 1841–1991*

(London, 1991); Mark Micale and Roy Porter (eds) *Discovering the History of Psychiatry* (Oxford, 1994). German Berrios and Hugh Freeman (eds) *150 Years of British Psychiatry, 1841–1991- vol. 2 – The Aftermath* (London, 1996); Dylan Tomlinson and John Carrier (eds) *Asylum in the Community* (London, 1996); German Berrios and Roy Porter (eds) *A History of Clinical Psychiatry: The Origin and History of Psychiatric Disorders* (London, 1996); Jo Melling and Bill Forsythe, *Insanity, Institutions and Society: New Approaches to the Social History of Insanity* (London, 1999).

16. Richard Hunter, *Psychiatry for the Poor. 1851 Colney Hatch Asylum. Friern Hospital 1973: A Medical and Social History* (London, 1974); Anne Digby, *Madness, Morality and Medicine: A Study of the York Retreat, 1796–1914* (Cambridge, 1985); Elizabeth Malcolm, *Swift's Hospital: A Story of St. Patrick's Hospital, Dublin, 1746–1989* (Dublin, 1989); Charlotte MacKenzie, *Psychiatry for the Rich: A History of the Private Ticehurst Asylum, 1792–1917* (London, 1992).

17. John Walton, 'Lunacy in the Industrial Revolution: A Study of Asylum Admissions in Lancashire, 1848–1850', *Journal of Social History*, 13 (1979), 1–22; Allan Beveridge, 'Madness in Victorian Edinburgh: A Study of Patients Admitted to the Royal Edinburgh Asylum under Thomas Clouston, 1873–1908 (part I)', *History of Psychiatry*, 6 (1995), 22–54; Laurence Ray, 'Models of Madness in Victorian Asylum Practice, *European Journal of Sociology*, 22 (1981), 229–64.

18. For a survey of the literature, see David Wright, 'Getting Out of the Asylum: Understanding the Confinement of the Insane in the Nineteenth Century', *Social History of Medicine*, 10 (1997), 137–55. See also Jonathan Andrews on Gartnavel Royal Asylum, Glasgow, and David Wright on the Buckinghamshire County Asylum and Pam Michael on the Denbigh Asylum in Jo Melling and Bill Forsythe (eds) *Insanity, Institutions and Society*, forthcoming.

19. Michael MacDonald, *Mystical Bedlam*; Roy Porter, *Mind Forg'd Manacles: A History of Madness in England from the Restoration to the Regency* (London, 1987).

20. Akihito Suzuki, 'Lunacy in Seventeenth- and Eighteenth-century England: Analysis of Quarter Sessions Records: Part I, *History of Psychiatry*, 2 (1991), 437–56; 'Part II', *History of Psychiatry*, 3 (1993), 29–44; Peter Rushton, 'Lunatics and Idiots: Mental Disability, the Community, and the Poor Law in North East England, 1600–1800', *Medical History*, 32 (1988), 34–50; Rushton, 'Idiocy, the Family and the Community in Early Modern North-east England', in David Wright and Digby (eds) *From Idiocy to Mental Deficiency*, Jonathan Andrews, 'Identifying and Providing for the Mentally Disabled in

Early Modern London', in Wright and Digby (eds) *From Idiocy to Mental Deficiency*, 65–92; Suzuki, 'The Household and the Care of Lunatics in Eighteenth-Century London,' in Peregrine Horden and Richard Smith (eds) *The Locus of Care: Families, Communities, Institutions and the Provision of Welfare Since Antiquity* (London, 1998), 153–75.

21. Akihito Suzuki, 'The Household and the Care of Lunatics in Eighteenth-Century London'; David Wright, 'Familial Care of "Idiot" Children in Victorian England'; Mathew Thomson, 'Community Care and the Control of Mental Defectives in Inter-War Britain', in Peregrine Horden and Richard Smith (eds) *The Locus of Care*, 153–75, 176–97, 198–218.

22. Mary-Ellen Kelm, 'Women, Families and the Provincial Hospital for the Insane, British Columbia, 1905–1915', *Journal of Family History*, 19 (1994), 177–93; Richard Adair, Joseph Melling and Bill Forsythe, 'Migration, Family Structure and Pauper Lunacy in Victorian England: Admission to the Devon County Pauper Lunatic Asylum, 1845–1900, *Continuity and Change*, 12 (1997), 373–401; David Wright, 'Families Strategies and the Institutional Committal of "Idiot" Children in Victorian England', *Journal of Family History*, 23, (1998), 190–208.

23. Jones, *Asylums and After*, 60, Table 4.1; 116, Table 7.2.

24. Finnane, *Insanity and the Insane in Post-Famine Ireland*, 19, chapter 1.

25. Jonathan Andrews and Iain Smith, *'Let There be Light Again': A History of Gartnavel Royal Hospital from its beginnings to the Present Day* (Glasgow, 1993), 3.

26. Jonathan Andrews and Iain Smith, 'The Evolution of Psychiatry in Glasgow During the Nineteenth and Early Twentieth Centuries', in Hugh Freeman and German Berrios (eds) *150 Years of British Psychiatry – Vol 2* (London, 1996), 313–14.

27. Finnane, *Insanity and the Insane in Post-Famine Ireland*, Table ; Jones, *Asylums and After*, Table 7.1, 116;

28. Twenty-eighth Report of the Commissioners in Lunacy, PP (1874) xxvii, 34.

29. Edward Higgs, *Making Sense of the Census: The Manuscript Returns for England and Wales, 1801–1901* (London, 1989), 74–6.

30. Poor Law Amendment Act, 4 & 5 William IV, c.76, s.45.

31. Pauline Prior, *Mental Health and Politics in Northern Ireland* (Aldershot, 1993), chapter one.

32. See, for comparison, Stephen Garton, *Medicine and Madness: A Social History of Insanity in New South Wales, 1880–1940* (Kensington, Aus., 1988); Wendy Mitchinson, 'The Toronto and Gladesville

Asylums: Humane Alternatives for the Insane in Canada and Australia?', *Bulletin of the History of Medicine*, 43 [1989], 52–72.

33. Finnane, *Insanity and the Insane in Post-Famine Ireland*, 72.

34. Twenty-eighth Report of the Commissioners in Lunacy, PP (1874) xxvii, 34.

35. Private Lunatic Asylums (Ireland) Act 1842, 5 & 6 Vict. c.27.

36. Hervey, Nicholas, 'A Slavish Bowing Down: the Lunacy Commission and the Psychiatric Profession, 1845–1860' in W.F. Bynum *et al.*. (eds) *The Anatomy of Madness, vol 2*, 98–131; Jonathan Andrews, 'They're in the Trade ... They "cannot interfere" – they say': The Scottish Lunacy Commissions and Lunacy Reform in Nineteenth Century Scotland', (London, Wellcome Institute Occasional Publications, 1998).

37. David Wright, 'Familial Care of 'Idiot' children',182.

38. Ellen Ross, 'Survival Networks: Women's Neighbourhood Sharing in London before World War I', *History Workshop*, 15 (1983), 4–27.

39. Mark Finnane, 'Asylums, Families and the State', *History Workshop Journal*, 20 (1985), 134–48.

40. Wright, 'Getting Out of the Asylum'.

41. (1855) 6 Cox C.C. 549; 25 L.T. 118, 24 L.J.R. (N.S.) M.C. 129. This case was distinguished in *R v. Porter* (1864) 33 L.J.R. (N.S.) M.C. 126; 10 L.T., N.S., 306; 10 Jur. N.S. 547; 12 W.R. 718; 4 N.R. 71; L & C 394; 9 Cox C.C. 449 and in *R. v. Smith and Smith* (1880) 14 Cox C.C. 398, on the basis that the latter cases involved the care of siblings. While held to be outside the statutory offence, *Rundle* was convicted for common assault of his wife.

42. For public county asylums, this provision dates to 1828: v. 9 Geo. IV, c. 40, ss. 39–40. In the private madhouse sector, this authority seems originally to have been based on the implied authority of the individual paying (or ceasing to pay) the bill for the lunatic's accommodation. In 1845, similar statutory provisions were enacted to those in the public asylum sphere: v. 8/9 Vict. c. 100, ss. 72, 75.

43. Lunacy Act 1890, 53 Vict., c. 5, s. 207(6).

44. See Bartlett, *The Poor Law of Lunacy* (London, 1999).

45. It remains a debatable point the degree to which such admissions are actually voluntary in a real sense, and how much the result of non-legal social control mechanisms, either within the psychiatric facility or in the community.

46. David Healy, 'Irish Psychiatry in the Twentieth Century', in Hugh Freeman and German Berrios (eds) *150 Years of British Psychiatry – Vol 2*, 274.

47. 8/9 Vict. c. 126, s. 71.

48. P. Bartlett, *The Poor Law of Lunacy*, (London, forthcoming 1999), ch. 4.

49. 25/26 Vict., c. 111, s. 8 allowed the transfer of the individuals. Their continuation as asylum inmates reflected a legal opinion of the Law Officers of the Crown, (PRO MH 51/760) and was given formal legislative authority in 1867: 31/32 Vict. c. 106, s. 23.

50. See *R v Hallstrom, ex p. W (No.2)* [1986] 2 ALL ER 306. This case only precluded requiring the return of the individual to hospital so that the confinement could be renewed; it did not preclude allowing the patient out on leave for the remainder of an existing section. The technique thus remains available until the expiry of the patient's existing period of confinement.

51. See section 34(2) of the Mental Health Act 1983.

52. David Wright, 'The Discharge of Pauper Lunatics in Mid-Victorian England', in Jo Melling and Bill Forsythe (eds) *Insanity, Society and Institutions* (London, 1999), in press.

53. Mental Health Act 1983, s. 117.

54. Stan Cohen, *Visions of Social Control* (Oxford, 1985).

55. Andrew Scull, Charlotte MacKenzie and Nicholas Hervey, *Masters of Bedlam: The Transformation of the Mad-Doctoring Trade* (Princeton N. J., 1996).

56. Janet Oppenheim, *Shattered Nerves: Doctors, Patients and Depression in Victorian England* (New York, 1991).

57. Virginia Berridge, 'Stamping out Addiction: the work of the Rolleston Committee, 1924–1926' and Brenda Parry-Jones and William Parry-Jones, 'British Contributions on the Eating Disorders: a Historical Perspective', in Hugh Freeman and German Berrios (eds) *150 Years of British Psychiatry, 1841–1991- vol. 2*, 18, 58.

58. See, for example, *W v. L* [1974] QB 711 (CA), where a wife's decision not to allow the confinement of her husband was overridden by the courts as unreasonable.

59. Kathleen Jones, *Asylums and After: A Revised History of the Mental Health Services* (London, 1993).

60. Peter Barham, *Closing Down the Asylum*.

61. Andrew Scull, *Decarceration: Community Treatment and the Deviant – A Radical View*, 2nd ed., (Oxford, 1984); See Anne Rogers and David Pilgrim, *Mental Health Policy in Britain: A Critical Introduction*, London, Macmillan, 1996, chapters 3–6; Simon Goodwin, *Comparative Mental Health Policy: From Institutional to Community Care* (London, 1997), 6–8.

62. Mark Micale, 'Hysteria and its Historiography – The Future Perspective', *History of Psychiatry*, 1 (1990), 37.

63. Mathew Thomson, '"Though ever the subject of psychological medicine": Psychiatrists and the Colony Solution for Mental Defectives',

in Hugh Freeman and German Berrios (eds) *150 Years of British Psychiatry – Vol 2* (London, 1996),130–43.

64. Mitchenson, 57.

CHAPTER TWO

1. This chapter is based on research carried out during a Leverhulme fellowship in 1996–97. A monograph study of perceptions of mental incapacity (rather than their care) will appear in due course. R. A. Houston, *Madness and its Social Milieu in Eighteenth-century Scotland*, forthcoming. I am grateful to the editors and to Jonathan Andrews for their comments on earlier drafts. The quotation in the title is from Signet Library (SL), Session Papers, vol. 58, case 30, 'Petition of Gilbert Lawrie . . .', 7–8.

2. These categories are proposed by M. Daunton, 'Introduction', in M. Daunton ed., *Charity, Self-interest and Welfare in the English Past* (London, 1996), 9–10.

3. J. Andrews and I. Smith (eds) *'Let there be light again'. A History of Gartnavel Royal Hospital from its Beginnings to the Present Day* (Glasgow, 1993); L. Rosner, *Medical Education in the Age of Improvement: Edinburgh Students and Apprentices, 1760–1826* (Edinburgh, 1991); G. B. Risse, *Hospital Life in Enlightenment Scotland* (Cambridge, 1986). England is better served. K. Jones, *Lunacy, Law, and Conscience, 1744–1845: The Social History of the Care of the Insane* (London, 1955); W. L. Parry-Jones, *The Trade in Lunacy: A Study of Private Madhouses in England and Wales in the Eighteenth and Nineteenth Centuries* (London, 1971); A. Fessler, 'The Management of Lunacy in Seventeenth Century England: An Investigation of Quarter-session Records', *Proceedings of the Royal Society of Medicine*, 49 (1956), 901–7; P. Rushton, 'Lunatics and Idiots: Mental Disability, the Community, and the Poor Law in North-east England, 1600–1800', *Medical History*, 32 (1988), 34–50; P. Rushton, 'Idiocy, the Family and the Community in Early Modern North-east England', in D. Wright and A. Digby (eds) *From Idiocy to Mental Deficiency: Historical Perspectives on People with Learning Disabilities* (London, 1996), 44–6;. A. Suzuki, 'Lunacy in Seventeenth- and Eighteenth-century England: Analysis of Quarter Sessions Records, Part I', *History of Psychiatry*, 2 (1991), 437–56; A. Suzuki, 'Lunacy in Seventeenth- and Eighteenth-century England: Analysis of Quarter Sessions Records, Part II', *History of Psychiatry*, 3 (1992), 29–44. This paper was substantially written before the publication of A. Suzuki, 'The Household and the Care of Lunatics in Eighteenth-century London', in P. Horden and R. Smith (eds) *The Locus of Care*.

Families, Communities, Institutions, and the Provision of Welfare since Antiquity (London, 1998), 153–75.

4. *An Introduction to Scottish Legal History* Stair Society 20 (Edinburgh, 1958), 170–3; P. Gouldesbrough, *Formulary of old Scots legal documents* Stair Society 36 (Edinburgh, 1985), 74; W. Bell, *Dictionary and Digest of the Law of Scotland* (Edinburgh, 1838), 112–13; D. M. Walker (ed.) *The Institutions of the Law of Scotland . . . by James, Viscount of Stair . . . 1693* (Edinburgh, 1981), 702–11. From the middle ages English law too distinguished those unfit to inherit on the basis of mental incapacity (idiocy) and lunacy. Rushton, 'Lunatics and Idiots', 36.

5. Jones, *Lunacy*, ix.

6. Jones, *Lunacy*, 2, 10.

7. Andrew Halliday argued that there was no true 'public' asylum in Scotland, even in the 1820s. A. Halliday, *A General View of the Present State of Lunatics, and Lunatic Asylums, in Great Britain and Ireland, and in some other kingdoms* (London, 1828), 30.

8. Paisley Main Library (PML), Town Hospital Minute Book, 1786–1801, 16 July 1793.

9. See also PML Town Hospital Minute Book, 1786–1801, 7 and 21 June 1791 (Loudon); 1801–19, 4 May 1807 (Wilson) and 7 January 1817 (Smith).

10. R. A. Houston, 'Fraud in the Scottish linen industry: Edinburgh's charity workhouse, 1745–58', *Archives* 21, 91 (1994), 43–56.

11. Lothian Health Board HB7/1/1, 23 April 1813, 20 May 1813.

12. Halliday, *A General View of the Present State of Lunatics*, 27.

13. Edinburgh's eighteenth-century madhouse was known as Bedlam. A new Bedlam was built next to the Charity Workhouse of Edinburgh (next to Greyfriars churchyard) in the early 1740s. Initially it had about a dozen inmates. There were 19 lunatics at the time of the annual report in summer 1749, 17 for 1750, 13 in 1751, and 18 in 1752. There were said to be about 40 inmates in early 1763. A. Birnie, 'The Edinburgh Charity Workhouse, 1740–1845', *Book of the Old Edinburgh Club*, 22 (1938), 38–55. Edinburgh City Archives (ECA), Edinburgh Charity Workhouse vol. 2, 25, 38, 47, 54–5. Scottish Record Office (SRO), SC39/36/6, John Rutherford (1763). Edinburgh also had a house of correction called Paul's Work which had housed furious people since the late seventeenth century. M. Wood, 'St Paul's Work', *Book of the Old Edinburgh Club*, 17 (1930), 49–75. This was one of only two such institutions know at this date and it is likely that this type of reformatory played a very limited role in Scottish care of the insane. R. Mitchison, 'North and South: the Development of the

Gulf in Poor Law Practice', in R. A. Houston and I. D. Whyte (eds) *Scottish Society, 1500–1800* (Cambridge, 1989), 208.

14. Halliday, *A General View of the Present State of Lunatics*, 28.

15. D. H. Tuke, *History of the Insane in the British Isles* (1882), 330 quoted in C. C. Easterbrook, *The Chronicle of Crichton Royal (1833–1936)* (Dumfries, 1940), 14. See also *Summary, showing, according to the returns from the parochial clergy in Scotland the number of lunatics in each presbytery* (House of Commons, 9 July 1817). SRO SC9/21/1.

16. P.P., 1816, VI, 399–400.

17. Sums given are per year and from parish funds unless otherwise stated. See J. Andrews, 'Identifying and Providing for the Mentally Disabled in Early Modern London', in D. Wright and A. Digby (eds) *From Idiocy to Mental Deficiency: Historical Perspectives on People with Learning Disabilities* (London, 1996), 82–4 for a seventeenth-century London comparison.

18. SL Session Papers, vol. 120, case 17, 'Petition of Gilbert Lawrie . . .', 3.

19. SL Session Papers, vol. 120, case 17, 'Petition of Gilbert Lawrie . . .', 4.

20. SL Session Papers, vol. 120, case 17, 'Petition of Gilbert Lawrie . . .', 7.

21. SL Session Papers, vol. 58, case 30, 'Petition of Gilbert Lawrie . . .', 7–8.

22. ECA St Cuthbert's Charity Workhouse Minutes, vol. 3, 2 July 1782.

23. A. T. Scull, *The Most Solitary of Afflictions. Madness and Society in Britain, 1700–1900* (London, 1993), 370.

24. C. Ryskamp and F. A. Pottle (eds) *Boswell: The Ominous Years, 1774–76* (London, 1963), 43.

25. Greater Glasgow Health Board, HB13/7/183.

26. SL Session Papers, vol. 260, case 1, 'Proof and exhibits', 41. Paterson was eventually cognosced and sent to Saughtonhall.

27. SL Session Papers, vol. 284, case 17, 'Petition of Miss Elizabeth Blair . . .', 6–7.

28. SRO SC36/74/10, Archibald Coats (1807).

29. Andrews, 'Identifying and providing for the mentally disabled', 73–4. See also J. M. McPherson, *The Kirk's Care of the Poor. With Special Reference to the North-east of Scotland* (Aberdeen, 1945), 140–1, 174–5, where examples are given of clothing purchase, payments for making chains, and (in 1805) the provision of a strait-waistcoat by parish kirk sessions.

30. A. M'Neel-Caird, *The Poor-Law Manual for Scotland* (Edinburgh, 1851), 17 (quotation), 20. A case of 1800 is set out at greater length

on p. 66 of the manual. See also A. M. Dunlop, *The Law of Scotland Regarding the Poor* (Edinburgh, 1854), 45–6. Dunlop quotes a Court of Session judgement of 1806 that an idiot could not normally acquire a settlement by residence because he was unable to work and was thus in receipt of relief. However, a later judgement found that the insane who had lucid intervals and so could work might obtain a settlement.

31. Mitchison, 'North and south', 219. Dunlop, *Law of Scotland Regarding the Poor*, 32–4 offers a concise statement of the historic principles.
32. ECA Kirk Treasurer's Accounts, vol. 3, 1663–93. In Scotland's towns, parish relief was normally supplemented by funds from a communal purse or 'common good' administered centrally. R. A. Houston, 'The economy of Edinburgh, 1694–1763: the evidence of the common good', in R. A. Houston *et al.* (eds) *Conflict and Identity in the History of Scotland and Ireland from the Seventeenth to the Twentieth Century* (Preston, 1993), 45–62.
33. R. A. Houston, *Social Change in the Age of Enlightenment. Edinburgh, 1660–1760* (Oxford, 1994), 234–89. Houston, 'Fraud in the Scottish linen industry', 43–56.
34. ECA, Kirk Treasurer's Accounts, vol. 4, 1694–1715.
35. H. Armet (ed.) *Extracts from the Records of the Burgh of Edinburgh, 1689–1701* (Edinburgh, 1962), 140.
36. ECA Obligations to Desist from Begging, 1743–58, 10.
37. Dumfries and Galloway Archives (DGA), GG2/1, 2 March 1775. GG2/2, 12 June 1782. Andrews, 'Identifying and Providing for the Mentally Disabled', 72–4 shows that London poor relief records are similarly sparse in mentions.
38. DGA GG2/1, 60. Her destination is unclear.
39. Even at reduced rates, Bedlam was twice the price of care in a workhouse. ECA St Cuthbert's Charity Workhouse Minutes, vol. 3, 2 July 1782.
40. I owe this information to Marion Stewart.
41. R. A. Cage, *The Scottish Poor Law, 1745–1845* (Edinburgh, 1981). See also Andrews, 'Identifying and Providing for the Mentally Disabled', 73–4.
42. R. Mitchison, 'The Making of the Old Scottish Poor Law', *Past & Present*, 63 (1974), 89–90. Mitchison, 'North and South', 214–20 charts the developing regional variations in the relief of the merely indigent during the eighteenth century.
43. SRO SC36/74/12, James Fullarton (1812).
44. SRO SC39/36/4, Charles Simpson (1753). CC8/7/119/2.
45. *The Edinburgh Weekly Journal*, vol. 2, no. 59, p. 3.
46. J. Kay, *A Series of Original Portraits and Caricature Etchings, by the*

late John Kay, miniature painter, Edinburgh; with biographical sketches and illustrative anecdotes 2 vols. (Edinburgh, 1838), vol. 1, 7–8, 184; vol. 2, 17–18.

47. SL Session Papers, vol. 507, case 40, 'Petition of Rev. John Thomson and others, members of the Kirk Session of Newbattle, 10 September 1818', 2–3. *Decisions of the First and Second Divisions of the Court of Session from [1808–1825]* 7 vols. (Edinburgh, second edition, 1815–28), 1815–19, no. 183, 558–561. Daft Jamie is used as a generic term in this case. It was later used of an imbecile murdered by the celebrated grave-robbers Burke and Hare.

48. P. G. B. McNeill (ed.), *The Practicks of Sir James Balfour of Pittendreich, reproduced from the printed edition of 1754* 2 vols. (Edinburgh, 1962–3), vol. 2, 514. See also *The Laws and Customs of Scotland in Matters Criminal*, in *The Works of that Eminent and Learned Lawyer, Sir George MacKenzie of Rosehaugh, advocate . . .* 2 vols. (Edinburgh, 1716, 1722), vol. 2, 59.

49. This had earlier happened to Jean Blair. SRO JC3/41, 13 March 1781.

50. SRO SC1/18/1, 16.

51. P.P., 1816, VI, 374. The early nineteenth century saw a lively debate about who should be responsible for pauper criminal lunatics: crown, parish of settlement, or parish where apprehended. M'Neel-Caird, *Poor-law Manual for Scotland*, 68–70. SL Session Papers, vol. 501, case 43, 'Petition of . . . the Commissioners of Supply of Wigton, 30 June 1817'. SL Session Papers, vol. 507, case 40, 'Petition of Rev. John Thomson and others, members of the Kirk Session of Newbattle, 10 September 1818'. Following a case of 1818, it was established that the pauper lunatic's parish of settlement was ultimately responsible for his care but until that was established the parish where he was apprehended should bear the burden of support. Dunlop, Law of Scotland regarding the poor, 31, 53–4. The case is discussed in *Decisions of the . . . Court of Session*, 1815–19, no. 183, 558–561. See also the case of James Fisher in ibid., 1822–25, no. 43, 174–8 (Commissioners of Supply of Wigtonshire v heritors and Kirk Session of St Quivox, 21 February 1823).

52. The development should not be seen as a simple indicator of 'progress'. The Scottish poor law was being re-interpreted around this time to exclude parish responsibility for the able-bodied poor, making some form of central provision for the criminal insane increasingly necessary. Mitchison, 'Old Scottish Poor Law', 88–92.

53. Parry-Jones, *Trade in Lunacy*, 36, 283. There is another, unverifiable, explanation: perhaps regions which for some reason had more insanity also had more extensive provisions.

54. R. K. Marshall, 'Wetnursing in Scotland, 1500–1800', *Review of*

Scottish Culture, 1500–1800, 1 (1984), 43–51. V. Fildes, *Wet Nursing: A History from Antiquity to the Present* (Oxford, 1988), 159, 161, 169. Private provision for the mentally incapable in eighteenth-century England was much denser in and around London than elsewhere; within London it was concentrated in and around Hoxton and Chelsea. I. Macalpine and R. Hunter, *George III and the Mad-business* (London, 1969), 323. Most private madhouses in the East Riding of Yorkshire during the nineteenth century clustered near Hull and this Riding had more provision than was the case in Devon, for example. J. A. R. and M. E. Bickford, *The Private Lunatic Asylums of the East Riding* (Beverley, 1976), 10–12. Glasgow had no significant private establishments until the 1830s and 1840s.

55. SRO SC39/36/1, Robert Porteous (1728).
56. Halliday, *A General View of the Present State of Lunatics*, 29–30.
57. Poor Law Enquiry Commission for Scotland. Communications. P.P., 1844 XXII, 949–60.
58. The reason may have been less sinister than it appears since virtually all Scottish poor relief was seen as a supplement to individual endeavour rather than as a dole which would provide total support. Mitchison, 'Old Scottish Poor Law', 58.
59. National Register of Archives for Scotland, 3503/1/21/1–15 [Tyninghame Estate Office, Dunbar: TD73/130/ bundle 21, item 1].
60. J. D. Comrie, *History of Scottish Medicine to 1800* (London, 1927), 136. J. E. Gibson, *A Medical Sketch of Dumfriesshire* (Dumfries, 1827), 53–5. Easterbrook, *The Chronicle of Crichton Royal*, 14–15. M. Williams, *History of Crichton Royal Hospital, 1839–1939* (Dumfries, 1989), 7. For part of the 1790s only four cells were available because a gentleman murderer called Douglas of Luce lived in one and his servant the other. Crichton Royal Hospital (CRH), Dumfries and Galloway Royal Infirmary, Minutes of the Weekly Meeting, 12 September 1795.
61. PML Town Hospital Minute Book, 1786–1801, 20 August 1792 and 3 February 1801.
62. ECA St Cuthbert's Charity Workhouse Minutes, vols. 1–4.
63. Macalpine and Hunter, *George III*, 323.
64. Parry-Jones, *Trade in Lunacy*, 7–8. Beveridge assumes this to be the case for Scotland though he cites only one example, that of James Boswell's brother John. A. Beveridge, 'James Hogg and abnormal psychology: some background notes', *Studies in Hogg and his World* 2 (1991), 91. In reality, however, Lieutenant John Boswell was sent to Newcastle for treatment. Ryskamp and Pottle, *Boswell: the ominous years*, 43–4, 49.
65. SRO C22/68, 603.

66. SL Session Papers, vol. 29, case 98, 'Memorials and answers for John Stark . . .', 1.
67. SRO SC54/2/36, Duncan Campbell (1726).
68. SRO SC36/74/13, James Couper (1816).
69. SRO SC67/57/3, 45–8, William Govan (1775). SC67/57/13, William Govan (1767). C22/77, 58. C22/82, 44.
70. SRO SC67/42/1, William Govan (1775).
71. SRO SC49/56/5, John Stewart (1806). C22/98, 161. CC8/6/84, Stewart v. Menzies (1807).
72. SRO C22/91, 193. CC9/7/79, 538.
73. SRO C22/112, 116.
74. SRO C22/96, 346.
75. SRO JC54/1, report for Forfar (1818).
76. Jolly may have had a special reason for taking on the unnamed patient. On 2 July 1798 his brother Alexander Jolly, episcopal minister of Fraserburgh, petitioned about his sister Ann who was a lunatic. Sunnyside Royal Hospital (Montrose) SR1/1.
77. SRO SC39/47/9, Francis Stuart (1816).
78. SRO SC49/57/5, Christian Graeme (1787). C22/83, 371.
79. There are many examples in the family papers. For instance, SRO GD155/453. James Maxtone and John Murray of Murrayshall (deponents in Christian's case) entered into a bond together in 1774 while John Murray had dealings with Thomas Graham of Balgowan.
80. SRO SC49/57/4, George Henderson (1782). Alexander Pirie may have followed a similar career to that of Francis Willis. Chosen to treat George III in 1788, Willis is credited with propagating the notion that madness was curable. He had come to medicine rather late in life. Born in 1718 he had taken an MA in theology at Oxford in 1740 and an MD there in 1759, thereafter establishing a reputation in Lincolnshire for treating insanity. Parry-Jones, *Trade in Lunacy*, 75. Macalpine and Hunter, *George III*, 269–74.
81. SRO SC54/2/36, Duncan Campbell (1726).
82. SRO SC39/47/6, Charles Irvine (1801). SC39/37/7, John Murray (1776). There is one case where a person may have been in a doctor's care. Jean Bannerman lodged with Mr John Troup in the parish of Fetteresso, Angus. Troup may be the John Troup who graduated MA from Marischal College in 1727 and became a Doctor of Medicine in 1770. The name is relatively uncommon but there is no certainty that this is the same person.
83. P.P., 1816, VI, 370. See also 372.
84. SRO SC39/47/9, David Cross (1818). The Spence referred to was presumably Dr Thomas Spens, one of two visiting physicians to the

Morningside Asylum. C. J. Smith, *Historic South Edinburgh* (Edinburgh, 1978), 195.

85. Lothian Health Board (LHB) HB7/1/1, Minute Book of the Association for Instituting a Lunatic Asylum, 1792–1816, 25 January 1813.

86. LHB HB7/1/1, 23 April 1813, 20 May 1813.

87. SRO SC1/18/1, 12.

88. Parry-Jones, *Trade in Lunacy*, 284.

89. SRO SC1/18/1, 11–12.

90. SRO SC39/36/1, Robert Porteous (1728).

91. SRO JC7/27, 334–8. The Dumfries quotation is from Williams, *History of Crichton Hospital*, 7, based on CRH Dumfries and Galloway Royal Infirmary, Annual Reports, 1785. This had been standard practice since at least 1779. CRH Dumfries and Galloway Royal Infirmary, Minutes of the Weekly Meeting, 11 and 21 October 1779. Easterbrook, *Chronicle of Crichton Royal*, 15. Not surprisingly, attendants at many English asylums were recruited from among the labouring classes for their size and strength. L. D. Smith, 'Behind closed doors: lunatic asylum keepers, 1800–60', *Social History of Medicine* 1, 3 (1988), 301–27. MacDonald comments on the low standard of early keepers at Glasgow Asylum. K. MacDonald, 'Keepers to carers', in J. Andrews and I. Smith (eds) *'Let There Be Light Again'. A History of Gartnavel Royal Hospital from its Beginnings to the Present Day* (Glasgow, 1993), 85.

92. SC39/36/6, John Rutherford (1763).

93. SRO SC39/36/4, James Arbuthnot (1752).

94. SRO SC39/36/4, Robert Gordon (1754).

95. SRO SC39/47/6, Charles Irvine (1801).

96. SRO SC39/47/3, Hugh Maxwell (1784).

97. SC39/47/7, David Balfour Hay, 1807. SC39/47/8, John Hay (1811). SC39/47/8, David Paterson (1811). Hughes set up his own small, select private madhouse at Inveresk sometime in 1815 or early 1816. SRO JC54/1, report for Edinburgh (1816), 15.

98. SRO SC39/47/9, David Cross (1818).

99. P.P., 1816, VI, 367–71.

100. SRO SC39/47/6, John Cunningham (1801). Andrews, 'Identifying and providing for the mentally disabled', 82–4 finds a number of women nursing idiots in early modern London, though this may be because the objects of their care were usually young children. There is some evidence for this in some of the Renfrewshire examples but the licensed madhouses of Midlothian dealt exclusively with adults, as did the public asylums of the early nineteenth century.

101. SL Session Papers, vol. 400, case 22, 'Answers for James Whyte . . .', 2 (1799).

102. For example SRO SC39/36/13, Agnes Wright (1795).
103. *Edinburgh Evening Courant*, no. 10,473, 2 March 1785.
104. The word 'patient' was only used by medical men or asylum keepers in court depositions, and in official surveys of private and public madhouses in the early nineteenth century. Most witnesses tended to describe a mentally incapable person as furious (or some colloquial equivalent) or idiotic or a sufferer.
105. For example, SRO SC36/74/10, Andrew Boyd (1808). SC39/47/3, Hugh Maxwell (1784). SC36/74/13, James Couper (1816).
106. SRO SC1/18/1, 11–12. See also R. Porter, 'Madness and Its Institutions', in A. Wear (ed.) *Medicine in Society: Historical Essays* (Cambridge, 1992), 288–9.
107. SRO SC5/24/2, Jean Bannerman (1755).
108. SL Session Papers, vol. 284, 'Petition of Miss Elizabeth Blair . . .', case 17, 9–10.
109. SRO SC39/36/4, James Arbuthnot (1752).
110. SRO SC39/36/4, James Arbuthnot (1752).
111. Bleeding was, of course, a standard treatment for maniacal and melancholic conditions, along with purging. W. Cullen, *First Lines of the Practice of Physic* 4 vols. (4th edition, 1784), vol. 4, 156–60, 173, 184–6.
112. Suzuki, 'Household and the care of lunatics', 157.
113. CRH Dumfries and Galloway Royal Infirmary, Minutes of the Weekly Meeting, 12 September 1795. *Dumfries Weekly Journal* 15 September 1795.
114. SRO SC15/66/2, Lewis Alexander Grant (1806).
115. Suzuki, 'Household and the care of lunatics', 154.
116. In the civil court cognitions male deponents outnumbered female by more than six to one. In a sample of 3,215 witnesses before the High Court of Justiciary between 1650 and 1760 the sex ratio was only slightly more balanced at 454 males per 100 females. R. A. Houston, *Scottish Literacy and the Scottish Identity* (Cambridge, 1985). For the reasons see *The Laws and Customs of Scotland in Matters Criminal*, vol. 2, 255–6. See also R. A. Houston, 'Women in the economy and society of Scotland, 1500–1800', in R. A. Houston and I. D. Whyte (eds) *Scottish Society, 1500–1800* (Cambridge, 1989), 118–47.
117. Rice, 'Madness and industrial society', 237, 268.

CHAPTER THREE

1. This work was carried out as a Wellcome University Award Holder, and I am grateful to the Wellcome Trust for their support in funding this project. My thanks to Peter Bartlett and David Wright for their

valuable comments, and to audiences in Warwick, Oxford, Manchester and Glasgow where sections of this article have been presented.

2. Including witnesses in infanticide trials which provide some of the best evidence of seventeenth- and eighteenth-century understandings of 'insanity of childbirth': see Mark Jackson, *New-Born Child Murder: Women, Illegitimacy and the Courts in Eighteenth-century England* (Manchester, 1996); Peter C. Hoffer and N.E.H. Hull, *Murdering Mothers: Infanticide in England and New England 1558–1803* (New York, 1981).

3. Studies of puerperal insanity are scarce, but see Nancy M. Theriot, 'Diagnosing Unnatural Motherhood. Nineteenth-Century Physicians and "Puerperal Insanity"', *American Studies*, 26 (1990), 69–88; Shelley Day, 'Puerperal Insanity: The Historical Sociology of a Disease', unpublished PhD thesis, University of Cambridge, 1985, and Irvine Loudon, 'Puerperal Insanity in the 19th Century', *Journal of the Royal Society of Medicine*, 81 (Feb. 1988), 76–9.

4. Observing descriptions of women's liability to become mentally disturbed following birth in the broader context of a range of potential complications, leads to qualification of Showalter's analysis, where female madness in the Victorian era has close connotations with their reproductive cycles and ideals of feminine behaviour: Elaine Showalter, *The Female Malady: Women, Madness and English Culture, 1830–1980* (New York, 1985).

5. See e.g. Janet F. Saunders, 'Institutionalised Offenders: A Study of the Victorian Institution and its Inmates, with Special Reference to Late Nineteenth Century Warwickshire', unpublished PhD thesis, University of Warwick, 1983, 173, where women's slightly raised 'proneness' to insanity is linked, as evidenced by the case notes of the Warwick County Asylum, to bearing numerous children, prolonged feeding, poor diet and exhaustion, rather than to their biological role *per se.*

6. Robert Gooch, *Observations on Puerperal Insanity* (London, 1820) (extracted from 6th volume of *Medical Transactions*, Royal College of Physicians, read at the College, 16 Dec. 1819).

7. *Lives of British Physicians* (London, 1830), 305–41 for the physician Henry Southey's sympathetic account of Gooch's life and work.

8. Esp. *Gooch on Some of the Most Important Diseases Peculiar to Women, with Other Papers*, with prefatory essay by Robert Ferguson (London, 1831); *A Practical Compendium of Midwifery; Being the Course of Lectures on Midwifery, and on the Diseases of Women and Infants, Delivered at St. Batholomew's Hospital by the Late Robert*

Gooch, M.D., prepared for publication by George Skinner (London, 1831).

9. *Lives of British Physicians*, 341.

10. Modern psychiatric textbooks explain how puerperal and lactational psychoses were thought to be specific entities during the nineteenth century, but later psychiatrists such as Bleuler and Kraepelin regarded puerperal psychosis as indistinct from other psychoses, a view still widely held today. No clear relationship has been established between psychosis and obstetric factors. Yet the occurrence of puerperal psychosis appears to be very much higher than for psychosis amongst non-puerperal women of the same age: Michael Gelder *et al.*, *Oxford Textbook of Psychiatry*, 3rd edn. (Oxford, 1996), 396–7. Ian Brockington and his colleagues have outlined the way in which nosology denied puerperal psychosis its identity: I.F. Brockington and R. Kumar (eds) *Motherhood and Mental Illness* (London and New York, 1982).

11. See e.g. W.F. Menzie, 'Puerperal Insanity: An Analysis of One Hundred and Forty Consecutive Cases', *American Journal of Insanity*, 50 (1893–94), 147–85, who used case records from the Rainhill Asylum, Liverpool to seek evidence of links with heredity and mental and physical predisposition.

12. Loudon, 'Puerperal Insanity', 76.

13. Francis H. Ramsbotham, *Principles and Practice of Obstetric Medicine and Surgery in Reference to the Process of Parturition*, 3rd edn. (London, 1851), 554.

14. Fleetwood Churchill, *On the Diseases of Women; Including those of Pregnancy and Childbed*, 4th edn. (Dublin, 1857), 738.

15. James Reid, 'On the Causes, Symptoms, and Treatment of Puerperal Insanity', *Journal of Psychological Medicine*, 1 (1858), 128–51, 284–94, quote on 134–5.

16. Gooch, *Observations on Puerperal Insanity*, 20–1.

17. F.W. Mackenzie, 'On the Pathology and Treatment of Puerperal Insanity: Especially in Reference to its Relation with Anaemia', *London Journal of Medicine*, 3 (1851), 504–21.

18. In representations in infanticide trials, medical witnesses, claimed the mother to be in a state of temporary insanity because of puerperal mania, blaming the condition in turn on an excessive flow of milk, suppression of the milk and lochia, or simply 'bad breasts': Roger Smith, *Trial by Medicine: Insanity and Responsibility in Victorian Trials* (Edinburgh, 1981), esp. chapter 7; J.P. Eigen, *Witnessing Insanity: Madness and Mad-Doctors in the English Court* (New Haven and London, 1995), esp. 142, 147–9; Nigel Walker, *Crime and Insanity in*

England, vol. 1: *The Historical Perspective* (Edinburgh, 1968), chapter 7 'Infanticide'; Hilary Marland, 'Murdering mothers revisited: infanticide, responsibility and puerperal insanity in nineteenth-century Britain', unpublished paper, History Seminar, University of Huddersfield, 11 Dec. 1997.

19. John B. Tuke, 'Cases Illustrative of the Insanity of Pregnancy, Puerperal Mania, and Insanity of Lactation', *Edinburgh Medical Journal*, 12 (1866–67), 1083–1101, quote on 1093.

20. A. Campbell Clark, 'Clinical Illustrations of Puerperal Insanity', *Lancet*, II (1883), 97–9, 180–1, 277–9, on 98.

21. For chloroform, see A.J. Youngson, *The Scientific Revolution in Victorian Medicine* (London, 1979), esp. chapter 3, and e.g. the *Association Medical Journal* (the precursor of the *British Medical Journal*) in 1853, when an intense debate followed the publication of John Snow's article 'On the Administration of Chloroform During Parturition', in June of that year (500–2).

22. Charles Kidd, 'On Chloroform and Some of its Clinical Uses', *London Medical Review or Monthly Journal of Medical and Surgical Science*, II (1862), 243–7, quote on 244.

23. E.g. A.T.H. Waters, 'On the Use of Chloroform in the Treatment of Puerperal Insanity', *The Journal of Psychological Medicine*, 10 (1857), 123–35.

24. Loudon, 'Puerperal Insanity', 77; Richard Gundry, 'Observations upon Puerperal Insanity', *Journal of Psychological Medicine*, 13 (1860), 414–25, on 415.

25. Gundry, 'Observations', 415.

26. General Report of the Royal Hospitals of Bridewell and Bethlem, and of the House of Occupations, for the year ending 31st Dec. 1845.

27. Annual Reports of the West Riding Lunatic Asylum. My thanks to Rob Ellis for generously sharing his data with me.

28. Figures dropped away again, with no admissions between 1868 and 1878 under the heading puerperal insanity. They then increased, accounting for around 5 to 10 per cent of female admissions during the 1880s.

29. See e.g. Eigen, *Witnessing Insanity*, 142, 147–8.

30. John Thomson, 'Statistical Report of Three Thousand Three Hundred Cases of Obstetricy', *Glasgow Medical Journal*, 3 (1855), 129–50.

31. Ibid., 143–5.

32. John Raymond (ed.) *Queen Victoria's Early Letters*, rev. edn. (London, 1963), 74.

33. Queen Victoria to the Princess Royal, 9 March, 1859, in Roger Fulford (ed.) *Dearest Child: Letters between Queen Victoria and the Crown Princess of Prussia, 1858–1861* (London, 1964), 165.

34. Judith Schneid Lewis, *In the Family Way: Childbearing in the British Aristocracy, 1760–1860* (New Brunswick, NJ, 1986), 213–16.

35. For the care of women during pregnancy, delivery and post-partum, and for the large amount of advice literature available on the subject, see Patricia Branca, *Silent Sisterhood: Middle-Class Women in the Victorian Home* (London, 1975), chapter 5. Thomas Bull's, *Hints to Mothers for the Management of Health during the Period of Pregnancy, and in the Lying-in Room; with an Exposure of Popular Errors in Connection with those Subjects* (London, 1837) was one such volume, which gave common sense advice on diet, exercise, avoidance of constipation, and deportment during delivery, based partly on his work at the Finsbury Midwifery Institution.

36. Michael Ryan, *A Manual of Midwifery and Diseases of Women and Children*, 4th edn. (London, 1841), 167.

37. Ibid., 334.

38. *A Practical Compendium of Midwifery*, 292–3.

39. *Lives of British Physicians*, 341.

40. W.S. Playfair, *A Treatise on the Science and Practice of Midwifery* (London, 1876), 226. See also Hilary Marland, 'Destined to a Perfect Recovery': The Confinement of Puerperal Insanity in the Nineteenth Century', in J. Melling and B. Forsythe (eds) *Insanity, Institutions and Society* (London and New York, 1999), 137–56.

41. W. Tyler Smith, 'Puerperal Mania' (Lecture XXXIX of 'A Course of Lectures on the Theory and Practice of Obstetrics'), *Lancet*, 18 Oct. 1856, 423–5, quote on 424.

42. Reid, 'On the Causes, Symptoms, and Treatment', 290.

43. Ramsbotham, *Principles and Practice*, 568.

44. *Some of the Most Important Diseases Peculiar to Women*, 79.

45. Smith, 'Puerperal Mania', 425.

46. *Annual Reports of the Cumberland & Westmorland Lunatic Asylum, 1863–1870.*

47. Tuke, 'Cases Illustrative', 1092. Many interested parties in Scotland were anxious to keep asylums as a last resort for various categories of insanity, and the notion of moral treatment was more pervasive and long-standing than in England; this may well have influenced the opinions of Scottish authorities on puerperal mania.

48. Campbell Clark, 'Clinical Illustrations', 180.

49. Ramsbotham, *Principles and Practice*, 567.

50. Reid, 'On the Causes, Symptoms, and Treatment', 289.

51. *Lancet*, 26 Dec. 1829, 436–7.

52. Smith, 'Puerperal Mania', 424. Smith also had some 'masterful' means of treating erotic and nervous symptoms of menopause, including injections of ice water into the rectum and vagina, and leeching the

labia and cervix: W. Tyler Smith, 'The Climacteric Disease in Women', *London Journal of Medicine* 1 (1848), 601–9.

53. Gooch, *Observations on Puerperal Insanity*, 22.
54. *A Practical Compendium of Midwifery*, 294.
55. Ibid., 290.
56. Gooch, *Observations on Puerperal Insanity*, 34–41.
57. Ibid., 41.
58. Thomas More Madden, 'On Puerperal Mania', *British and Foreign Medico-Chirurgical Review*, 48 (1871), 477–95, 485.
59. Gundry, 'Observations', 422.
60. Reid, 'On the Causes, Symptoms, and Treatment', 293.
61. Ramsbotham, *Principles and Practice*, 561.
62. William Thackeray to his mother, Sept. 1842, in Gordon N. Ray (ed.) *The Letters and Private Papers of William Makepeace Thackeray*, 4 vols. (London, 1945), vol. 2, 81.
63. George H. Savage, *Insanity and Allied Neuroses: Practical and Clinical* (London and New York, 1884), 376–7.
64. Ibid., 377.
65. Gundry, 'Observations', 414–15.
66. Warwick County Record Office, CR/1664/654: Warwick County Lunatic Asylum, Admissions Register, Female Patients, 1886–1890; Loudon, 'Puerperal Insanity', 77.
67. Menzie, 'Puerperal Insanity', 147.
68. Campbell Clark, 'Clinical Illustrations'; idem, 'Aetiology, Pathology, and Treatment of Puerperal Insanity', *Journal of Mental Science*, 33 (1887), 169–89, 372–9, 487–96.

CHAPTER FOUR

1. Acknowledgements: This chapter is based on research funded by the Wellcome Trust. The authors are grateful to Neil Evans and Dai Michael for comments and suggestions.
2. *Ninth Report of the Commissioners in Lunacy*, (P.P., 1854–55, XVII), 575.
3. P. Rushton, 'Lunatics and Idiots: Mental Disability, the Community and the Poor Law in North-East England, 1600–1800', *Medical History*, 32 (1988), 34–50. A. Suzuki, 'Lunacy in Seventeenth- and Eighteenth-Century England: Analysis of Quarter Sessions Records', *History of Psychiatry*, 2 (1991), 437–56; 3 (1992), 29–44.
4. D. Wright, 'Getting Out of the Asylum: Understanding the Confinement of the Insane in the Nineteenth Century', *Social History of Medicine*, 10 (1997), 137–55.
5. T. G. Davies, 'Mental Mischief: Aspects of Nineteenth Century

Psychiatric Practice in Parts of Wales', in H. Freeman and G. E. Berrios (eds) *150 Years of British Psychiatry Volume 2, The Aftermath,* (London, 1996), 367–82.

6. County Lunatic Asylums Act, 1828, 9 Geo. IV, c. 40, s. 36
7. Poor Law Amendment Act, 1842, 5 & 6 Vict., c. 57, s. 6.
8. *Tenth Annual Report of the Poor Law Commissioners,* (P.P., 1844, XIX), 31.
9. *Thirteenth Report of the Commissioners in Lunacy,* (P.P., 1859(2), XIV), 608.
10. *Further Report of the Commissioners in Lunacy,* (P.P., 1847–48, XXXII), 650–1, 656.
11. *Fourteenth Report of the Commissioners in Lunacy,* (P.P., 1860, XXXIV), 398–9, Appendix G3. Memorandum of a Visit to Pauper Patients in the Island of Anglesey
12. Denbighshire Record Office [DRO], QSD/AL/1/1–27. There are no returns for the years 1832, 1838, 1847 and 1857. For 1845, only the returns for the Denbighshire parishes in the Conway Union exist. For other years, the returns of some parishes or unions are missing. References to these returns are cited in the form DRO, L[unacy]R[eturn], [Parish and/or Union], [Year(s)]. Duplicate copies of the returns are sometimes bound into the correspondence files in the MH 12 series in the PRO.
13. J. and S. Rowlands, *The Surnames of Wales,* (Birmingham, 1996), frontispiece, 4, 47.
14. See H. R. Davies, 'Automated Record Linkage of Census Enumerators Books and Registration Data: Obstacles, Challenges and Solutions', *History and Computing,* 4(1992), 16–26.
15. Twenty one parishes failed to make a return in 1829. DRO QSD/AL/ 3/2, A Return of the Parishes in the County of Denbigh which have not complied with the Provisions of the 9th Geo. IV, c. 40, sec. 36, and the reasons for such neglect so far as the same are known to the Clerk of the Peace, 4 March 1830.
16. For example, the entry for Ellin Jones was crossed out by the Overseer of Llannefydd as she 'lives with her father at Tan y Graig, Nantglyn [Parish]'. DRO, LR, Llannefydd, 1840,
17. DRO, LR, Ruthin Union, 1843. No return survives for the Ruthin Union in the 1842 series.
18. Metropolitan Commissioners on Lunacy, *Supplemental Report Relative to the General Condition of the Insane in Wales,* (P.P., House of Lords, 1844, XVI), 318–19.
19. Ibid., 306.
20. DRO, LR, St Asaph Union, 1851–53.

21. Metropolitan Commissioners on Lunacy, *Supplemental Report*, (P.P., House of Lords, 1844, XVI), 334–5.
22. DRO, LR, Ruthin Union, 1853–56.
23. Metropolitan Commissioners on Lunacy, *Supplemental Report*, (P.P., House of Lords, 1844, XVI), 319; DRO, LR, Ruthin Union, 1852.
24. Metropolitan Commissioners on Lunacy, *Supplemental Report*, (P.P., House of Lords, 1844, XVI), 319; DRO, LR, St Asaph Union, 1846.
25. PRO MH 19/168, Correspondence Poor Law Board and Commissioners in Lunacy 1847- 1858, Copy of Report by J. Gaskell, 28 November 1858, received by Poor Law Board 24 December 1858
26. Lunatic Asylums Amendment Act, 1853, 16 & 17 Vict. c. 97.
27. PRO MH 19/168, Report by J. Gaskell.
28. *Sixteenth Report of the Commissioners in Lunacy*, (P.P., 1862, XXIII), 77–8.
29. Metropolitan Commissioners on Lunacy, *Supplemental Report*, (P.P., House of Lords, 1844, XVI), 322.
30. DRO, LR, Llanrwst, 1841; Llanrwst Union, 1843–44, 1846, 1848, 1850–51, 1854–56.
31. DRO PD 2/5/2, Overseers Accounts, Aberchwiler, 28 March 1836; DRO, LR, Aberchwiler, 1828–29, 1831, 1833–37, 1839
32. Metropolitan Commissioners on Lunacy, *Supplemental Report*, (P.P., House of Lords, 1844, XVI), 330.
33. Paupers Removal Act, 1861, 24 & 25 Vict., c. 55, s. 6, 9.
34. *Sixteenth Report of the Commissioners in Lunacy*, (P.P., 1862, XXIII), 77.
35. DRO PD 27/1/28, Vestry Minutes, Eglwysbach, 1825–1890 , 25 May 1865.
36. *Eighteenth Report of the Commissioners in Lunacy*, (P.P., 1866, XXXII), 29.
37. S. A. Williams, 'Care in the Community: Women and the Old Poor Law in Early Nineteenth Century Anglesey', *Llafur*, 6(1995), 30–43.
38. DRO, LR, Wrexham, 1831.
39. DRO, LR, Ruabon, 1831.
40. P. Bartlett, The Poor Law of Lunacy: The Administration of Pauper Lunatics in Mid-nineteenth Century England with Special Emphasis on Leicestershire and Rutland, Unpublished PhD thesis, University of London, 1993, 79.
41. DRO, LR, St Asaph Union, 1846.
42. DRO, LR, Wrexham Union, 1842.
43. DRO, LR, Denbigh, 1841.
44. See e.g. H. Land, 'Who Cares for the Family?', *Journal of Social Policy*, 7 (1978), 257–84.
45. See M. A. Crowther, 'Family Responsibility and State Responsibility

in Britain before the Welfare State', *Historical Journal*, 25 (1982), 131–45. Obligations under Scottish law were wider.

46. For other studies of the family's role in caring for lunatics and idiots see R. Adair, J. Melling and B. Forsythe, 'Migration, Family Structure and Pauper Lunacy in Victorian England: Admissions to the Devon County Pauper Lunatic Asylum, 1845–1900', *Continuity and Change*, 12(1997), 373–401; D. Wright, 'Familial Care of 'Idiot' Children in Victorian England', in P. Horden and R. Smith, (eds) *The Locus of Care: Families, Communities, Institutions and the Provision of Welfare Since Antiquity*, (London, 1998), 176–97.

47. A.D. Rees, *Life in a Welsh Countryside* (Cardiff, 1961). E. Davies and A.D. Rees (eds) *Welsh Rural Communities*, (Cardiff, 1960).

48. Metropolitan Commissioners on Lunacy, *Supplemental Report*, (P.P., House of Lords, 1844, XVI), 317–18; DRO, LR, Denbigh, 1840–41; St Asaph Union, 1842–44, 1846, 1849–53.

49. DRO, LR, Wrexham Union, 1844.

50. DRO, LR, Wrexham Union, 1843.

51. DRO, LR, Llanfair Dyffryn Clwyd, 1837.

52. DRO, LR, Betws-yn-Rhos, 1828, 1836–37, 1839–40, St Asaph Union, 1842–44, 1846, 1849.

53. C. Philo, 'Journey to Asylum: A Medical-geographical Idea in Historical Context', *Journal of Historical Geography*, 21(1995), 148–68.

54. See P. Michael and D. Hirst, 'Establishing the 'Rule of Kindness': The Foundation of the North Wales Asylum, Denbigh', in J. Melling and W. Forsythe (eds) *Insanity, Institutions and Society*, forthcoming.

55. *Fourteenth Report of the Commissioners in Lunacy*, (P.P., 1860, XXXIV), 398–9.

56. Metropolitan Commissioners on Lunacy, *Report to the Lord Chancellor*, (P.P., House of Lords, 1844, XVI), 205.

57. Metropolitan Commissioners on Lunacy, *Supplemental Report*, (P.P., House of Lords, 1844, XVI), 318. DRO, LR, Derwen, 1840, Ruthin Union, 1843–44, 1846.

58. Metropolitan Commissioners on Lunacy, *Supplemental Report*, (P.P., House of Lords, 1844, XVI), 335–41.

59. Ibid., 339

60. Ibid., 340.

61. Ibid., 338.

62. DRO, LR; Metropolitan Commissioners on Lunacy, *Supplemental Report*, (P.P., House of Lords, 1844, XVI), 339.

63. J. Walton, 'Casting Out and Bringing Back in Victorian England: Pauper Lunatics, 1840–70', in W.F. Bynum, R. Porter and M. Shep-

herd (eds) *The Anatomy of Madness: Essays in the History of Psychiatry. Vol. 2: Institutions and Society*, (London, 1985), 132–46.

64. Metropolitan Commissioners on Lunacy, *Report to the Lord Chancellor*, (P.P., House of Lords, 1844, XVI), 205.

65. National Library of Wales [NLW] MSS, 3149, William Day Papers, Correspondence with Unions and Circulars, item 1073.

66. PRO MH/12/161131, Poor Law Union Files, St Asaph, Letter from William Day to George Cornewall Lewis, 5 April 1841. Emphasis in original.

67. DRO, LR, Denbigh, 1828–1836.

68. DRO, PD 24/1/131, Vestry Minutes, Denbigh, 29 January 1827.

69. Ibid., 29 May 1828.

70. Ibid., 5 February 1829.

71. DRO, LR, Denbigh, 1829, DRO, PD 24/1/131, Vestry Minutes, Denbigh, 2 January 1830. No record of Smith's committal survives among the remaining papers of the Chester Asylum.

72. Ibid., 2 January 1830.

73. Ibid., 22 December 1831.

74. Ibid., 25 May 1833.

75. Ibid., 5 December 1833.

76. Ibid., 6 February 1834.

77. Ibid., 14 January 1836.

78. Ibid., 4 May 1837.

79. 1851 Census for Denbigh.

80. 1881 Census for Denbigh

81. Rees, *Life in a Welsh Countryside*; Davies and Rees (eds) *Welsh Rural Communities*; I. Emmet, *A North Wales Village*, (London, 1964).

CHAPTER FIVE

1. F. Rice, 'Madness and Industrial Society: A Study of the Origins and Early Growth of the Organisation of Insanity in Nineteenth Century Scotland. c1830–70', unpublished PhD thesis, University of Strathclyde, 1981.

2. A. S. Presly, *A Sunnyside Chronicle, 1781–1981. A History of Sunnyside Royal Hospital* (Dundee, 1981); J. Andrews and I. Smith (eds) *'Let there be light again.' A History of Gartnavel Royal Hospital from its Beginnings to the Present Day* (Glasgow, 1993); A. Beveridge, 'Madness in Victorian Edinburgh: A Study of Patients Admitted to Royal Edinburgh Asylum under Thomas Clouston, 1873–1908, part 2', *History of Psychiatry*, 6 (1995), 113–56; A. Beveridge and M. Barfoot, 'Madness at the Crossroads: John Home's letters from the

Royal Edinburgh Asylum, 1886–1887', *Psychological Medicine*, 20 (1990), 263–84 and M. S. Thompson, 'The Mad, the Bad and the Sad: Psychiatric Care at the Royal Edinburgh Asylum 1811–1894', unpublished PhD thesis, University of Boston, 1985.

3. G. Doody, 'Fife and Kinross District Asylum', Unpublished M.Sc. thesis, University of Edinburgh, 1992.

4. Although an unpublished study of the Scottish 'trade in lunacy' was undertaken by Parry-Jones and Sturdy in 1996.

5. W. Ll. Parry-Jones, 'The Model of the Geel Lunatic Colony and its Influence on the Nineteenth Century Asylum System in Britain', in A. Scull (ed.) *Madhouses, Mad-doctors and Madmen: The Social History of Psychiatry in the Victorian era* (London, 1981), 201–17.

6. P. McCandless, 'Build, build! The Controversy over the Care of the Chronically Insane in England, 1855–1870', *Bulletin of the History of Medicine*, 53 (1979), 558.

7. Royal (Chartered) asylums were established long before the legislation of 1857, and for many years received both pauper and private patients, the former being maintained either through charitable funds or admitted on reduced rates. District asylums were public institutions erected and managed by the District Boards of Lunacy, created in 1857. They were intended for the reception of pauper patients where such provision was not otherwise available. Parochial asylums were erected out of taxes levied upon parishes, managed by parochial boards, but licensed by the Board of Lunacy. They received paupers suffering from all forms of insanity. Certain wards in poorhouses also accommodated insane patients, having been granted licenses from the Board of Lunacy for the reception solely of harmless patients not amenable to curative treatment.

8. The Commission was established 'to inquire into the condition of Lunatic Asylums in Scotland, and the existing law in reference to Lunatics and Lunatic Asylums in that part of the United Kingdom'. Report of Royal Commission (1857), [2148. Session 1] v.1.293

9. Report of the Royal Commission (1857), 196.

10. General Board of Commissioners in Lunacy for Scotland (GBCLS) 3rd AR (1861), main report pxxxvii.

11. An Act for the Regulation of the Care and Treatment of Lunatics, and for the Provision, Maintenance and Regulation of Lunatic Asylums, in Scotland. 25th August 1857 [20 and 21 Victoria cap 71]

12. Ibid.

13. GBCLS 3rd AR (1861), main text, piv.

14. The Report of the Royal Commission contained the declaration that 'we shall take the liberty, in accordance with the usual phraseology, of employing the terms 'insane persons' or 'lunatic' as applying to

them all, unless where a different meaning is indicated.' Report of the Royal Commission (1857), 3.

15. GBCLS 33rd AR (1891), main report, pxxxv.

16. H.Marr, 'John Fraser's obituary', *Journal of Mental Science*, 293 (1925), 191.

17. GBCLS 32nd AR (1890),119.

18. Ibid.

19. GBCLS 18th AR (1876) main report, ii.

20. Before the introduction of this grant-in-aid, each parish had borne the entire maintenance costs of their insane paupers. Smaller, impoverished parishes were often barely able to provide for their paupers. The Act of 1875 (modified in 1889) provided for an annual Parliamentary grant, whereby half the cost of upkeep for each pauper patient was paid to the parish so encouraging officials to register weak-minded, chronic cases.

21. In the earlier years, many parish officials expressed resentment at the additional workload required. There was clear evidence of hostility at the degree of control exerted by Commissioners in an area once considered the responsibility of the parish – the care and control of insane paupers. Among a number of parish officials there appears to have been a lack of understanding of the characteristics of lunacy, with many sharing the belief that all insane persons should be confined in asylums. This was reinforced when they came into contact with certain patients who were of disturbing appearance and behaviour. Further, the bias of the Board of Supervision (the controlling body of all parochial boards) in favour of lunatic wards was strongly pronounced, particularly in the early years of the Board of Lunacy. This was not altogether unexpected, as poorhouses were controlled by the Board of Supervision and asylums and boarding-out by the Board of Lunacy. In addition, patients in lunatic wards required little supervision from inspectors of poor, in contrast to the heavy workload involved in visiting the boarded-out.

22. See D. Cameron, 'Admissions to Scottish Mental Hospitals in the Last Hundred Years', *British Journal of Preventive and Social Medicine*, 8 (1954), 180–6 for a useful discussion of this.

23. GBCLS 30th AR (1888), main report, x. In Shetland, for example, 54 per cent of their pauper insane were boarded-out, contrasted to only 8 per cent in Nairn.

24. In the same year, 1616 private patients were accommodated in royal and district asylums and 157 in private madhouses. GBCLS 35th AR (1893), main report, x.

25. GBCLS 18th AR (1876) and 50th AR (1908).

26. By the turn of the century, almost 80 per cent (394) of patients in

Fifeshire were located in an area of 6 miles by 15 miles. Only two other colonies exceeded these proportions; Dun-sur-Auron, in France, with 500 patients, and Gheel in Belgium, the first and largest colony of its kind, with 1983 patients scattered over an area of 40 square miles, among a general population of approximately 7000.

27. The system of boarding-out pauper children throughout Scotland is examined by H. Macdonald, 'Care of Children under the Scottish Poor Law', unpublished PhD thesis, University of Glasgow, 1994.

28. On a visit to Kennoway in 1994, several villagers reminisced about the time when patients lived among them.

29. GBCLS 36th AR (1894), main report, xliv.

30. GBCLS 32nd AR (1890), 110.

31. In 1877, the Board of Lunacy prohibited any increase in the number of lunatics boarded at Kennoway; a similar prohibition was enforced in 1885 at Balfron, Stirlingshire, and the possibility of doing so for other villages was considered.

32. GBCLS 55th AR, (1913), 167.

33. GBCLS 8th AR (1866), 240.

34. G.Gibson, 'The Boarding-out System in Scotland', *American Journal of Psychiatry*, 71 (1925), 256.

35. GBCLS 24th AR (1882), 156.

36. GBCLS 45th AR (1903), 149. Of those classified as suffering from acquired forms of insanity, 72 per cent had dementia, 13 per cent delusional insanity, 7 per cent chronic mania, 4 per cent melancholia and 4 per cent had various forms of degenerative disease.

37. GBCLS 16th AR (1874).

38. GBCLS 24th AR (1882).

39. T. W. L. Spence, 'The Present Position of the Insane Poor under Private Care in Scotland', *Poor Law Magazine*, 12 (1902), 625.

40. Figures for the year 1858 are shown separately, being the first year of boarding-out. Source of data: GBCLS AR, 1858–1913, *passim.*

41. Spence, 'The Present Position of the Insane Poor', 636.

42. GBCLS 20th AR (1878), 99. The particular identification of the Highlands and Islands as districts of 'low morality' serves to emphasise an apparent prejudice among Lowland Commissioners for the mode and values of life in these areas.

43. GBCLS 1st AR (1859),195.

44. GBCLS 35th AR (1893),109.

45. Ibid.

46. GBCLS 22nd AR (1880),126.

47. GBCLS 38th AR (1896),122.

48. GBCLS 24th AR (1882),156.

49. Lawson's short assessment of the 'Importance of personal character

and influence of the guardian' outlines the desired characteristics of guardians, and is worth noting. GBCLS 31st AR (1889), 138.

50. Anon, 'Colonisation of Lunatics by the Legislature', *Medical Critic and Psychological Journal*, 2 (1862), 441.
51. See for example, comments in GBCLS AR (1859–1862) *passim.*
52. GBCLS 23rd AR (1881), 123.
53. Ibid.
54. Source of data: GBCLS AR (1861–1911) *passim.*
55. GBCLS 49th AR (1907), 153.
56. Noted, for example, in GBCLS 35th AR (1893) and 45th AR (1903).
57. GBCLS 45th AR (1903) Such continuity was most famously observed at Gheel, where families automatically took over care of a patient when the elderly guardian was no longer capable.
58. The Act of 1862 sanctioning special licenses for guardians and the government grant-in-aid of 1875 being the only notable legislation after the Lunacy (Scotland) Act, 1857.
59. In 1906, for example, the proportion of deaths among patients resident in royal and district asylums was 10 per cent, while that in private dwellings was only 3.9 per cent. GBCLS 49th AR (1907), main report, xxi. Commissioners regarded this low rate as particularly impressive in view of the wide age range of patients and their tendency to suffer from mental conditions which lowered physical vitality.
60. GBCLS 33rd AR (1891), *passim.*
61. T. S. Clouston, 'Lunacy Administration of Scotland,' in G. Alder Blumer and A. B. Richardson (eds) *Commitment, Detention, Care and Treatment of the Insane* (Baltimore, 1893), 186–97.
62. GBCLS 56th AR (1914), main report, lxxii.
63. A. R. Turnbull, 'Some Remarks on Boarding-out as a Mode of Provision for Pauper Insane', *Journal of Mental Science*, 34 (1888), 371.
64. W. L. Lindsay, 'The Family System as Applied to the Treatment of the Chronic Insane', *Journal of Mental Science*, 16 (1871), 517.
65. Royal Commission on the Care and Control of the Feeble-minded (1908), 45.
66. M. Morel, 'The Present State and Future Prospects of Psychological Medicine. An Address', *Journal of Mental Science*, 10 (1865), 339.
67. GBCLS 19th AR (1877), 119.
68. GBCLS 38th AR (1896), 134.
69. Reported in Anon, 'Gheel in the North', *Journal of Mental Science*, 11 (1866), 284.
70. J. B. Tuke, 'The Cottage System of Management of Lunatics as

Practised in Scotland, with suggestions for its elaboration and improvement', *Journal of Mental Science*, 15 (1870), 529.

71. GBCLS 25th AR (1883), 170.
72. The proceedings of the International Congress held at Edinburgh on Home Relief are discussed in the *Poor Law Magazine*, (1903) 8, 409–13.
73. GBCLS 51st AR (1909), 151–2.
74. Ibid.
75. A. Burnett, untitled, *American Journal of Insanity*, 52 (1895), 576.
76. D. H. Tuke, 'Boarding-out of Pauper Lunatics in Scotland', *Journal of Mental Science*, 35 (1889), 511.
77. Between 1859 and 1913, removal due to these risks was reported on less than 20 occasions, out of an average boarded-out population of approximately 2500 patients. GBCLS AR *passim*.
78. GBCLS 51st AR (1909), 158.
79. GBCLS 35th AR (1893), 95.
80. M.Foucault, *Madness and Civilisation* (London, 1967).
81. Editorial. 'Objections to the Boarding-out System', *Journal of Mental Science*, 42 (1896), 352.
82. A. Scull, *'The Most Solitary of Afflictions. Madness and Society in Britain, 1700–1900'* (New Haven, 1993), 372.
83. J. F. Sutherland, *'The Insane Poor in Private Dwellings'*, (Edinburgh, 1897), 59.
84. C. Riggs, 'The Boarding-out System in Scotland', *American Journal of Insanity*, 52 (1895), 328–9.
85. F. Jolly, 'On the Family Care of the Insane in Scotland', *Journal of Mental Science*, 21 (1875), 60.
86. Chancery patients were seen quarterly by Visitors who could insist on their removal, if improper treatment was evident. To Bucknill, Chancery patients experienced 'untold blessing' when boarded in private dwellings. J. C. Bucknill, *The Care of the Insane and their Legal Control* (London, 1880), xxii.
87. J. Stallard, 'Pauper Lunatics and their Treatment', *Transactions of the National Association Promotion of Social Science*, 70 (1869), 470.
88. GBCL 43rd AR (1889).
89. GBCLS 22nd AR (1880),134.
90. Clouston, 'Lunacy Administration of Scotland'.
91. In this environment, too, recommendation for the establishment of convalescent homes for the insane poor fell on a receptive audience. See for example, the suggestions by H. Hawkins, 'A Plea for Convalescent Homes in Connection with Asylums for the Insane Poor', *Journal of Mental Science*, 16 (1871), 107–16.

92. D. Henderson, *The Evolution of Psychiatry in Scotland* (Edinburgh, 1964), 98.

CHAPTER SIX

1. M. Foucault, *Histoire de la folie à l'âge classique*, 2nd ed. (Paris, 1972). See also *idem, Discipline and Punish: The Birth of the Prison* (Harmondsworth, 1979).
2. A. Scull, *The Most Solitary of Afflictions: Madness and Society in Britain, 1700–1900* (New Haven, 1993); Scull, *Social Order/Mental Disorder* (London, 1989).
3. M. MacDonald, *Mystical Bedlam: Madness, Anxiety, and Healing in Seventeenth-Century England* (Cambridge, 1981).
4. R. Porter, *Mind-Forg'd Manacles: A History of Madness in England from the Restoration to the Regency* (London, 1987), 136–47 and 187–228. In the American context, Nancy Tomes represents this direction of research. See N. Tomes, *The Art of Asylum-Keeping: Thomas Story Kirkbride and the Origin of American Psychiatry* (Cambridge, 1984; paperback rept. with new introduction, Philadelphia, 1994).
5. R. Castel, *The Regulation of Madness: The Origin of Incarceration in France*, translated by W.D. Harris (Oxford, 1988). Y. Ripa, *Women and Madness: The Incarceration of Women in Nineteenth-Century France*, trans. by C. du Peloux Menagé (Cambridge, 1990).
6. P. E. Prestwich, 'Family Strategies and Medical Power: "Voluntary" Committal in a Parisian Asylum, 1876–1914', *Journal of Social History*, 27(1994), 799–818. This direction of investigation has been suggested by N. Tomes, 'The Anatomy of Madness: New Directions in the History of Psychiatry', *Social Studies of Science*, 17(1987), 358–71. Likewise, in the non-institutional context, Ruth Harris has perceptively shown that late nineteenth-century psychiatrists provided women with the power to redress injuries done to them by their husbands and lovers, and, at the same time, imposed on them inferior 'feminine' role. See R. Harris, *Murderers and Madness: Medicine, Law, and Society in the fin de siècle* (Oxford, 1989), 155–242.
7. E. Lunbeck, *The Psychiatric Persuasion: Knowledge, Gender and Power in Modern America* (Princeton, 1994), 96.
8. For medical penetration into the family, see J. Donzelot, *The Policing of Families*, trans. by R. Hurley (London, 1979). See also A. Suzuki, 'Framing Psychiatric Subjectivity: Doctors, Patients, and Record-Keeping at Nineteenth-Century Bethlem', in B. Forsythe and J. Melling, *Insanity, Institutions, and Society*, forthcoming.
9. For literature on the history of community care, see K. Jones,

Asylums and After: A Revised History of the Mental Health Service (London, 1993), 125–40. W. Ll. Parry-Jones, 'The Model of the Geel Lunatic Colony and Its Influence on the Nineteenth-Century Asylum System in Britain', in A. Scull (ed.) *Madhouses, Mad-Doctors, and Madmen: the Social History of Psychiatry in the Victorian Era* (London, 1981), 201–17.

10. My understanding of the public and private spheres have been shaped by the works of Jürgen Habermas and French historians of the ancien régime. See J. Habermas, *The Structural Transformation of the Public Sphere: An Inquiry into a Category of Bourgeois Society*, trans. by T. Burger (Cambridge, 1989). D. Goodman, 'Public Sphere and Private Life: Toward a Synthesis of Current Historiographical Approaches to the Old Regime', *History and Theory*, 31(1992), 1–20. Its gender connotations, which have been studied in detail by Leonore Davidoff and Catherine Hall in general and Elaine Showalter in the context of Victorian psychiatry, are largely left unexplored in this paper. See L. Davidoff and C. Hall, *Family Fortunes: Men and Women of the English Middle Class 1780–1850* (London, 1992). E. Showalter, *The Female Malady: Women, Madness and English Culture, 1830–1980* (London, 1987).

11. For the range of the power of the commission, see A. Highmore, *A Treatise on the Law of Idiocy and Lunacy* (London, 1807). J. Elmer, *An Outline of the Practice in Lunacy, under Commissions in the Nature of Writs de Lunatico Inquirendo* (London, 1844). For the outline of commission *de lunatico inquirendo*, see 'Chancery Lunatics' in D. H. Tuke (ed.) *A Dictionary of Psychological Medicine*, 2 vols. (London: J. & A. Churchill, 1892). R. Neugebauer, 'Mental Handicap in Medieval and Early Modern England', in D. Wright and A. Digby (eds) *From Idiocy to Mental Deficiency: Historical Perspectives on People with Learning Disabilities* (London, 1996), 22–43. M. MacDonald, 'Lunatics and the State in Georgian England', *Social History of Medicine*, 2(1989), 299–313. I thank Peter Bartlett for letting me consult his unpublished paper, 'Legal Madness in the Nineteenth Century'.

12. The only study which has used some reports of the commission of lunacy is P. McCandless, 'Liberty and Lunacy: the Victorians and Wrongful Confinement', in A. Scull (ed.) *Madhouses, Mad-Doctors, and Madmen*, 339–62. From 1833, two physicians and one lawyer were appointed as visitors to inspect Chancery Lunatics. Sir John Bucknill and Sir James Crichton-Brown were among the most prominent of them. See 'From Disciple to Critic: Sir John Charles Bucknill (1817–1897)', in A. Scull, C. Mackenzie, and N. Hervey, *Masters of Bedlam: Transformation of the Mad-Doctoring Trade* (Princeton,

1996), 187–225; M. Neve and T. Turner, 'What the Doctor Thought and Did: Sir James Crichton-Brown (1840–1938)', *Medical History*, 39(1995), 399–432.

13. For debates over asylumdom and alternative care systems, see Scull, *The Most Solitary of Afflictions* and Parry-Jones, 'The Model of the Geel Lunatic Colony'. For the opposition to 'home treatment' on the basis of medical-scientific convenience, see B.A. Morel, 'The Present State and Future Prospects of Psychological Medicine', *Journal of Mental Science*, 10 (1864–5), 338–42.

14. See, for example, Scull, *The Most Solitary of Afflictions*, 293–4 and 309–10. Porter, *Mind Forg'd Manacles*, 137–8. In the 1860s, a husband-hunting young woman wrote in her diary: '[Mr. West is] worth about £500–1,000 a year and expectations, but unfortunately there's madness in the family, which is rather a drawback.' A. C. Miles, *Every Girl's Duty: The Diary of a Victorian Debutante*, ed. with a Commentary by Maggy Parsons (London, 1992), 24.

15. C. MacKenzie, *Psychiatry for the Rich: A History of Ticehurst Private Asylum* (London, 1992); N. Hervey, 'Lunacy Commission 1845–1860, with Special Reference to the Implementation of Policy in Kent and Surrey', Unpublished PhD thesis, University of Bristol, 1987. For rather isolated examples of confined lunatics à la Mrs Rochester, see cases of George Smith and Brent Spencer, discussed below.

16. *The Times*, 23 Oct. 1839, p. 6, col.4. Richard Jones, a gardener to Lord Portsmouth, testified that 'I never saw any money with his lordship; he has borrowed money of me'. *A Genuine Report of the Proceedings on the Portsmouth Case, under a Commission Issued by His Majesty* (London, n.d.), 15 and 36.

17. *The Times*, 29 July 1830, p. 4, col.3. Being in a licensed house itself did not affect the person's capacity to sign contract, etc. This paradox was pointed out by William Griggs, a former-inmate of Kensington House: 'What, bring deeds to a person for his signature confined as a lunatic, and to a madhouse too? This smuggling is really too bad. . . . Now, Mr. Wright, if you are actually mad, how dare any one presume to get your signature, knowing it must be illegal; and if you are not mad, you ought to be with your family.' William Griggs, *Lunacy and Liberty. A Letter to the Lord Chancellor* (London, 1832), 12. 'Mr. Wright' in the quote above is Charles Wright, whose commission of lunacy was reported in *The Times*, 5 Dec. 1832, p. 2, col.6.

18. *The Times*, 4 July 1832, p. 6, cols.2–3.

19. *The Times*, 2 April 1841, p. 6, cols.2–3. Likewise, when John Nicholas Durand ordered six watches, each of which costs 35 and 45 guineas, under the delusion that he possessed an immense property of £20,000,000, they were not delivered, since the accompanying clerk

informed the watch-seller of his disease. *The Times*, 26 Jan. 1836, p. 7, cols.1–2.

20. *The Times*, 7 Nov. 1837, p. 6, cols.1–2.
21. *The Times*, 16 Jan. 1844, p. 5, cols.4–5.
22. *The Times*, 6 July 1832, p. 3. col.6 & p. 4, cols.1–2. Windus's advice was followed, and it was directed that 'she would not be present at the large parties without some person being present to control her conduct. After that she was very seldom present at the large parties, and never without control.'
23. For the importance of religious gathering as a public space and the ambiguity of gender distinction, see Davidoff and Hall, *Family Fortunes*, 107–48.
24. *The Times*, 16 Jan. 1844, p. 5, cols.4–5.
25. *The Times*, 9 Sept. 1841, p. 6, col.4.
26. *The Times*, 5 July 1832, p. 5, cols.4–5.
27. *The Times*, 13 Dec. 1842, p. 3, col.2.
28. *The Times*, 16 Jan. 1844, p. 5, col.4. The governess testified that 'on one occasion she ran into a cutler's shop and tied up her garter before all the young men, and would frequently do so in the street without regard to any one.' Ibid. Likewise, when the commissioners examined Sarah Eliason, an alleged lunatic, in her carriage, 'the circumstance soon attracted a crowd, who began to manifest some symptoms of a determination to know "the rights" of the matter.' *The Times*, 8 Aug. 1823, p. 2, col.5.
29. *The Times*, 27 March 1841, p. 7, col.4.
30. *The Times*, 4 Feb. 1842, p. 6, col.4.
31. The *locus classicus* of watching insane patients for entertainment and moral lesson was the Bethlem Hospital. See J. Andrews, A. Briggs, R. Porter, P. Tucker, and K. Waddington, *The History of Bethlem* (London, 1997), 178–99.
32. G.M. Burrows, *A Letter to Sir Henry Halford, Bart, K.C.H* (London, 1830), 9–10.
33. Ibid., 10.
34. *The Mysteries of the Madhouse; or Annals of Bedlam by a Discharged Officer of Twenty Years' Experience* (London, 1847), 11–12. The investigating crowd in the fiction was, however, in the end rather easily duped into believing the insanity of the man, as in the case of Davies.
35. The three-volume letter-books of Middleton are held in City of Westminster Library (WBA 796), with index compiled by G.F. Osborn in 1978. There are referred to as WCL HNMLB, with volume and page numbers.
36. Middleton to Miss Gale, 9 Oct 1816, WCL HNMLB, vol.1, 82. He

also wrote to the mother herself that he was ready to receive 'you under our roof'. Middleton to the mother, 15 Oct 1816, WCL HNMLB, vol.1, 90–91.

37. Middleton to Miss Gale, 25 Oct 1816, WCL HNMLB, vol.1, 98.

38. Middleton to Mrs Cator, 29 Oct 1816, WCL HNMLB, vol.1, 113–14.

39. Ibid., 114. John Perceval criticized exactly this kind of self-serving logic of his family, whom he had trusted at the beginning of his disease. J. Perceval, *Perceval's Narrative: a Patient's Account of His Psychosis 1830–1832*, ed. by G. Bateson (Stanford, 1961), 74 and 138, and *passim.*

40. When the mother died, she wished Sarah 'to take charge of him in the same manner as she had herself', and the father left the same request at his deathbed. The father even wished Sarah never to marry during George's life, thinking George would not live long as his health then seemed precarious. *The Times*, 7 August 1826, p. 3, cols.1–4.

41. *The Times*, 7 August 1826, p. 3, cols.1–4. One cannot exclude the possibility that all these evidences were faked to put Sarah in a favourable light and to win the case. My impression is that those evidences were more or less genuine, not least because there was no evidence put forward against the kindness of the family.

42. *The Times*, 7 August 1826, p. 3, cols.1–4. The room where George was kept was, however, the best room on the first floor of the house.

43. *The Times*, 7 August 1826, p. 3, cols.2–4.

44. *The Times*, 7 August 1826, p. 3, col.2, an extract from *The Birmingham Journal*, 11 Feb. 1826.

45. Although George Smith seems to have been relatively calm and well at the Asylum, he soon died there.

46. *The Times*, 12 August 1826, p. 3, col.3. At the beginning of the trial, it was predicted that several other actions would depend upon the result of the trial Smith v. Hodget. I could not trace the results of the other law suits related with George Smith, which might have been dropped.

47. *The Times*, 11 August 1826, p. 2, col.6 – p. 3, col.1.

48. *The Times*, 7 August 1826, p. 3, col.3; 11 August 1826, p. 3, col.2.

49. *The Times*, 7 August 1826, p. 3, col.4.

50. *The Times*, 7 August 1826, p. 3, col.3; 11 Aug 1826, p. 3, col.2. Of course, the two accounts of the scene are very different. Almost certainly the magistrates' one obviously exaggerated the alarm and hesitation of the family, while the servant's one exaggerated the kindness and integrity of the family.

51. *The Times*, 11 August 1826, p. 3, col.2.

52. *The Times*, 19 August 1844, p. 6, col.6. The commission was unoppo-

sed, but the mother was present at the examination and made some interruption during the examination, which prompted remonstrance from the commissioner.

53. *The Times*, 7 August 1826, p. 3, col.1; 11 August 1826, p. 3, col.4.
54. Even the Commissioners in Lunacy, with its power to inspect all institutionalised lunatics in England (except Bethlem Hospital, which came under Lunacy Commission's surveillance from 1852), could not obtain the power to visit single lunatics in private lodgings.
55. *The Times*, 7 August 1826, p. 3, col.1; 11 August 1826, p. 3, col.4.
56. See Highmore, *A Treatise on the Law of Idiocy and Lunacy*, 239–43; *Elmer, An Outline of the Practice in Lunacy*, 1–2.
57. The intervention into domestic affairs from outside the nuclear household was commonplace, and close neighbourly and kinship surveillance of domestic relations were fairly common, as Lawrence Stone has argued from evidences of disputes over marriage. See L. Stone, *The Road to Divorce: England 1530–1987* (Oxford, 1990).
58. Newton Fellowes, a brother of the fourth Earl of Portsmouth twice asked for commission in order to nullify the Earl's marriage and to secure his inheritance of the Earl's estate. Mr Bellamy, a brother-in-law of Rev. Edward Frank, started the commission to discontinue the Reverend's marriage with an openly adulterous wife. George Davenport's father-in-law asked for a commission to withdraw his daughter from the marriage with a man whose religious zeal seems to have been excessive. *A Genuine Report of the Proceedings on the Portsmouth Case, under a Commission Issued by His Majesty* (London, n.d.); *The Times*, 5 August 1825, p. 2, col.5; *The Times*, 10 Feb. 1838.
59. It is almost certain that their real motive was to claim their own rights to the property (of about £100,000) and to prevent the property from going to his wife and the wife's child (not Robinson's own), which Robinson himself seems to have 'desired'. *The Times*, 11 Feb 1840, p. 7, col.2; 17 Feb 1840, p. 3, col.4.
60. *The Times*, 26 Aug. 1831, p. 3, col.6; 27 Aug., p. 4, col.1; 29 Aug., p. 6, col.5; 31 Aug., p. 4, col.2; 1 Sept., p. 4, col.2; 2 Sept., p. 6, cols.2–3; 5 Sept., p. 6, col.3.
61. The commission for Lord Portsmouth in 1823, the cost was about £25,000, and that for Edward Davies in 1829 cost about £4,000, about one-fourth of the entire value of his property. *2 Hansard*, 22(1830), 1148–54; 23(1830), 547–8. See also *The Times*, 18 Dec., 1829, p. 3, cols.2–3. 'An Act to Diminish the Inconvenience and Expense of Commissions in the Nature of Writs De Lunatico Inquirendo' 3 & 4 W.IV, cap. 36. See also *3 Hansard*, 1(1831), cols.1840–43; 2(1831), 838–42; 15(1833), 550–8.

62. *The Times*, 10 Feb., 1838, p. 5, col.5.
63. *The Times*, 16 Feb., 1842, p. 6, col.6.

CHAPTER SEVEN

1. Andrew Scull, *The Most Solitary of Afflictions: Madness and Society in Britain, 1700–1900* (New Haven, 1993) (first published as *Museums of Madness* 1979); W.F. Bynum and Roy Porter, see, amongst others, *The Anatomy of Madness* (3 vols) (London, 1985–87) and Elaine Showalter, *The Female Malady: Women, Madness and English Culture, 1830–1980* (London, 1987).

2. See for example Charlotte MacKenzie, 'Social Factors in the Admission, Discharge, and Continuing Stay of Patients at Ticehurst Asylum, 1845–1917' in W.F. Bynum, Roy Porter, and Michael Shepherd (eds) *The Anatomy of Madness: Essays in the History of Psychiatry, vol.2* (London, 1986); Patricia Prestwich, 'Family Strategies and Medical Power: 'Voluntary' Committal in a Parisian Asylum, 1876–1914', *Journal of Social History* 27 (1994) or Dennise Jodelet, *Madness and Social Representations: Living with the Mad in One French Community* (Exeter, 1991).

3. The asylum originally served the counties of Galway, Roscommon, Sligo, Leitrim and Mayo. In 1855 a new asylum was built at Sligo which took the patients of that county along with those from Leitrim, and in 1866 another such institution opened at Castlebar, for the Mayo patients.

4. Scull, *Solitary of Afflictions* p. 1.

5. *Commissioners for Inquiring into the Condition of the Poorer Classes in Ireland, First Report*, 1835 (369) XXXII, 1.

6. Mel Cousins, *The Irish Social Welfare System: Law and Social Policy* (Dublin, 1995),13.

7. In 1836, the Commissioners' Report on Irish Poverty had recommended that asylums be brought under the direct control of the Poor Law Commissioners, but this advice was rejected on the grounds that the insane required specialist attention. Thus the Irish Poor Law System, formed by the Poor Relief Act of 1838, made no specific provision for lunatics. In that same year however (1838) the so-called 'Dangerous Lunatics' Act' was passed (se below) which, in contrast to other British lunacy legislation, linked the prison and asylum systems together under the control of the Lord Lieutenant's Office.

8. Ruth Barrington, *Health, Medicine and Politics in Ireland, 1900–1970* (Dublin, 1987), 5.

9. The role of the Lord Lieutenant is crucial to an understanding of governmental attitudes towards the asylums. In nineteenth century

Ireland, in direct contrast to the decentralising process in local government in England, local power bases were consistently undermined. Because of broader political tensions, there was a desire to centralise power as far as possible, so that the Boards of Governors in each asylum (drawn in Ballinasloe mainly from the local landowing gentry and business community, and solely Protestant) simply implemented decrees from Dublin.

10. Quoted in Helen Burke, *The People and the Poor Law in 19th Century Ireland* (Dublin, 1987), 2.
11. Joseph Robins, *Fools and Mad: A History of the Insane in Ireland* (Dublin, 1986), 72.
12. Ibid.
13. I Vic. Cap xxvii, 1838.
14. Minutes of the Board of Guardians, Connaught District Lunatic Asylum, November 26, 1833.
15. Ibid, Jan. 24, 1834.
16. Ibid, Feb. 25, 1834.
17. Ibid, May 7, 1835.
18. Ibid, July 3, 1835.
19. Ibid.
20. Sixteenth Report on the District, Criminal and Private Lunatic Asylums in Ireland, Dublin, 1867.
21. Fifteenth Report, 15.
22. For some inmates at least, residence in the asylum was favoured over the workhouse, despite a certain stigma attaching itself to lunacy. Robins, *Fools and Mad*, 110.
23. Sixteenth Report, p. 35.
24. Mark Finnane, *Insanity and the Insane in Post-Famine Ireland* (London, 1981) p. 27.
25. Nineteenth Report, p. 5.
26. Ibid, 30–1.
27. Twenty-third Report, 88–9.
28. There were 1,084 beds at Ballinasloe, 419 at Castlebar, and 636 at Sligo.
29. Account Book, Connaught District Lunatic Asylum, year ending 31 March 1846.
30. Committal Warrants for 1879, Ballinasloe Asylum.
31. David Wright, 'Getting Out of the Asylum: Understanding the Confinement of the Insane in the Nineteenth Century', *Social History of Medicine*, 10:1, (1997), 137–55.
32. The Great Famine of 1845–50 was responsible for greatly accelerated emigration from Ireland, in addition to population decline through famine-related mortality. Ireland was a 'demographic freak' in nine-

teenth century Europe, with a population decline of 45 per cent between 1841 and 1901 – a loss of almost four million people. Barrington, *Health, Medicine and Politics*, 2.

33. A series of Land Acts at the end of the nineteenth century saw the large-scale transfer of property from landlords to their tenants.

34. Male Case Book, no. 3376, 67.

35. This runs contrary to the official perspective of the hospital authorities. Concerned at the large increase in the asylum population, the government commissioned a report on 'the alleged Increasing Prevalence of Insanity in Ireland'. The opinion of the RMS at Ballinasloe was that 'The question of heredity as a cause comes so frequently before us that there can be no doubt of its being a very general cause of insanity in this district', 189.

36. No. 3315, 29

37. Changes in the system of Irish land inheritance after the Great Famine of 1845–1850 meant that the family farm now generally passed in the male line. As such, it was largely among the male patients that apparent cases of wrongful incarceration in order to gain property occurred. One interesting female instance at Ballinasloe is to be found not among the asylum records themselves, but in fiction. Edith Somerville and Martin Ross (authors of the *Irish R.M.*) wrote *The Real Charlotte* in 1894, a novel of overwhelming ambition. The titular heroine, Charlotte Mullen, has designs on amongst other things, the house and land of Julia Duffy, a minor Ascendancy character. Knowing Julia to be physically weak, Charlotte goads her into undertaking a journey in midsummer to plead with her landlord, precipitating a collapse which allows Charlotte to 'have her removed to Ballinasloe asylum' There, in common with the majority of real-life single patients in the 1890s, she died.

38. No. 3353, 54.

39. No. 3282, 10

40. All quotes taken from case notes.

41. No. 3413, 91

42. 3286, 13.

43. Ibid, April 16, 1901

44. Ibid, September 11, 1901.

45. 'Complains of not being let out but very doubtfully anxious to go: Has no plans for the future and would probably be at once back in if let out.' May 31, 1904.

46. Correspondence with the asylum authorities reveals a good deal regarding the attitudes of relatives. For analysis of letters in Canada and America see Mary-Ellen Kelm, 'Women, Families and the Provincial Hospital for the Insane, British Columbia, 1905–1915', *Journal*

of Family History, 19 (1994), 177–193, and Nancy Tomes, *A Generous Confidence: Thomas Story Kirkbride and the Art of Asylum-Keeping, 1840–1883* (Cambridge, 1985), 92–103.

47. Case no. 3347, 49.
48. Yannick Ripa, *Women and Madness: the Incarceration of Women in Nineteenth-Century France* (Cambridge, 1990), 3.
49. Section 10 of the 30 and 31 Vic., c. 118 (1867). In 1894, 'the Irish Court of Appeal ruled that there was no absolute right of a relative or friend to remove a lunatic from an asylum' (Finnane *Insanity and the Insane*, 120).
50. Case no. 3507, 141.
51. Case no. 3415, 92.
52. Case no. 3347, 49. He had worked as a clerk in Dublin for two years.
53. Case no. 3306, 23.
54. See for example case nos. 3348 and 2789. All official business in the asylum was conducted through English, including the assessments of patients, despite the fact that the west of Ireland had a high cocentration of monoglot Irish speakers throughout the nineteenth century. The nurses acted as interpreters for the physician and other senior staff, few of whom spoke Irish.
55. Case no. 2964, 13.
56. Verbal abuse, from the fishmongers at Billingsgate market.
57. Case no.3348, 51.
58. No.3353, 54.
59. No.3281, 9.
60. No. 3385, 74.

CHAPTER EIGHT

1. J. Walton, 'Casting out and bringing back in Victorian England: Pauper Lunatics, 1840–1870' in W. Bynum, R. Porter, M. Shepherd (eds) *The Anatomy of Madness: Essays in the History of Psychiatry Vol. 2 Institutions and Society* (London, 1985), 132–46. D. Wright, 'Getting Out of the Asylum: Understanding the Confinement of the Insane in the Nineteenth Century', *Social History of Medicine* 10 (1) (1997), 137–55. 'The Discharge of Pauper Lunatics from County Asylums in mid-Victorian England' in J. Melling and B. Forsythe (eds) *Accommodating Madness: Insanity, institutions and society*, forthcoming.
2. L. Smith, 'The County Asylum in the Mixed Economy of Care, 1808–48' in Melling and Forsythe, *Accommodating Madness*, forthcoming. A. Suzuki, 'Lunacy in Seventeenth and Eighteenth-Century England: Analysis of Quarter Session Records' *History of Psychiatry*,

2 (1991), 437–57 and 3 (1992), 29–44, provides an illuminating discussion of the role of family in relation to the institutions of the old Poor Law and the legal system, see particularly 439–51.

3. R. Wall, 'Historical Developments of the Household in Europe' in E. van Imhoff, A. Kuijsten, P. Hooimeijer and L. van Wissen (eds) *Household Demography and Household Modelling* (New York, 1995), particularly 36–7, 46–7, for example.

4. J. Walton, 'Lunacy in the Industrial Revolution: A Study of Asylum Admissions in Lancashire, 1848–50' *Journal of Social History*, 13 (1979), 6–7, 18–19 and *passim*. Walton was particularly concerned to redress the exaggerated emphasis on calculative family behaviour which he found in M. Anderson, *Family Structure in Nineteenth-Century Lancashire* Cambridge University Press (1971) Cambridge, as well as the analogous perspective on family tolerance which was provided by A. Scull, *Museums of Madness: The Social Organization of Insanity in Nineteenth-Century England* (London, 1979).

5. See the essays gathered in P. Horden and R. Smith (eds) *The Locus of Care* (London, 1998) for a recent summation of such scholarship. Also A. Beveridge, 'Madness in Victorian Edinburgh: A Study of Patients Admitted to the Royal Edinburgh Asylum under Thomas Clouston, 1873–1908: Part I' *History of Psychiatry* 4 (1995), 21–54, especially 28–38 for an analysis of socio-demographic characteristics of admissions to a Scottish institution and J. Andrews, 'Raising the tone of asylumdom' in Melling and Forsythe (eds) *Accommodating Madness*, forthcoming, for Glasgow.

6. G.N. Grob, 'The Social History of Medicine and Disease in America' *Journal of Social History*, 10 (1977), 391–409. C.M. McGovern, 'The Community, the Hospital, and the Working Class Patient: the Multiple Uses of Asylum in Nineteenth-Century America' *Pennsylvania History*, (1987), 17–33, especially 26–9. A. Scull, 'Psychiatry and Social Control in the Nineteenth and Twentieth Centuries' *History of Psychiatry* 2, (1991), 149–69, especially 156–61.

7. R. Smith, 'Charity, Self-interest and Welfare: Reflections from Demographic and Family History' in Daunton (ed.) *Charity, Self-interest and Welfare in the English Past* (London, 1996), 23–4, 27 and *passim* follows Blaug, Sokoll and Laslett and others in challenging this image of the care systems developed around the nineteenth-century Poor Law. See also B. Reay, 'Kinship and Neighbourhood in Nineteenth-Century Rural England: the Myth of the Autonomous Nuclear Family' *Journal of Family History* 21, 1 (1996), 87–104, provides an excellent analysis of the micro-history of family kinship networks and the utilisation of Poor Law resources. Wright, 'Getting out', similarly

argues for a long-term perspective on the development of lunatic asylums.

8. S. King, 'Reconstructing Lives: the Poor, the Poor Law and Welfare in Calverley, 1650–1820' *Social History*, 22 (3, (1997), 318–38, and especially 319–23, offers a more critical view of the old Poor Law than that given by Smith and many other demographic historians. King's suggestion that the northern counties experienced a much more Spartan pauper regime than those found in the south of England may weaken Smith's assumption that welfare provisions meet popular demand.

9. R. Adair, J. Melling and B. Forsythe, 'Migration, Family Structure and Pauper Lunacy in Victorian England: Admissions to the Devon County Pauper Lunatic Asylum, 1845–1900', *Continuity and Change* 12 (3), (1998) 373–401.

10. M. Strathern, 'The Place of Kinship: Kin, Class and Village Status in Elmdon, Essex' in A.P. Cohen (ed.) *Belonging: Identity and Social Organisation in British Rural Cultures*, (Manchester, 1982) 72–100, particularly 74–8, remains a stimulating anthropological account which provided the companion study to J. Robin's classic *Elmdon: Continuity and Change in a North-west Essex Village, 1861–1964* (Cambridge, 1980).

11. M. Foucault, *Madness and Civilisation: A History of Insanity in the Age of Reason* (New York, 1985).

12. P. Bartlett, 'The Poor Law of Lunacy: The Admission of Pauper Lunatics in Mid-Nineteenth Century England with Special Reference to Leicestershire and Rutland', (unpublished PhD thesis, University College, London, 1993). D. Garland, *Punishment and Welfare: A History of Penal Strategies*, (Aldershot, 1985) which is critically assessed and adapted in M. Thomson, 'Sterilisation, Segregation and Community Care: Ideology and Solutions to the Problem of Mental Deficiency in Inter-war Britain' *History of Psychiatry* 3, (1993), 473–98, particularly 475–85.

13. N. Finzsch and R. Jutte (eds) *Institutions of Confinement: Hospitals, Asylums and Prisons in Western Europe and North America, 1500–1950* (Cambridge, 1996), including the essays by Finzsch, Dinges and Wetzell. See A. de Swaan, *In Care of the State: Health Care, Education and Welfare in Europe and the United States in the Modern Period* (Cambridge, 1988) for an attempt to historicise rational choice models of welfare development by the application of the Elias methodology to poor law and other social reforms.

14. Bartlett, 'The Poor Law'; R. Smith, *Trial by Medicine: Insanity and Irresponsibility in Victorian Trials*, (Edinburgh, 1981).

15. Suzuki, 'Lunacy in Seventeenth and Eighteenth-century England',

provides an illuminating example of how fragmentary legal sources might be deployed to cast light on motivation as well as the charges incurred by the parishes for the maintenance of the insane.

16. J. Melling, R. Adair and B. Forsythe, '"A Proper Lunatic for Two Years": Pauper Lunatic Children in Victorian and Edwardian England. Child admissions to the Devon County Asylum, 1845–1914', *Journal of Social History*, 30 (2) (1997), 371–405.

17. R. Porter, *Mind-Forg'd Manacles: A History of Madness in England from the Restoration to the Regency* (Harmondsworth, 1990), 229. Suzuki, 'Lunacy in the Seventeenth and Eighteenth-century . . . Part I', 437–9 provides a comment on this point.

18. For the history of the Devon Asylum and Bucknill in its early years, L. Brizendine, 'British Psychiatric Reform 1830–1860: A Socio-historical Study of Devon County Lunatic Asylum and John Charles Bucknill', unpublished D.Med. thesis, Yale University, 1981.

19. 8 and 9 Vict. Cap. 126, 16 and 17 Vict. Cap. 97, 53 Vict cap. 5

20. 4 and 5 William 4 cap. 76

21. R. Adair, B. Forsythe and J. Melling, 'A Danger to the Public? Disposing of the Pauper Lunatic in Victorian and Edwardian England: the Exminster Asylum, 1845–1914' *Medical History*, 42 (1998), 1–25, provides an assessment based on Plympton St Mary, where we calculate that between 22 and 29 per cent of admissions to the Devon Asylum originated in the Union workhouse.

22. N. Walker and S. McCabe, *Crime and Insanity in England. Volume 2: New Solutions and New Problems* (Edinburgh, 1973), 9.

23. Report of the Commission Appointed by the Secretary of State For The Home Department To Inquire Into The Subject of Criminal Lunacy PP 1882 vol. xxxii, 11

24. Fourteenth Annual Report Lunacy Commission, PP 1860 vol. xxxiv, 105; *46th Annual Report Lunacy Commission* PP 1892 vol. xl, 140–1

25. In 1909 the charge was fourteen shillings per week, for example.

26. A. Scull, C. Mackenzie and N. Hervey, *Masters of Bedlam: The Transformation of the Mad-doctoring Trade*, (Princeton, 1996) is illustrated by the most famous of all criminal lunatic celebrities, Richard Dadd, whose portrait of the noted psychiatrist Morison is set against a dramatic landscape portraying a barred asylum.

27. A. Suzuki, 'Framing Psychiatric Subjectivity: Doctor, Patient, and Record-keeping in Bethlem in the Nineteenth Century' in Melling and Forsythe, *Institutions*, argues for a decisive appropriation of this form of detective role by psychiatrists in general cases at Bethlem in the 1850s.

28. Bucknill, *Journal of Mental Science*, 16 (1856), 252–3.

29. Bucknill, *Journal of Mental Science*, 16 (1856) 245–53.

30. Smith, *Trial By Medicine*, 123.

31. 5th Annual Report Lunacy Commission PP 1850 vol.xxiii, 17

32. J. Saunders, 'Institutionalised Offenders: A Study of the Victorian Institution and its Inmates with Special Reference to Late Nineteenth-century Warwickshire', (unpublished PhD thesis, University of Warwick, 1983, 248–50.

33. 43rd Annual Report Lunacy Commission PP 1889 vol. xxxviii.

34. Subject of course to the supply-side constraints in provision which asylums themselves often faced within a couple of decades of opening. If Broadmoor filled to capacity and if the offence was not regarded as particularly heinous then an individual might well be directed to a county asylum such as Exminster.

35. Devon record Office [hereafter DRO] 3769a/ H9 cases 2217, 2218, 4337.

36. DRO 3769a/H9 case 2233

37. DRO 3769a/ H9 case 442

38. DRO 3769a/ H9/1 case 443

39. Care of Lunatics Who Are Paupers Or Criminals Act 1808 48 Geo. 3 c. 96 s. xxvii

40. DRO Axminster Guardians Minute Books 27 September 1844, 11 July 1845.

41. Insane Prisoners Act 3 and 4 Vict. c. 54 s. 2.

42. DRO Axminster Guardians 3 June 1880.

43. DRO St. Thomas Guardians 5 December 1856.

44. DRO St. Thomas Guardians Minute Books 21 October 1859.

45. Criminal Lunatics Act 1884 47 and 48 Vict. c. 64 s. 10.

46. A. Scull, *The Most Solitary of Afflictions*, 1; also J. Walton, 'Casting Out and Bringing Back', especially 133–8.

47. R. Smith, 'Charity, Self-interest and Welfare', pp. 23–4, 27–8. P. Horden and R. Smith, 'Introduction' to *The Locus of Care* (London, 1998); cf. Hunt, 'Paupers and Pensioners', 407–30 and King, 'Reconstructing Lives', 318–38, especially 320. King stresses the importance of alternatives to 'harsh communal welfare', particularly kinship ties.

48. L.J. Ray, 'Models of Madness in Victorian Asylum Practice', *European Journal of Sociology*, 22 (1981), 30–2 and *passim*, for example, provides a critical response to the bleak images of incarceration offered by Scull but also argues that eugenicist ideology provided the asylum superintendents with the professional rationale for mere warehousing large numbers of the insane.

49. R. Hodgkinson, *The Origins of the National Health Service: The Medical Services of the New Poor Law* (London, 1967), 164, 179, 578.

50. 8th Annual Report Lunacy Commission PP 1854 vol. xxix pp. 38–9.

51. N. Hervey, 'The Lunacy Commission 1845–1860: with special refer-

ence to the implementation of policy in Kent and Surrey', (unpublished PhD thesis, University of Bristol, 1987), 269.

52. Devon Quarter Sessions Minute Book 1/30 Epiphany Sessions 1852, 488.

53. J. Bucknill, *Journal of Mental Science*, 15 (1855) 116, 120.

54. C.A. Conley, *The Unwritten Law: Criminal Justice in Victorian Kent*, (Oxford, 1991) 68–135, offers a methodology for deriving evidence of such abuse by inference from legal and other sources.

55. DRO EAC 3769a H9 case 4258 admitted 1872.

56. DRO EAC 3769a H9/1 case 494 admitted 1848.

57. DRO EAC 3769a/H9 case 4903 admitted 1876.

58. DRO EAC 3769a/ H9 case 4293 admitted 1872, for example.

59. DRO Devon County Pauper Lunatic Asylum Visiting Justices' Minute Book Devon Quarter Sessions 147/1 2nd May 1854.

60. DRO EAC 3769a H9/1 case 431 Jane M. aged six, admitted 1847; case 441 Giles H. aged twelve, admitted 1847.

61. J. Melling *et al.*, ' 'A Proper Lunatic for Two Years', 371–405.

62. DRO EAC 3769a/H9 case 4955 admitted 1876.

63. DRO EAC 3769a H9/1 case 526 admitted 1848.

64. DRO Quarter Sessions Minute Book 1/30, 1852 Epiphany Sessions.

65. DRO Medical Cases Book: Admissions 3769a/ H9/8 case 8115.

66. Brizendine, 'British Psychiatric Reform 1830–1860', 56–7.

67. DRO Annual Report Visitors and Medical Officer 1854 DQS 117/5.

68. 30th Annual Report of the Lunacy Commission PP 1876 vol xxxiii, 77.

69. DRO Devon County Lunatic Asylum Visiting Justices' Minute Book Quarter Sessions 147/1 5 August 1845, 27 October 1845.

70. 49th Annual Report of the Lunacy Commission, PP 1895 vol. liv p. 221.

71. 19th Annual Report of the Lunacy Commission, PP 1865 vol. xxi pp. 41–2.

72. Melling *et al.*, "A Proper Lunatic", for Barnstaple cases.

73. Wright, 'Getting out', for a literature review.

74. Adair *et al.*, 'Migration, Family structure'.

75. J.C. Bucknill and D.H. Tuke *A Manual of Psychological Medicine*, (Philadelphia,1858), 267–8 for discussions of medico-legal aspects of insanity and also 322–3 for hereditarianism; C. Mackenzie, *Psychiatry for the Rich: A History of Private Ticehurst Asylum 1792–1917* (London, 1992), 19–20, for more affluent classes. Psychiatrists were able to use the implication of hereditarian infection to discredit the unwelcome testimony of family members, see Scull, 'Psychiatry and Social Control', 160–2.

76. Strathern, 'Elmdon', 85, for attitudes expressed in the 1950s-60s.

77. DRO EAC 3769a H9/1 case 429 admitted 1847.
78. DRO EAC 3769a/H9 cases 4351[admitted 1872], 4362 [admitted 1872], 4430 [admitted 1873]. Includes the case of the epileptic John R. aged seven who was reported to have slashed at village children before being sent to Exminster.
79. DRO Exminster Admissions Certificates hereafter EAC 3769a H9 case 471 admitted 1847.
80. DRO EAC case 2251 admitted 1860.
81. DRO EAC cases 2308, 4885 admitted 1861 and 1876 respectively.
82. DRO EAC 3769a H9 case 4260 admitted 1872.
83. DRO EAC 3769a H9 case 5038 admitted 1877.
84. DRO EAC 3769a H9 case 9856 admitted 1902.
85. DRO EAC 3769a H9/1 case 450 admitted 1847
86. DRO EAC 3769a/ H9 case 10047 admitted 1903.
87. DRO EAC 3769a H9/1 case 72 admitted 1845, case 416 admitted 1847.
88. DRO EAC 3769a/ H9 cases 4827 admitted 1875, 5055 admitted 1877.
89. DRO EAC cases 2362 admitted 1861, 2261.
90. DRO EAC 3769a H9/1 case 512 admitted 1848.
91. DRO EAC 3769a /H9 cases 2365 admitted 1861, 4309 admitted 1872 respectively.
92. Select Committee of The House of Commons on the Lunacy Laws P.P., 1877, vol.xiii, 91, evidence of J. Bucknill.
93. As we have noted, solitary householders in fact formed a disproportionately small number of those admitted to the Devon Asylum.
94. Bucknill and Tuke *A Manual of Psychological Medicine*, 525.
95. DRO EAC 3769a / H9 case 473 admitted 1847.
96. DRO Devon County Pauper Lunatic Asylum Visiting Justices' Minute Book Devon Quarter Sessions 147/6 1 November 1904, 134.
97. DRO EAC 3769a /H9 case 4316 admitted 1872.
98. DRO EAC 3769a/ H9 case 9802 admitted 1902.
99. DRO St. Thomas General Committee Minute Book 1836–1842 Book, 29 August 17 1841.
100. DRO Okehampton Board of Guardians Minute Books 7 January 1865.
101. DRO Exeter Corporation of the Poor Minute Books, 16 January 1866.
102. DRO Axminster Board of Guardians Minute Books 28 November 1851, 17 July 1902.
103. DRO EAC 3769a H9/1 case 498 admitted 1848; DRO St. Thomas Board of Guardians 16 March 1888.
104. EAC DRO 3769a/ H9 case 8170 admitted 1894.
105. DRO EAC 3769a H9/1 case 469 admitted 1847, for John W. who had

been passed over in the election as pastor for his chapel; and case 447 admitted 1847, Charlotte H. who was servant to a minister and talked 'long and enthusiastically on religious topics' prior to attacks of bitter depression. William W., case 472 admitted 1846, was likewise 'unhappy in mind and depressed in spirit . . . and is discontented with his life.'

CHAPTER NINE

1. See for example A. Alaszewski, *Institutional Care and the Mentally Handicapped: The Mental Handicap Hospital* (London, 1986); J. Ryan and F. Thomas, *The Politics of Mental Handicap* (London, 1990); M. Potts and R. Fido, *A Fit Person to be Removed* (Plymouth, 1991).

2. See, for example, M. Thomson, 'Family, Community and State: the Mirco Politics of Mental Deficiency' in A. Digby and D. Wright (eds) *From Idiocy to Mental Deficiency* (London, 1996)

3. See J. Collins, *The Resettlement Game* (London, 1993), J. Sinson, *Group Homes and Integration of Developmentally Disabled People* (London, 1993)

4. See J. Finch, 'Community Care: Developing non-sexist alternatives', *Critical Social Policy*, 9 (1984), 7–18.

5. M. Thomson ,'The Problem of Mental Deficiency in England and Wales 1913–1946' Unpublished D.Phil. Thesis, University of Oxford, 1992.

6. A Note on Terminology: the question of what terminology to use is a difficult one. Few groups can have had as many labels as people who are now labelled as having a learning disability. In this chapter we use contemporary labels, such as idiot, imbecile, mental defective, for historical accuracy. However, we are aware that many people with learning disabilities find these labels offensive and we therefore use quotation marks to indicate their historical specificity.

7. A.F. Tredgold, *A Text Book of Mental Deficiency* (amentia) 7th edition 1947, 442.

8. A.F. Tredgold's standard text book *Mental Deficiency* was first published in 1908. It went into eight editions, and was in use in mental handicap nursing courses as late as the 1970s. Tredgold had himself given evidence to the Royal Commission, and was firmly committed to controlling heredity of 'psychopathic and inefficient stocks'. The information in this paragraph is taken from 470–81 of the 7th edition.

9. Report of Royal Commission on the Feeble Minded 1908 vol. viii,

10. Quoted in G. Jones *Social Hygiene in Twentieth Century Britain* (London, 1986).

11. Idem., 33.

12. Mental Deficiency Committee (Wood Report), Part 3: The Adult Defective (HMSO, 1929) p. 71.

13. F.C. Shrubsall and A.C. Williams 'Mental Deficiency Practice', 1932, 177.

14. Idem., 445.

15. The National Association for the Care and Control of the Feeble Minded was reconstituted as the Central Association for Mental Welfare as a result of provisions of the 1913 Act. The Act allowed for local voluntary committees to ascertain the existence of mental defectives, and refer them to the statutory authorities for certification and classification. The CAMW published a journal *Studies in Mental Inefficiency*, later entitled *Mental Welfare*,

16. Figures extracted from Annual Reports of Board of Control, presented in Tredgold, *Mental Deficiency*, 488.

17. Figures quoted in Tredgold, *Mental Deficiency*, 482.

18. Lewis was a member of the Eugenics Society and it was a considerable coup for the Society that its members were so well represented. The Report's findings were strongly influenced by eugenic ideas.

19. See for example Caradog Jones *Social Survey of Merseyside* begun in 1929 and published in 1934, Tomlinson's *Investigation into Social Problem families in Luton* (Luton, 1947).

20. Report of the Interdepartmental Committee on Mental Deficiency Part IV 'Investigation into the incidence of Mental Deficiency in six areas' 1925–27 by E.O. Lewis MA.

21. See, for example, Pat Thane, *Origins of the Welfare State* (London, 1982); Fiona Williams, *Social Policy: A Critical Introduction* (Cambridge, 1989); Anne Digby, *British Welfare Policy: Workhouse to Workforce* (London, 1989).

22. See, for example, Bulmer 1987, Alaszewski 1991, Lewis 1994.

23. Walker 1996, 205.

24. R. Means and R. Smith, *Community Care: Policy and Practice* (London, 1994) pp. 2 and 3.

25. Peter Rushton, 'Idiocy, the Family and the Community in Early Modern North East England' in David Wright and Anne Digby (eds) *From Idiocy to Mental Deficiency*, 44–64.

26. Jonathan Andrews 'Identifying and providing for the mentally disabled in early modern London' in Wright and Digby, *From Idiocy to Mental Deficiency*, 65–92.

27. Ibid., 74.

28. Oonagh Walsh, 'Madness and Society in 19th Century Ireland', unpublished paper, 1997; Lorraine Walsh, 'The Role of Charity within the Development of the Early 19th Century Scottish Institutions for the Insane – Dundee Royal Lunatic Asylum', unpublished paper,

1997; David Wright, 'The National Asylum for Idiots, Earlswood, 1847–1886', unpublished D.Phil. thesis, University of Oxford, 1993; Janet Saunders, 'Quarantining the Weak-Minded: Psychiatric Definitions of Degeneracy and the Late-Victoria Asylum' in *The Anatomy of Madness. Essays in the History of Psychiatry, Vol. 3.*

29. Mathew Thomson 'Family, Community and State: the Micropolitics of Mental Deficiency' in Wright and Digby, *From Idiocy to Mental Deficiency*, 207–30.

30. E. Fox, 'Community Schemes for the Social Control of Mental Defectives', *Mental Welfare*, 21 (1930), 71.

31. See, for example, Walmsley's account of the implementation of the Mental Deficiency Acts in Bedfordshire, in Dorothy Atkinson, Mark Jackson and Jan Walmsley (eds) *Forgotten Lives*, (Kidderminster, 1997).

32. Most of the findings presented here have been put together from records in the Buckinghamshire and Somerset County Record Offices, as well as national collections in the Public Record Office and Wellcome Institute. As Thomson's work indicates, the preservation of records relating to mental deficiency has been somewhat ad hoc. Some CROs have extensive collections, others, such as the London Metropolitan Archives, have the legacy of decisions made by past archivists – in London's case just 55 case files. Where records exist there are problems of access and confidentiality. The recording practices of past Clerks to Mental Deficiency Committees were uninformed by modern ideas about confidentiality, hence minutes and other official papers are littered with names, addresses and other details which make the subjects readily identifiable. Further, some CROs also have collections of correspondence about individuals deemed 'subject to be dealt with' under the 1913 Act. These are if anything more informative than the official minutes, but raise further problems relating to confidentiality. We are grateful to the archivists concerned that they have accepted our affirmations that we will respect the spirit of the law relating to access to medical or personal records, and hence we have altered any details which might make individuals known to a wide readership.

33. Board of Control 12th Annual Report 1925. Somerset also had the third highest ascertainment rate of all Local Authorities in that year.

34. More information appertaining to Somerset will be found in Dorothy Atkinson 'Learning from Local History: Evidence from Somerset' in Atkinson *et al.* (eds) *Forgotten Lives: Exploring the History of Learning Disability* (Kidderminster, 1997).

35. Report on the Care of Idiots (1900) Somerset Boards of Guardians.

36. Somerset CRO, letter dated 19th May 1900.

37. South Western Counties' Association for the Care of the Feeble minded 'Appeal for funds to establish a feeble minded colony', 1912.
38. Ibid., 113.
39. Ibid., 114.
40. Ibid. p. 111.
41. 1926 Conference of the Central Association for Mental Welfare: from the opening address of the chairman, Sir Leslie Scott.
42. Somerset Mental Deficiency Committee Minutes, May 1920 Somerset CRO.
43. Ruth Darwin: 'The Proper Care of Defectives Outside Institutions': conference paper at the 1926 Conference on Mental Welfare.
44. Board of Control Annual Report 1926.
45. Somerset CRO: Mental Deficiency Sub Committee Report 1927.
46. Somerset CRO Mental Deficiency Sub Committee Report 1927.
47. Ibid.
48. Somerset Association for Mental Welfare 13th Annual Report. 1927 Somerset CRO.
49. Somerset Association for Mental Welfare 13th Annual Report 1927, Somerset CRO.
50. 'Mental Defectives on Licence', Report of the Executive Sub Committee of the Somerset Mental Deficiency Committee, June 1925 Somerset CRO.
51. Bucks CRO, Bucks Voluntary Association for the Care of the Mentally Defective Minute Book Vol. 1.
52. Bucks CRO, Bucks Voluntary Association for the Care of the Mental Defective Minute Book Vol. 3.
53. Bucks CRO Report of VAMD AGM in Bucks Herald 21/4/1935.
54. Bucks CRO Annual Reports of Bucks VAMD 1924, 1925.
55. Bucks CRO Report of 1935 AGM of VAMD, Bucks Herald 21/4/ 1935.
56. Bucks VAMD Minute Book Volume 1 Report of half yearly meeting of General Committee 21/10/1919.
57. Bucks CRO Minutes of Bucks VAMD Vol. 1 19/9/1916.
58. Unlike Somerset, Bucks was late in setting up its own colony Before that time a good deal of energy had to be expended in finding beds for certified defectives.
59. Bucks CRO VAMD Minute Book Vol. 2 21/10/1919.
60. Bucks CRO Bucks VAMD Annual Report 1923.
61. Bucks CRO VAMD Minute Book Vol. 4 Feb. 1923.
62. Bucks CRO VAMD Minute Book Vol. 1 16/10/1917.
63. Bucks CRO VAMD Minute Book Vol. 1 21/10/1919.
64. Bucks CRO VAMD Minute Book Vol. 3 April 1925.

65. S. Rolph, *The History of Community Care for People with Learning Difficulties in Norfolk.*

66. M. Thomson, 'The Problem of Mental Deficiency in England and Wales, 1913–46', unpublished D.Phil. Thesis, University of Oxford, 148.

CHAPTER TEN

I would like to thank the Wellcome Trust for funding this research (project grant 038059/Z/93) and the participants of a conference at the University of Exeter where an earlier draft was given as a paper.

1. Caring for People: Community Care in the Next Decade and Beyond, (Cmd. 849, London, 1989), 3, 4, 13, paras. 1.1, 1.9, 2.21.

2. A. Walker (ed.) *Community Care: The Family, the State and Social Policy* (Oxford, 1982); G. Parker, *With Due Care and Attention: A Review of Research on Informal Care* (London, 1990); R. Means and R. Smith, *Community Care: Policy and Practice* (London, 1994), 17–45.

3. J. Finch and D. Groves, 'Community Care and the Family – A Case for Equal Opportunities?', *Journal of Social Policy*, 9:4 (1980), 487–511; R. Parker, 'Elderly People and Community Care: The Policy Background', in I. Sinclair *et al.* (eds) *The Kaleidoscope of Care: A Review of Research on Welfare Provision for Elderly People* (London, 1990), 5–22.

4. J. Lewis and H. Glennerster, *Implementing the new Community Care* (Buckingham, 1996).

5. K. Jones, *Mental Health and Social Policy, 1845–1959* (London, 1960), 178–203.

6. A. T. Scull, *Decarceration: Community Treatment and the Deviant – A Radical View* (Englewood Cliffs, 1977, second edn., 1984), 135–53; V. Navarro, *Class Struggle, The State and Medicine: An Historical and Contemporary Analysis of the Medical Sector in Great Britain* (Oxford, 1978), 138–40.

7. P Sedgwick, *Psycho Politics* (London, 1982), 192–4; J. Busfield, *Managing Madness: Changing Ideas and Practice* (London, 1986), 326–30. See also K. Jones, *Asylums and After: A Revised History of the Mental Health Services: From the Early 18th Century to the 1990s* (London, 1993), 148–56.

8. C. Webster, *The Health Services Since the War: Volume 1: Problems of Health Care: The National Health Service Before 1957* (London, 1988), 222; C. Webster, *The Health Services Since the War: Volume 2: Government and Health Care. The National Health Service 1958–1979*

(London, 1996); C. Unsworth, *The Politics of Mental Health Legislation* (Oxford, 1987).

9. H. Freeman, 'Mental Health Services in an English County Borough Before 1974', *Medical History*, 28 (1984), 111–28.

10. C. Ham, *Policy-Making in the National Health Service: A Case Study of the Leeds Regional Hospital Board* (London, 1981).

11. M. Thomson, 'Social Policy and the Management of the Problem of Mental Deficiency in Inter-War London', *London Journal*, 18: 2 (1993), 129–42.

12. See for example, R. Porter, 'Madness and its Institutions', in A. Wear (ed.) *Medicine and Society: Historical Essays* (Cambridge, 1992), 277–301.

13. 3 & 4 Geo. V, Mental Deficiency Act, 1913, ch. 28, Part II, Section 30; 17 & 18 Geo. V, Mental Deficiency Act, 1927, ch. 33; Jones, *Mental Health and Social Policy, 1845–1959*, 70–80.

14. 53 & 54 Vict., Lunacy Act, 1890, ch. 5; 20 & 21 Geo. V, Mental Treatment Act, 1930, ch. 23; Jones, *Mental Health and Social Policy, 1845–1959*, 93–146; Busfield, *Managing Madness*, 330–8.

15. M. Thomson, 'Sterilization, Segregation and Community Care; Ideology and Solutions to the Problem of Mental Deficiency in Inter-War London', *History of Psychiatry*, III (1992), 473–98.

16. Board of Education and Board of Control, Report of the Mental Deficiency Committee (London, 1929), Part III, 26, 42–3, 53–60, 91–5, paras. 25, 45, 56–65, 100.

17. 9 & 10 Geo. VI, National Health Service Act, 1946, Part III, section 28, Part V, Section 51.

18. Public Record Office, Kew (hereafter PRO) MH 134/80: Ministry of Health, circular 91/49, Mental Deficiency Acts 1913–38: Provision of Occupation Centres, 26/9/49.

19. P.P. 1952–53, XIII (Cmd. 8933), Annual Report of the Ministry of Health, 1952, 92–5.

20. P.P. 1953–54, XV (Cmd. 9321), Annual Report of the Ministry of Health, 1953, 139. See also Webster, *Government and Health Care*, 7–10.

21. Unsworth, *Politics of Mental Health Legislation*, 260; Jones, *Asylums and After*, 148–56.

22. Jones, *Asylums and After*, 159–65.

23. Scull, *Decarceration*, 135–53, 171; Busfield, *Managing Madness*, 326–30, 345–6; Webster, *Government and Health Care*, 110–21.

24. Royal Commission on the Law Relating to Mental Illness and Mental Deficiency 1954–1957 (Cmnd. 169) (London, 1957), 17–18, 101, 203, 206–7, paras. 47–8, 294, 592, 598–601.

25. 7 & 8 Eliz. II, Mental Health Act, 1959, Part II, Sections 6–13;

Unsworth, Politics of Mental Health Legislation, 14–15, 231, 247, 261–2.

26. Ministry of Health, On the State of the Public Health, 1957 (London, 1958), 123–4; Ministry of Health, On the State of the Public Health, 1958 (London, 1959), 121.

27. PRO MH 134/14: 'Mental Health Visits', 6/8/59; ibid., A. G. Rose to F. D. Riddett, 26/11/59.

28. PRO MH 134/15: 'Mental Health Services. Local Health Authorities Requiring "Stimulation"', 14/6/60; ibid., Ministry of Health to PROs, 15/9/60. See also Busfield, *Managing Madness*, 346–9; Webster, *Government and Health Care*, 120.

29. P.P. 1961–62, XXXI (Cmnd. 1604), A Hospital Plan for England and Wales, 5, 9–12, 278–9, paras.16–18, 31–4,. appendix D. See also Unsworth, *Politics of Mental Health Legislation*, 262; Webster, *Government and Health Care*, 109–10, 736.

30. P.P. 1962–63, XXXI (Cmnd. 1973), Health and Welfare: The Development of Community Care. Plans for the Health and Welfare Services of the Local Authorities in England and Wales, iii, 1–3, 16–19, 44–5, 366–7. See also Webster, *Government and Health Care*, 126.

31. PRO MH 134/20: D. M. O'Brien to the Deputy Secretary, 1/8/62; ibid., drafts of ten year plans.

32. Health and Welfare, 2, 24.

33. P.P., 1966–67, LVIII (Cmd. 3022), Health & Welfare: The Development of Community Care, Revision to 1975–76 of Plans for the Health and Welfare Services of the Local Authorities in England and Wales, 1–2, 26, 412–13, paras. 1–7, 100.

34. Ministry of Health, *On the State of the Public Health, 1962* (London, 1963), 143.

35. Ministry of Health, *On the State of the Public Health, 1964* (London, 1965), 139–40; Ministry of Health, *On the State of the Public Health, 1965* (London, 1966), 164–9.

36. P.P., 1968–69, XXXII (Cmd. 4100), Annual Report of the DHSS, 1968, p. 21.

37. P.P., 1967–68, XXXII (Cmnd. 3703), Report of the Committee on Local Authority and Allied Personal Social Services, 30, 90–6, 107–17, paras. 76, 293–309, 337–65.

38. M. Bayley, *Mental Handicap and Community Care: A Study of Mentally Handicapped People in Sheffield* (London, 1973), 342–4; Finch and Groves, 'Community Care and the Family', 489–90.

39. P.P., 1970–71, XX (Cmd. 4683), Better Services for the Mentally Handicapped, 13, 18, 43, paras. 55, 80, 198. See also Webster, *Government and Health Care*, 402–5.

40. DHSS, *Health and Personal Social Statistics for England (with Summary Tables for Great Britain), 1975* (London, 1976), 122, table 7.6.

41. P.P., 1974–75, XI (Cmnd. 6233), *Better Services for the Mentally Ill*, ii-iii, 11, 14–17, 83, paras. 2.1, 2.8, 2.17, 11.1. See also Sedgewick, *Psycho Politics*, 193–4; Busfield, *Managing Madness*, 349–50; Webster, *Government and Health Care*, 646–7.

42. H. G. Orme and W. H. Brock, *Leicestershire's Lunatics: The Institutional Care of Leicestershire's Lunatics During the Nineteenth Century* (Leicester, 1987), 5–9, 30, 49; J. Welshman, 'Eugenics and Public Health in Britain, 1900–40: Scenes from Provincial Life', *Urban History*, 24: 1 (1997), 56–75.

43. Leicestershire Record Office (hereafter LRO): minutes of the mental health services sub-committee, 18/7/47, 27.

44. LRO: minutes of the mental health services sub-committee, 16/3/49, 612.

45. LRO: minutes of the mental health services sub-committee, 12/3/58, 135, E. K. Macdonald, 'Informal Admission of Patients to Mental Deficiency Hospitals and Certified Institutions; Review of Guardianship Cases', 10/3/58.

46. LRO: minutes of the mental health services sub-committee, 12/11/58, 236, E. K. Macdonald, 'Mental Health Services. Admission of Patients to Hospital', 3/11/58; *idem.*, 'Training of Mental Defectives in Leicester', 3/11/58.

47. LRO: minutes of the mental health services sub-committee, 20/4/49, 627.

48. LRO: minutes of the Health Committee, 29/5/59, 19/6/59, 6, 19, G. C. Ogden, 'Mental Health Service', 17/6/59.

49. LRO: Health Committee minutes, 'Development of Local Authority Health and Welfare Services: Summary of Ten Year Plan', 22/8/62; ibid., L. W. Faulkner to G. C. Ogden, 9/10/62; LRO: Council minutes, 30/10/62, 241–63.

50. P.P. 1962–63, XXXI (Cmnd. 1973), *Health and Welfare*, 122–3.

51. P.P. 1966–67, LVIII (Cmnd. 3022), *Health & Welfare*, 102–3.

52. Leicester Health Committee, *Annual Report of the MOH, 1960* (Leicester, 1961), 28–37.

53. Leicester Health Committee, *Annual Report of the MOH, 1965* (Leicester, 1966), 19.

54. LRO: minutes of the mental health services sub-committee, 12/12/62, 291–2.

55. Leicester Health Committee, *Annual Report of the MOH, 1969* (Leicester, 1970), 5.

56. Leicester Health Committee, *Annual Report of the MOH, 1970* (Leicester, 1971), 22–3.

57. K. Jones, 'Problems of Mental After-Care in Lancashire', *Sociological Review*, 2 (1954), 34–56.

58. Jones, *Mental Health and Social Policy, 1845–1959*, 164–5.

59. N. O' Connor and J. Tizard, *The Social Problem of Mental Deficiency* (London, 1956), 141–65.

60. J. Tizard and J. C. Grad, *The Mentally Handicapped and their Families: A Social Survey* (Oxford, 1961), 106–13, 120–31. See also J. Tizard, *Community Services for the Mentally Handicapped* (London, 1964), 144–76.

61. G. F. Rehin and F. M. Martin, 'Some Problems for Research in Community Care', in H. Freeman and J. Farndale (eds) *Trends in the Mental Health Services: A Symposium of Original and Reprinted Papers* (Oxford, 1963), 290–302. See also J. Grad and P. Sainsbury, 'Evaluating a Community Care Service', in Freeman and Farndale (eds) *Trends in the Mental Health Services*, 303–17.

62. H. Freeman, 'Local Authority Services', in Freeman and Farndale (eds) *Trends in the Mental Health Services*, 318–33.

63. C. Colwell and F. Post, 'Community Needs of Elderly Psychiatric Patients', in Freeman and Farndale (eds) *Trends in the Mental Health Services*, 251–60.

64. Library of the London School of Economics and Political Science (hereafter LSE), Richard Titmuss Papers, 3/383: R. Titmuss, 'Community Care of the Mentally Ill' (n.d.).

65. LSE, Richard Titmuss Papers, 2/104: R. Titmuss, 'Community Care as Challenge', newspaper cutting, 12/5/59.

66. R. M. Titmuss, 'Community Care – Fact or Fiction?', in Freeman and Farndale (eds) *Trends in the Mental Health Services*, 221–5.

67. R. M. Titmuss, 'Care – or Cant?', *Spectator*, 6925, 17/3/61, 354–6; *ibid.*, 351–2.

68. LSE, Richard Titmuss Papers, 2/104: R. Titmuss, 'Planning for Ageing – Some Notes'; R. M. Titmuss, 'Planning for Ageing and the Health and Welfare Services', in *idem.*, *Commitment to Welfare* (New York, 1968), 91–103.

69. R. M. Titmuss, 'Social Work and Social Service: A Challenge for Local Government', *Journal of the Royal Society of Health*, 86: 1 (1966), 19–21, 32.

70. Ministry of Health *et al.*, *The Field of Work of the Family Doctor: Report of the Sub-Committee* (London, 1963), 22, 54, 57.

71. R. M. Titmuss, 'Role of the Family Doctor Today in the Context of Britain's Social Services', *Lancet* (1965), I, 1–4.

72. Busfield, *Managing Madness*, 350–3.

CHAPTER ELEVEN

1. D. Pilgrim and A. Rodgers, *A Sociology of Mental Health and Mental Illness* (London, 1993).
2. K. Jones, *A History of the Mental Health Services* (London, 1972).
3. A. Scull, *Decarceration: Community Treatment and the Deviant* (New Jersey, 1977).
4. M. Finnane, *Insanity and the Insane in Post-Famine Ireland* (London, 1981).
5. P. Prior, *Mental Health and Politics in Northern Ireland* (Aldershot, 1993).
6. J. Whyte, *Interpreting Northern Ireland* (Oxford, 1991).
7. F. Gaffikin and M. Morrissey, *Northern Ireland: The Thatcher Years* (London, 1990).
8. D. Birrell and A. Murie, *Policy and Government in Northern Ireland* (Dublin, 1980).
9. K. McCoy 'Integration: A Changing Scene' in *Perspectives on Integration*, DHSS(NI) (Belfast, 1993).
10. Department of Health and Social Services (Northern Ireland), *People First: Community Care in Northern Ireland for the 1990s*,(Belfast, 1990).
11. M. Smyth and J. Campbell, 'Social Work, Sectarianism and Anti-Sectarian Practice in Northern Ireland', *British Journal of Social Work*, 22, 77–92.
12. J. Campbell and J. Pinkerton, 'Embracing Change as Opportunity: Reflection on Social Work From a Northern Ireland Perspective', in B. Lesnik (ed.) *Change in Social Work* (Aldershot, 1997).
13. J. Campbell and M. Donnelly, 'Mental Health Service Users' Views of a Community Mental Health Social Work Team in Belfast', *Social Services Research*, 1 (1996), 1–14.
14. Prior, *Mental Health Policy and Politics in Northern Ireland*, 134–41.
15. Department of Health and Social Services (Northern Ireland), *Health and Wellbeing into the Millennium, Regional Strategy 1997–2001* (Belfast, 1996), 90.
16. J. Rafferty, 'The Decline of Asylum or the Poverty of the Concept?', in D. Tomlinson and J. Carrier (eds) *Asylum in the Community* (London, 1996).
17. M. Byrne, 'Mental Health Social Work in Northern Ireland – What does the Future Hold?', in R. Manktelow, J. Campbell and J. Park (eds) *Social Work and Mental Health: Proceedings of the Third Conference* (Belfast, 1997).
18. Western Health and Social Services Board, *Report into the Brian Doherty Case* (Fenton Report), (Derry, 1995).

19. HMSO, *Northern Ireland Review Committee on Mental Health Legislation* (MacDermott Report), (Belfast, 1981).
20. *Well into the Millennium*, 90.
21. S. Onyet, A. Heppleston and D. Bushness, *The Organisation and Operation of Community Mental Health Teams in England* (London, 1994).
22. Department of Health and Social Services (Northern Ireland), *Report of the Chief Inspector of Social Services*, (Belfast, 1995).
23. Prior, 'Mental Health Policy and Politics in Northern Ireland', 137.
24. Clinical Standards Advisory Group, Schizophrenia, 1 (London, 1995).
25. M. Donnelly, S. McGilloway, N. Mays, et al., *Opening New Doors: An Evaluation of Community Care for People Discharged from Psychiatric and Mental Handicap Hospitals*, (Belfast, 1994).
26. M. Donnelly and S. McGilloway, *Don't Look Away: Homelessness and Mental Health in Belfast*, (Belfast, 1996).
27. H. A. Lyons, 'Psychiatric Sequalae of the Belfast Riots, *British Journal of Psychiatry*, 118 (1971), 265–73.
28. G.C. Loughry, P. Bell, M.Kee, R.J. Roddy et al., 'Post-Traumatic Stress Disorder and Civil Violence in Northern Ireland, *British Journal of Psychiatry*, 153 (1988), 554–60.
29. E. Cairns and R. Wilson,'Mental Health Aspects of Political Violence in Northern Ireland', *International Journal of Mental Health*, 18 (1989), 38–56.
30. J. Benson, 'The Secret War in the Disunited Kingdom: Psychological Aspects of the Ulster Conflict', *Group Analysis*, 28 (1995), 47–62.
31. J. Darby and A. Williamson (eds) Violence and the Social Services in Northern Ireland (Dublin 1978).
32. Smyth and Campbell, 'Social Work, Sectarianism and Anti-Sectarian Practice in Northern Ireland', 83.
33. A. Healy 'Systemic Therapy in a Culture of Conflict: Developing a Therapeutic Conversation', *Child Care in Practice*, 3, 68–86.
34. M. Gibson 'The Kegworth Experience' in *NISW Journeys of Discovery: Creative Learning from Disasters* (London, 1996), 56–72.
35. D. Bolton 'When a Community Grieves: the Remembrance Day Bombing, Enniskillen', ibid, 73–89.
36. Command Paper 3883 (*The Agreement*) (Belfast, 1998), 1.
37. Department of Health and Social Services (Northern Ireland), *Report on a Developmental Project to Examine and Promote the Further Development of Services to Meet the Social and Psychological Needs of Individuals Affected by Civil Unrest in Northern Ireland*, (Belfast, 1998).
38. Department of Health and Social Services (Northern Ireland), *Wellbeing Into the Future*, 36

CHAPTER TWELVE

1. J. Busfield, *Men, Women and Madness: Understanding gender and mental disorder* (Basingstoke, 1996). P. Lelliott, A. Sims and J. Wing, 'Who Pays for Community Care? The Same Old Question', *British Medical Journal*, 307, (1993), 991–4. D. Pilgrim, 'Mental Health Services in the Twenty-first Century: The User-Professional Divide', in J. Bornea, C. Pereira, D. Pilgrim *et al.* (eds) *Community Care: A reader* (Milton Keynes, 1993).
2. P. Campbell, 'Mental Health Services: The User's View', *British Medical Journal*, 306 (1993), 848–50; D. Pilgrim and A. Rogers, *A Sociology of Mental Health and Illness* (Buckingham, 1993).
3. Lelliott *et al.*, *Who Pays for Community Care? The Same Old Question*, National Schizophrenia Fellowship, *Window Dressing : A Report from the National Schizophrenia Fellowship* (London, 1992).
4. M. Goldacre, V. Seagroatt and K. Hawton, 'Suicide after discharge from psychiatric inpatient care', *Lancet*, 342 (1993), 283–6; Royal College of Psychiatrists, *Community Supervision Orders: Discussion Document* (London, 1993).
5. Health Committee (House of Commons), 'Better Off in the Community? The Care of People Who are Seriously Mentally Ill', First Report, Volume 1 (London, 1994).
6. T. Groves, 'Closing Mental Hospitals', *British Medical Journal*, 306 (1993), 471–2. S.J.H. Dencker, K. Dencker, 'Does Community Care Reduce the Need for Psychiatric Beds for Schizophrenic Patients?', *Acta Psychiatrica Scandinavica*, 89 (Suppl 382) 1994, 74–9.
7. D. Carson, (ed.) *Risk Taking in Mental Disorder: Inter-disciplinary Conference Proceedings* (Southampton, 1990). H. Prins, in D. Carson (ed.) *Risk Taking in Mental Disorder* (1990). D. Pilgrim and A. Rogers, 'Two notions of risk in mental health debates', in T. Heller, J. Reynolds, R. Gomm *et al.* (eds) *Mental Health Matters* (Basingstoke, 1996).
8. *Daily Telegraph*, 17 Jan. 1998, 1.
9. D. Goldberg, P. Huxley, *Mental Illness in the Community* (London, 1980); D. Strathdee, R.M.A. Brown and R.J. Doig, 'Psychiatric Clinics in Primary Care: The Effect on General Practitioner Referral Patterns', *Social Psychiatry and Psychiatric Epidemiology*, 25 (1990), 95–100.
10. Department of Health, *The Health of the Nation: Key Area Handbook: Mental Illness*, (London, 1993).
11. D. Hunter, 'The Move to Community Care with Special Reference to Mental Illness' in E. Beck, S. Lonsdale, S. Newman and D. Patterson, (eds) *In the Best of Health?* (London, 1992).

12. S. Goodwin, *Comparative Mental Health Policy* (Aldershot, 1997); Busfield, *Men, Women and Madness: Understanding Gender and Mental Disorder*; Pilgrim and Rogers, *A Sociology of Mental Health and Illness*.

13. DHSS, Health and Personal Social Services Statistics for England & Wales (London, 1969). Department of Health, Mental Health in England (London, 1995).

14. Mental Health Foundation, *Creating Community Care : Report of the Mental Health Foundation Inquiry into Community Care for People with Severe Mental Illness* (London, 1994).

15. Pilgrim, *Mental Health Services in the Twenty-first Century: The User-Professional Divide*; Lelliott *et al.*, ibid.

16. Goodwin, *Comparative Mental Health Policy*.

17. Campbell, *Mental Health Services: The User's View*.

18. DHSS, *Health and Personal Social Services Statistics for England & Wales* (London, 1986). Department of Health, *Mental Health in England*.

19. Department of Health, *Mental Health in England*.

20. DHSS, *Health and Personal Social Services Statistics for England & Wales*; S. Payne, 'The rationing of psychiatric beds: changing trends in sex-ratios in admission to psychiatric hospital', *Health and Social Care in the Community*,3 (1995), 289–300.

21. Department of Health, *Mental Health in England*.

22. S. Payne, 'Psychiatric Care in the Community: Does it Fail Young Men?', *Policy and Politics*, 24 (1996), 193–205.

23. Payne, 'The Rationing of Psychiatric Beds', 298.

24. *British Medical Journal* Clunis inquiry cites 'catalogue of failure', *British Medical Journal*, 308 (1994), 613; Mental Health Act Commission, *Fifth Biennial Report of the Mental Health Act Commission 1991–1993* (London, 1993).

25. Payne, 'Psychiatric care in the community: Does it fail young men?'.

26. K. Abel, M. Buszewicz, S. Davison *et al.* (eds) *Planning Community Mental Health Services for Women* (London, 1996).

27. J. Finch, D. Groves, (eds) *A Labour of Love: Women, Work, and Caring* (London, 1983); D. Gittins, *The Family in Question* (Basingstoke, 1993); H. Graham, 'The Concept of Caring in Feminist Research : The Case of Domestic Service', *Sociology*, 25 (1991), 61–78.

28. M. Fisher, 'Man-made Care – Community Care and Older Male Carers', *British Journal of Social Work*, 24 (1994), 659–80; S. Arber and J. Ginn, 'Gender Differences in Informal Caring', *Health & Social Care In The Community*, 3 (1995), 19–31.

29. Pilgrim, 'Mental Health Services in the Twenty-first Century'; Lelliott *et al.*, 'Who Pays for Community Care?'.
30. P. Bean and P. Mounser, *Discharged from Mental Hospitals* (Basingstoke, 1993).
31. P. Barham, *Closing the Asylum: The Mental Patient in Modern Society* (Harmondsworth, 1992).
32. R. Barton, *Institutional Neurosis* (London, 1959).
33. Bean and Mounser, *Discharged from Mental Hospitals*; Campbell, *Mental Health Services: The User's View.*
34. Department of Health, *Mental Health in England.*
35. F. Creed, D. Black, P. Anthony *et al.*, 'Randomised Controlled Trial of Day Patient versus Inpatient Psychiatric Treatment', *British Medical Journal*, 300 (1990), 1033–37.
36. D. Hollander, R. Tobiansky, 'Crisis in Admission beds', *British Medical Journal*, 301 (1990), 664.
37. E. Murphy, 'Community Care I: Problems', *British Medical Journal*, 295 (1987), 1505–8; E. Fottrell, 'Asylum for Psychiatric Patients in the 1990s', *Lancet*, 335 (1990), 468.
38. T. Kendrick, B. Sibbald and J. Addington-Hall, 'General Practice: Distribution of Mental Health Professionals Working on Site in English and Welsh General Practices', *British Medical Journal*, 307 (1993), 544–6.
39. D. Goldberg, 'The Assault on Psychiatry', *Lancet*, 327 (1986), 1143–4.
40. P. Tyrer, 'Who is Failing the Mentally Ill?', *British Medical Journal*, 341 (1993), 1199.
41. M. Kastrup, 'Effectiveness of Treatment Strategies for the Chronic Mentally Ill', in H. Freeman and J. Henderson, *Evaluation of Comprehensive Care of the Mentally Ill* (London, 1991); Tyrer, *Who is Failing the Mentally Ill?*
42. D. Pilgrim, 'Rhetoric and Nihilism in Mental Health Policy: A Reply to Chapman *et al.*', *Critical Social Policy*, 34 (1992), 106–3, 109.
43. L. Prior, 'Community versus Hospital Care: The Crisis in Psychiatric Provision', *Social Science and Medicine*, 32 (1991), 483–9.
44. J. Busfield, 'Managing Madness: Changing Ideas and Practice', in J. Bornea, C. Pereira, D. Pilgrim and F. Williams, *Community Care: A Reader.* First ed. (Milton Keynes, 1993), 227–34.
45. P. Tyrer, 'Psychiatric Clinics in General Practice: An Extension of Community Care', *British Journal of Psychiatry*, 145 (1984), 9–14. P. Tyrer, S. Merson and N. Ghandi, 'Home Treatment for Psychiatric Disorder', *British Medical Journal*, 307 (1993), 200–201. Kendrick *et al.*, 'General Practice: Distribution of Mental Health Professionals Working on Site in English and Welsh General Practices'.
46. G. Jackson, R. Gater, D. Goldberg, *et al.*, 'A New Community Mental

Health Team Based in Primary Care: A Description of the Service and Its Effect on Service Use in the First Year', *British Journal of Psychiatry*, 162 (1993), 375–84. D.P. Goldberg, 'Integrating Mental Health in Primary Care', in H. Freeman and J. Henderson, *Evaluation of Comprehensive Care of the Mentally Ill* (London, 1991), 115–25.

47. Goldberg, *Integrating Mental Health in Primary Care.*
48. L. Sayce, T.K.J. Craig, A.P. Boardman, 'The Development of Community Mental Health Centres in the UK', *Social Psychiatry and Psychiatric Epidemiology*, 26 (1991), 14–20.
49. K. Wooff, D.P. Goldberg and T. Fryers, 'Patients in Receipt of Community Psychiatric Nursing Care in Salford 1976–82', *Psychological Medicine*, 16 (1986), 407–14; K. Wooff and D.P. Goldberg, 'Further Observations of the Practice of Community Care in Salford: Differences Between Community Psychiatric Nurses and Mental Health Social Workers', *British Journal of Psychiatry*, 153 (1989), 30–7; J. Shanks, 'Services for Patients with Chronic Mental Illness: Results of Research and Experience' in H. Freeman and J. Henderson, *Evaluation of Comprehensive Care of the Mentally Ill* (London, 1991).
50. C. Dean and E. Gadd, 'Home Treatment for Acute Psychiatric Illness', *British Medical Journal*, 301 (1990), 1021–3. C. Dean, J. Phillips, E.M. Gadd *et al.*, 'Comparison of Community Based Services With Hospital Based Service for People with Acute, Severe Psychiatric Illness', *British Medical Journal*, 307 (1993), 473–6. M. Muijen, J. Marks, J. Connolly *et al.*, 'Home Based Care and Standard Hospital Care for Patients with Severe Mental Illness: A Randomised Controlled Trial', *British Medical Journal*, 304 (1992), 749–54.
51. Dean and Gadd, *Home Treatment for Acute Psychiatric Illness.*
52. A. Rushton, 'Community-based Versus Hospital-based Care for Acutely Mentally Ill People – Literature Review', *British Journal of Social Work*, 20 (1990), 373–83.
53. Audit Commission for Local Authorities in England and Wales, *Making a Reality of Community Care* (London, 1986).
54. Cmnd 849, *Caring for People: Community Care into the Next Decade and Beyond* (London, 1989).
55. DHSS, *Community Care: Agenda for Action: A Report to the Secretary of State for Social Services (the Griffiths report)* (London, 1988).
56. P. Tyrer, J. Morgan, E. Vanhorn *et al.* 'A Randomized Controlled-Study of Close Monitoring of Vulnerable Psychiatric-Patients', *Lancet*, 345 (1995), 756–9.
57. M. Marshall, A. Lockwood and D. Gath, 'Social Services Case-management for Long-term Mental Disorders: A Randomised Controlled Trial', *Lancet*, 345 (1995), 409–12.

58. P. Fennell, 'Community Care, Community Compulsion and the Law' in M. Watkins, N. Hervey, J. Carson and S. Ritter (eds) *Collaborative Community Mental Health Care* (London, 1996).
59. L. Sayce, 'The Development of Community Care' in MIND, *1994 Directory of Health Services* (London, 1994).
60. Ibid.
61. P.H. Dick, T. Durham, C. McFee, M. Primrose, S. Mitchell and I.K. Crombie, 'Unnecessary Hospitalisation in a Psychiatric Rehabilitation Unit', *British Medical Journal*, 304 (1992), 1544.
62. Audit Commission, *Finding a Place: A Review of Mental Health Services for Adults* (London, 1994).
63. Tyrer *et al.*, *A Randomized Controlled-Study of Close Monitoring of Vulnerable Psychiatric-Patients*.
64. J. Allsop, *From Seamless Service to Patchwork Quilt?* In D. Gladstone (ed.) *British Social Welfare: Past, Present and Future* (London, 1995).
65. C. Paton, 'Present Dangers and Future Threats: Some Perverse Incentives in the NHS Reforms', *British Medical Journal*, 310 (1995), 1245–8.
66. Lelliott *et al.*, *Who Pays for Community Care?*; Mental Health Foundation, *Creating Community Care*.
67. Lords Hansard Text, 11/2/1998, Col 1239.
68. J. Ussher, *Women's Madness: Misogyny or Mental Illness?* (Hemel Hempstead, 1991); H. Meltzer, B. Gill and M. Pettigrew, *OPCS Surveys of Psychiatric Morbidity in Great Britain Report No 1: The Prevalence of Psychiatric Morbidity Among Adults Aged 16–64 Living in Private Households in Great Britain* (London, 1995).
69. Ussher, *Women's Madness*.
70. Goldberg and Huxley, *Mental Illness in the Community*; Busfield, *Men, Women and Madness: Understanding Gender and Mental Disorder*.
71. Strathdee *et al.*, 'Psychiatric Clinics in Primary Care: The Effect on General Practitioner Referral Patterns'.
72. Tyrer, *A Randomized Controlled-Study of Close Monitoring of Vulnerable Psychiatric-Patients*. G. Jackson, R. Rater, D. Goldberg, D. Tantam, L. Loftus and H. Taylor, 'A New Community Mental Health Team Based in Primary Care: A Description of the Service and its Effect on Service Use in the First Year', *British Journal of Psychiatry*, 162 (1993), 375–84.
73. M. Sheppard, 'General Practice, Social Work and Mental Health Sections: The Social Control of Women', *British Journal of Social Work*, 21 (1991), 663–83.
74. Ibid, 672.
75. Shanks, 'Services for Patients with Chronic Mental Illness'; Jackson *et*

al., 'A New Community Mental Health Team Based in Primary Care'; Wooff *et al.*, 'Patients in Receipt of Community Psychiatric Nursing Care in Salford 1976–82'.

76. K. Darton, J. Gorman and L. Sayce, *Eve Fights Back* (London, 1994).
77. K. Abel, M. Buszewicz, S. Davison, S. Johnson and E. Staples, *Planning Community Mental Health Services for Women* (London, 1996).
78. Hollander and Tobiansky, *Crisis in Admission Beds*; Fennell, *Community Care, Community Compulsion and the Law*.
79. Mental Health Act Commission, *Fifth Biennial Report*; Health Committee, *Better off in the Community*.
80. *British Medical Journal*, Clunis inquiry cites 'catalogue of failure', 77.
81. Health Committee, *Better Off in the Community*, xii.
82. Lelliott *et al. Who Pays for Community Care?.*
83. Mental Health Act Commission, *Fifth Biennial Report.*
84. D. Melzer, G. Hogman, A.S. Hale and S.J. Malik, 'Community Care for Patients with Schizophrenia One Year after Discharge', *British Medical Journal*, 303 (1991), 1023–26.
85. Royal College of Psychiatrists, *Community Supervision Orders: Discussion Document* (London, 1993).
86. National Schizophrenia Fellowship (NSF) *Window Dressing: A Report from the National Schizophrenia Fellowship* (London, 1992).
87. Mental Health Act Commission, *Fifth Biennial Report.*
88. Hollander and Tobiansky, 'Crisis in Admission beds'.
89. Payne, 'Psychiatric Care in the Community'.
90. Wooff *et al.*, 'Patients in Receipt of Community Psychiatric Nursing Care in Salford 1976–82'; Hollander and Tobiansky, 'Crisis in Admission beds'.
91. P. Moodley and R.E. Perkins, 'Routes to Psychiatric In-patient Care in an Inner London Borough,' *Social Psychiatry and Psychiatric Epidemiology*, 26 (1991), 47–51.
92. 'Inquiry into schizophrenic's care "inadequate"' in *Guardian*, 22 July 1995, 5.
93. Fennell, *Community Care, Community Compulsion and the Law.*
94. Royal College of Psychiatrists, *Community Supervision Orders*
95. Fennell, *Community Care, Community Compulsion and the Law.*
96. Ibid.
97. Ibid.
98. J. Ritchie, D. Dick and R. Lingham, *The Report of the Inquiry into the Care and Treatment of Christopher Clunis* (London, 1984).
99. K. Harrison, 'Growing opposition to "Uncontroversial" Bill', *Open Mind*, 74 (1985), 5.
100. *British Medical Journal*, Clunis inquiry cites 'catalogue of failure'.

101. *OpenMind*, 'Care not Coercion', 77 (1995), 4–5.
102. E. Francis, 'Community Care, Danger and Black People', *OpenMind*, 80 (1996), 4–5.
103. Department of Health (1996) The Government's Expenditure Plans 1997–97 to 1998–99.
104. Ibid.
105. *British Medical Journal*, Clunis inquiry cites 'catalogue of failure'.
106. Abel et al., *Planning Community Mental Health Services for Women*.
107. Carson, *Risk Taking in Mental Disorder*.

Index